Prenatal Diagnosis

Prenatal Diagnosis

The human side
(2nd edition)

Edited by

Lenore Abramsky
Genetic Associate, North Thames Perinatal Public Health Unit,
Kennedy-Galton Centre, North West London Hospitals NHS Trust,
Harrow, UK

Jean Chapple
Consultant in Perinatal Epidemiology, Westminster Primary Care Trust,
London, UK

Published in 2003 by:
Nelson Thornes Ltd
Delta Place
27 Bath Road
CHELTENHAM
GL53 7TH
United Kingdom

03 04 05 06 07 08 / 10 9 8 7 6 5 4 3 2 1

A catalogue record for this book is available from the British Library

ISBN 0 7487 6555 7

Illustrations by Acorn Bookwork
Page make-up by Acorn Bookwork

Printed and bound in Spain by GraphyCems

CONTENTS

CONTRIBUTORS

Lenore Abramsky
Genetic Associate and Honorary Lecturer, Imperial College, North Thames Perinatal Public Health Unit, Kennedy-Galton Centre, North West London Hospitals NHS Trust, Harrow, Middlesex, UK

Shamoly Ahmed
Research Associate, Department of Midwifery, City University, London, UK

Susan Bewley
Clinical Director Women's Services and Consultant Maternal–Fetal Medicine, Guys and St Thomas' Hospitals NHS Trust, London, UK

Sally Boxall
Consultant Nurse in Prenatal Diagnosis and Family Support, Princess Anne Hospital, Southampton, UK

Elizabeth M. Bryan
Paediatrician, Multiple Births Foundation, Hammersmith and Queen Charlotte's NHS Trust, London, UK

Jean Chapple
Consultant in Perinatal Epidemiology and Honorary Senior Lecturer, Imperial College; Public Health Directorate, Westminster Primary Care Trust, London, UK

Elizabeth Daly-Jones
Senior Ultrasonographer, Hammersmith and Queen Charlotte's NHS Trust, London, UK

Christine Garrett
Consultant in Clinical Genetics and Honorary Senior Lecturer, Imperial College; North West Thames Regional Genetics Service, Kennedy-Galton Centre, North West London Hospitals NHS Trust, Harrow, Middlesex, UK

Josephine M. Green
Senior Lecturer and Deputy Director, Mother and Infant Research Unit, University of Leeds, UK

Rachel Grellier
Research Fellow, School of Health and Social Studies, University of Warwick, UK

James B. Haddow
Partner, Petruccelli, Martin & Haddow, LLP, Portland, Maine, USA

Ray Hall
Member of ARC (Antenatal Results and Choices)

Jean Hollingsworth
Ultrasound Services Manager, Hammersmith and Queen Charlotte's NHS Trust, London, UK

Alison Lashwood
Consultant Nurse in Genetics and Preimplantation Diagnosis, Clinical Genetics Department, Guy's Hospital, London, UK

Lyn Margerison
Specialist Health Visitor in Genetics, North West Thames Regional Genetics Service, Kennedy-Galton Centre, North West London Hospitals NHS Trust, Harrow, Middlesex, UK

Jonathan Montgomery
Professor of Health Care Law, University of Southampton, UK

Margaretha van Mourik
Senior Genetic Counsellor, Regional West of Scotland Genetic Service, Duncan Guthrie Institute of Medical Genetics, Yorkhill, Glasgow, UK

Jane Sandall
Professor of Midwifery and Women's Health, King's College, London, UK

Wendy Solomou
Research Associate, Centre for Family Research, University of Cambridge, UK

Helen Statham
Senior Research Associate, Centre for Family Research, University of Cambridge, UK

Lucy Turner
Sister, Fetal Medicine Unit, Hammersmith and Queen Charlotte's NHS Trust, London, UK

Jennifer Wiggins
Genetic Counsellor, Hammersmith and Queen Charlotte's NHS Trust, London, UK

PREFACE

The first edition of this book evolved out of a conference held because of our conviction that prenatal screening and diagnostic techniques provide carers with a two-edged sword which can do both good and harm – often at the same time to the same person.

The conference (The human side of prenatal diagnosis) dealt with emotional, ethical and legal issues in prenatal screening and diagnosis. It took place in March 1992 at the Institute of Obstetrics and Gynaecology in London and was attended by obstetricians, paediatricians, geneticists, midwives and ultrasonographers from the North West Thames Health Region. The demand for places at the conference far exceeded the number of places available and many of those who attended expressed the hope that we would be organizing similar conferences in the future. This strengthened our belief that many carers working in the maternity services were deeply concerned about the human issues raised by the new technologies and encouraged us to work towards publication of the first edition of this book. In the years since the first edition came out, these issues have been the subject of much media attention – some of it thought provoking and important, some of it sensational and filled with inaccuracies. There has been an increase in public awareness, in the number of pregnancies subjected to prenatal screening and diagnosis, and in the number of health care workers involved in delivering these programmes. This has lead to an even greater need for an accessible book on the subject.

Prenatal diagnosis and the possibility of selective termination of affected pregnancies is part of a wider move towards reproductive choice. Like contraception and assisted conception, it can make a major difference to the lives of some people. However, it is important to remember that the whole idea of reproductive choice is bound by culture. In our culture, we tend to view choice as a good thing; we look upon it as our right to choose our occupation, our partner, the place where we live, the books that we read and the way that we vote. In some cultures these choices are not thought to be desirable and may not be allowed. Even within one cultural or social group, individuals may differ greatly in their views about choice, including reproductive choice.

Those who believe that reproductive choice in the form of contraception is good may still feel that termination of pregnancy is unacceptable. Even those who feel that termination of pregnancy is acceptable will find that the termination of a wanted pregnancy is emotionally traumatic. What about the many women who are pregnant with normal, healthy babies who are made anxious by screening and diagnostic tests or those who lose healthy babies due to prenatal diagnostic tests? These are some of the costs of prenatal diagnosis.

We could, of course, make a very long list of the benefits of prenatal diagnosis, such as not having to suffer with a baby who is dying from Tay–Sachs disease or to receive the agonizing news that a much wanted newborn baby has Down syndrome.

We do not want to present arguments for or against carrying out prenatal diagnosis. The technology is here, has grown rapidly since the first edition was published in 1994 and will continue to grow. We want to inspire people to think about the consequences of all the tests being offered. We want them to consider how they can maximize the benefits of those tests while minimizing any harm. We want people to ask themselves why they are offering particular tests and whether they are doing it in the best possible way. We want them to reconsider how test results are passed on to women and their families and to think about whether follow-up support is adequate for couples and staff.

While updating the book for this new edition, we have taken the opportunity to add chapters that were noticeably lacking from the first edition. We have looked at the issue of continuing a pregnancy after prenatal diagnosis of an anomaly. We have looked more closely at the issue of prenatal diagnosis in a multi-cultural society, and we have added a chapter on legal issues in the United States.

Communication technology has advanced enormously since the first edition of this book came out. This has implications for both pregnant couples and their carers. Couples faced with a diagnosis are quite likely to go straight to the Internet to find out more about the condition; some of the information will be high quality while some will be misleading. Carers need to be aware of how to access information so that they can find it themselves and so that they can guide parents who are trying to find out more. With this is mind, we have included information about useful websites in this edition.

Most of the contributors to this volume live and work in the United Kingdom, so much of the research and experiences cited are British. However, the issues are the same in any land and any culture in which prenatal screening and diagnosis is practised. The methods of dealing with the problems raised will differ over time and between cultures, but the problems themselves will be as constant as life and death, joy and sorrow.

The aim of this book is not to pass on a large body of information; it is to make people think about issues that are vital to the emotional health of pregnant women, their partners and families, workers in the maternity services and society as a whole.

Lenore Abramsky
Jean Chapple
London 2003

ACKNOWLEDGEMENTS

We dedicate this book to our children: Sasha, Kolya and Tanya Abramsky and Jamie and Nick Chapple. It was they who taught us the joys and challenges of parenthood. This, and the experiencing of our own pregnancies, enabled us to examine the issues in prenatal diagnosis from a personal perspective as well as from a professional viewpoint. Of course, the pregnancy experiences and parenting were shared with our husbands, Jack Abramsky and Syd Chapple, who have always been supportive whether it be as fathers or as partners of women temporarily unbalanced by the need to finish editing a book!

As with the first edition, we are incredibly grateful to all the authors. They produced excellent contributions and kept to the tight deadline set. We would also like to thank our many colleagues with whom we discussed the issues; they helped us to clarify our ideas and suggested sources of information and expertise.

Finally, we would not even have conceived the idea of this book were it not for the thousands of couples who have generously shared with us their feelings, thoughts and fears – giving us some insight into the emotional processes activated by the various stages of prenatal diagnosis, from the mere thought of considering screening to dealing with the consequences of receiving a diagnosis of fetal abnormality.

The cover illustration is by courtesy of Dr Darren K Griffin and Helen Tempest. Cell and Chromosome Biology Group, Department of Biological Sciences, Brunel University, Uxbridge, Middlesex, UB8 3PH.

The publisher would like to thank the *British Medical Journal* for permission to reproduce Figure 4.1 on page 48.

William Morris 1834–96

One of these cloths is heaven, and one is hell,
Now choose one cloth for ever; which they be,
I will not tell you, you must somehow tell
Of your own strength and mightiness.

Percy Bysshe Shelley 1792–1822

Alas! that all we loved of him should be,
But for our grief, as if it had not been,
And grief itself be mortal!

1 ETHICAL ISSUES IN PRENATAL DIAGNOSIS

Susan Bewley

INTRODUCTION

Prenatal diagnosis is the identification of diseases of the fetus. It may be made non-invasively (by ultrasound for structural defects) or invasively (by a needling technique to obtain a sample of amniotic fluid, placenta or fetal blood). Invasive techniques carry a risk of fetal loss or damage.

Prenatal diagnosis can have three purposes:

1 to inform and prepare parents for the birth of an affected infant;
2 to allow *in utero* treatment or delivery at a specialist centre for immediate postnatal treatment;
3 to allow termination of an affected fetus.

Current practice of prenatal diagnosis has all three purposes, but termination dominates management. In most societies, diseases of neonates and children are considered afflictions, and many tolerate abortion. However, there is no consensus on this.

WHY MUST WE CONSIDER ETHICS?

Ethics has to be considered in relation to prenatal diagnosis:

- to decide whether an action is right or wrong;
- to guide us in the future when a similar situation occurs;
- for society to come to an agreed compromise about what is and is not allowed.

Law sets the limits of acceptable behaviour, and there may be a conflict between law and ethics. A particular action in one situation may be lawful, but morally wrong, just as there can be right or good acts that are illegal. Some of the areas of ethical concern in prenatal diagnosis are introduced below.

ETHICAL ISSUES IN PRENATAL DIAGNOSIS

'Rights' of the fetus

What is the moral status of the embryo, fetus or newborn? Is there a difference between diagnosing cystic fibrosis in a preimplantation embryo or at 10 weeks' gestation? Do the unborn, who have no voice, have rights that should be protected? Is there a right to live whatever disease a fetus has? Some argue that fetuses cannot have rights, at least not until they are born and individuals. If that were so, would there be no moral difference between kicking a pregnant and non-pregnant woman in the abdomen?

When is abortion permissible?

Is abortion for congenital abnormality permissible? If so, why? If abortion is tolerated, how serious does the abnormality have to be? What is the difference between aborting for spina bifida, thalassaemia, cleft lip, club foot, sex or eye colour? How late can it be performed? Is there a difference between abortion for Down syndrome discovered at 10, 20, 30 weeks or at birth? If abnormal fetuses can be killed, is euthanasia, or the deliberate killing of neonates, children or adults also acceptable? Should doctors be allowed to give lethal injections to infants with anencephaly or severe complications of prematurity or the brain dead?

How does termination for abnormality square with respect for disabled adults?

Does abortion of an abnormal fetus degrade or affect adults with the same disease? If the law makes a difference between a third trimester fetus with and without spina bifida and hydrocephalus (i.e. one can be killed and the other cannot), does that send a message to the disabled that they are worth less than the able bodied? Is it wrong for parents to bring sick children into the world? Are parents who do not abort fetuses with chronic conditions that shorten life and cause suffering (such as beta thalassaemia) cruel? They could, after all, have an abortion and try again for a healthy child. If they do not wish to, should society pay the cost of their choice?

Are the risks acceptable?

Are there risks to the mother or fetus that are unacceptable? Some conditions, such as diaphragmatic hernia, can be operated on *in utero*. The fetus has to be removed from the womb for the operation. The mother requires several major operations and the fetus may be born prematurely. Increasingly, these treatments will move from the experimental to the clinical arena. Should there be limits to the risks taken?

Who decides?

Who is the patient/client: the mother, parents, family, future person or future society? If a family have genetic counselling and one member is gently pressurized into testing for linkage studies, is that just the family's business? Should the counsellor take sides, see each person individually, or accept the consensus opinion? Is it different if the pressure is extremely strong, or if the family member is a child, or a 13-year-old, or mentally ill, or just weak-willed? Who decides whether to test or not? Is it the parent, the counsellor, the operator or a combination of all? If there is a disagreement about testing, whose view prevails? If an explicit request is made for sex selection so that a first-born male can inherit a title, who says yes or no? What if a mother refuses life-saving treatment for her fetus? If the fetus will die or be damaged if a woman does not agree to treatment, such as a transfusion for Rhesus disease, or a caesarean section for fetal distress, should she be forced to help her fetus, or be punished? If not, why not, as the same refusal after birth can be overruled?

Are there unintended future effects?

Are conflicts of interest inevitable? Can looking after the genetic health of a family oppress individuals? Does prenatal diagnosis affect parent–child relationships? Can we show an improvement when the mother is reassured and the child is really wanted? Does choosing the quality of fetus make it a consumer object? As more and more genetic tendencies are elucidated, why not choose a fetus that is unlikely to get hypertension and diabetes in later life, and who will be guaranteed to be handsome, athletic and ambitious? Does screening of the general pregnant population increase maternal anxiety? Do ultrasound and serum screening (for Down syndrome) make women obsessed about certain diseases out of proportion to the range of potential problems?

Confidentiality and ownership of information

When can or should confidentiality be broken? If a person refuses to let siblings know that they are at risk of carrying abnormal genes, such as Fragile X, and these could be passed on to innocent, as yet unconceived, fetuses, should we not break confidentiality to prevent harm? Why protect people who are so unconcerned for their family members? What if the putative father is not the genetic father? Does a man have a right to know that the fetus is not his if this is discovered during the course of prenatal diagnosis? Who owns genetic information? If genetic information is common amongst family members, do they not have an interest or even right to know each other's results?

This list is not exhaustive, and new technologies will continue to pose more dilemmas. There are no easy definitive answers to the questions. Arguments about the moral status of the fetus, the permissibility of abortion, and the nature of the doctor–patient relationship (or genetic professional and client) lie at the heart of many of the ethical issues in prenatal diagnosis. The aim of this chapter is to analyse ethical disagreements, with particular reference to prenatal diagnosis. Some theoretical concepts will be explained and then practical suggestions made for dealing with conflicts.

PHILOSOPHICAL ETHICS

Approaches

There are several approaches to ethics:

Descriptive

We can measure ethical beliefs at a certain time in a certain place. Some beliefs appear to be universal (murdering your neighbour is wrong) whilst others are not (abortion ranges from being considered murder to a form of contraception). We may be able to measure what our present beliefs are, but this is not helpful in determining what they should be.

Intuitive

In a new situation we might react intuitively to decide whether something is right or wrong. Intuitions may be worth attending, in that they have evolved over the years, and be quicker than thought processes, but they are not infallible. Overcoming 'gut reactions' is part of professional training.

Rational argument

Philosophers, lawyers and politicians are experts in arguing (but are not always rational!). Philosophers practice the skills and test the logic of arguments. They do not all agree, so we do not have to automatically accept what they say.

If intuition comes into conflict with rational argument, then one must give way. Either the intuition is suppressed or dogged irrationality prevails, and each is potentially hazardous. Alternatively, the discrepancy can be examined in detail to find the flaw in the intuition or the arguments.

The tools

Philosophers use various tools to examine arguments:

- analysis of words and issues;
- drawing of distinctions;
- using logic;
- trying thought experiments to test theory.

Philosophers point out that two people may be using the same word in a different sense and mistakenly think they are talking about the same thing. Being precise about the definitions of words clarifies much conflict. There may be different implications of terms such as 'rights' and 'responsibilities' (see moral frameworks below). They may distinguish two situations that appear superficially similar but are actually different, and show how the difference is morally relevant.

Although philosophers can be vexing when they use unreal examples (what if a Martian requested prenatal diagnosis to abort on the basis of skin colour?), the purpose of thought experiments is to test a theory or belief. This is similar to scientific experiments, where observations are made to confirm or refute hypotheses. Imagining an unreal situation frees us from everyday prejudices and allows logical thought. If the result of the thought experiment is uncomfortable or unacceptable, maybe there was something wrong with the original intuition or underlying theory.

The components of moral acts

The key to those actions that have ethical significance lies in the interplay of a moral agent performing an action on an object of moral significance. The action could be a prenatal diagnosis consultation, an abortion or a promise of confidentiality. The interplay is depicted in Figure 1.1.

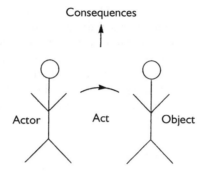

Figure 1.1 The components of moral acts

Moral frameworks

There are three main theoretical moral frameworks that underpin discussions of morality. They can be envisaged as three viewpoints on any moral action, looking primarily at the actor, the object or the consequences of the act.

1. Duty-based (conscience and motives paramount)
This is broadly speaking the religious framework, although there are secular versions. It concerns itself with the motivation and intentions of the actor. It is God who will judge the contents of our hearts, although it may be individual conscience in a secular version. We have duties or obligations to others. Any rights they have stem secondarily from our duty. Thus, the 'right to life' only stems from the duty not to kill. This duty exists whatever the other person says about it, even if they have no voice. Rights in this morality thus do not have much force, although they are persuasive rhetorical devices.

2. Goal-based (morality objectively determined by outcome)
This is the consequentialist or utilitarian approach developed in the nineteenth century ('the greatest happiness for the greatest number'). Actions have consequences and outcomes. There is nothing inherently right or wrong in any particular action. It does not depend on the intention of the actor; it depends only on the outcome. Humans are motivated by pleasure and increasing it is the purpose of morality. We should all be acting so as to maximize good outcomes. A major criticism of utilitarianism is that one may be sacrificed for the good of many. Also, no one has inherent value. It depends on qualities the person or thing possesses, such as sentience, the ability to feel pain or pleasure or make choices, intelligence, etc. (Indeed, it might be species prejudice to give more value to a human fetus than an adult monkey if it has more of the relevant qualities.)

3. Rights-based (rights providing protection)

This has largely developed from the political arena ('all men are equal and have certain inalienable rights'). People have inherent rights. Duties towards them stem secondarily from their rights. This is a most powerful interpretation of rights. For example, if people have a right (to vote, or be educated) that is not being fulfilled, there is a strong claim on others to do something to rectify the situation. These sorts of strong rights have certain characteristics: that they can be waived (you do not have to use your vote), that they can only be held by those capable of making autonomous choices (they are meaningless otherwise), and that they trump other moral considerations. If a woman has this kind of right to prenatal diagnosis (stemming from some basic right to reproduction) doctors are obliged to do it.

Few people are total purists, and the theories are being constantly modified and refined. In real life, features of all these moralities seem to co-exist. There is an uncomfortable amalgam of parts of all. Maybe that is because we live in a pluralistic society, or because we humans have incompatible parts to our characters or internal psychology. It is not possible to look from all directions at once. There is an underlying fundamental struggle between these philosophies. Each version is put forward as a total explanation for our everyday beliefs, and tries to incorporate its critics. So, when a problem is analysed from each point of view, different answers may emerge.

Illustration of the different moral theories

Let me try to illustrate the way the different fundamental approaches to a moral problem work: firstly, how taking the different viewpoints might explain the morality of an action; secondly, how changing one fact may change the rightness or wrongness of an action, but differently for each morality.

It is worth imagining that the theories are like different political parties trying to attract voters. Three philosophers representing each of the theories are trying to win your intellectual vote or allegiance. They all agree that murder is wrong, but for different reasons. I am going to use the example of killing an adult human for the time being so as not to confuse it with the issue of abortion or prenatal diagnosis yet. I shall give their general explanations and then change one fact to show how the moral judgement might change.

Mr X stabbed the postman who then died. Three philosophers agree that it was wrong and that Mr X should be punished. Why?

Philosopher 1 – Duty

It was wrong because X had a duty not to harm or kill others. He formed an evil motive, carried it out, and is a wicked person for doing so. By contrast, if X made a genuine mistake, reasonably thinking the postman was a cardboard cut out, not a person, then he would be blameless. The knife would have killed the postman, but X would not have murdered him, in that he had formed no intention. (The goal and right philosopher might still hold that it was wrong.)

Philosopher 2 – Goal

It was wrong because people want to live, and carry out their plans and desires. The benchmark of moral value is the maximization of happiness or welfare. Mr X may have enjoyed killing him but the postman suffered the loss of his life, his family are distraught, and everyone in the neighbourhood is now terrorized. The world is a worse off place for this murder, and therefore it was wrong. By contrast, if Mr X surreptitiously killed Adolf Hitler just as he was rising to power and changed the course of history for the better, then it would have been a right action. Note that it would not be a wrong action that was justified, but actually right. (The duty and right philosopher would still hold that it was wrong.)

Philosopher 3 – Right

The postman had a right to live that was inalienable. He was the only person who could waive this right. He did not agree or consent to being killed. Mr X violated his right to live, and therefore committed a wrong. By contrast, if the postman had asked Mr X to do it, having carefully considered and chosen death, there would be nothing wrong in the action. (The duty philosopher would still hold that it was wrong. The goal philosopher would determine whether, overall, the harms of allowing killing with consent outweighed the benefits of such a policy, before deciding whether it was right or wrong.) The three moral theories are summarized in Figure 1.2 and Table 1.1.

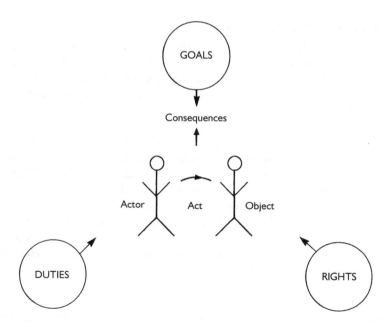

Figure 1.2 Summary of moral frameworks

Table 1.1 Summary of moral frameworks

Theory	Duty	Goal	Right
History	Traditional	Nineteenth century	Twentieth century
Central value	Inherent moral worth	Maximization of welfare	Autonomous choice
Keywords	Duty, obligation, responsibility	Welfare, utility, happiness, usefulness	Right, choice, autonomy
Abortion	Usually wrong; might be right if 'lesser of two evils'	Right if mother's preference; Might be obligatory if abnormality present	Always right as mother's right to choose
Psychology	Superego	Id	Ego

There are important theoretical battles being waged over the different theories of ethics. Although over-simplified, these thumbnail sketches may help untangle the arguments put forward for different aspects of prenatal diagnosis. The actual situation is much more complicated, as each theory contains elements of the others, and there are a range of views within the theories.

To return to prenatal diagnosis; if the knife is changed for a sampling needle or suction cannula and the postman for a fetus, how and why does the morality change? First, do fetuses count at all? It is useful to consider what gives an object moral worth or status.

MORAL STATUS

Who has moral status or moral value?

Adult humans normally have full moral status whereas property, such as a chair, does not. People are protected by this; one cannot be harmed, killed or incarcerated without good reason, but there is nothing wrong in selling or burning an old chair. What is the morally relevant difference between a person and a chair?

What makes us important?

If we agree that people have moral status and chairs do not, does that help determine whether fetuses have moral status? The answer will depend on the qualities that are considered to be those that give adult humans moral value. What qualities give status? It could range from merely being human (in which case all humans from conception may have full moral status), to having the ability to make autonomous choices (in which case many humans, such as fetuses and children, may not have it). Or it may be something else or something in between. If it were usefulness or pleasure to others, a Chippendale chair might have more value than fetuses and many humans.

Range of status

There may also be a range of status, from none to full. For instance, animals (generally) have some moral status. A horse can be bought and sold (like property), but we think it is wrong to throw one alive on a bonfire (unlike the chair).

Where do other objects of moral value fit in Table 1.2, and why? Do gametes, fetuses, children, incompetent adults, dying and dead humans have none, some or full moral status? Do adult humans all have equal full moral status, or do some (such as the brain dead) have less than others?

Table 1.2 Range of moral status

Full moral status	Some moral status	No moral status
Adult humans	Animals	Property/plants

There is a time before we exist (except as twinkles in our parents' eyes). How do we progress from non-existence to full status? Is it a sudden change at conception or birth? Or a gradual change, with increasing development of the fetus and child? Do future, potential generations count, and how much?

FETAL MORAL STATUS

There are three possibilities:

1. A fetus has full moral status. Its life cannot wantonly be put in danger (so invasive testing is not usually justified), and it has a right not to be killed (so abortion is wrong; indeed it is murder). This is an extreme deontological or duty-based view, corresponding to the Catholic position.
2. A fetus has no moral status. In this case, it does not enter the moral arena at all (unless its parents wish to endow it with some sentimental protection). If a mother wishes to have a termination, no wrong is committed. This would be an extreme view. If a third trimester fetus had no status, why should a newborn have any? It would be very difficult to see why there should be anything wrong with infanticide (of normal or abnormal babies), apart from the effect on third parties.
3. The fetus has some moral status, but not as much as adults. Now a complex balancing act will have to be performed when there is a conflict of interests or rights. If a fetus has more moral status as pregnancy progresses, then justifications for abortions will have to increase with gestation. And it is possible that while some abortions will be right, others will be wrong and unjustified killings (which may still not amount to murder, as it is killing of something less than an adult). Moderate deontologists (duty-based) would hold this view. Utilitarians tend to accord the fetus some status, but may do it through the eyes of the mother. If she wishes to have the fetus it is valued, but if not, then it is not. This is actually a view that gives the fetus no inherent worth, and would thus belong to (2) above. Utilitarians may also suggest viability as the time when the fetus can be treated as a patient, but again, this suggests that it has no inherent worth.

ABORTION

There are a wide variety of opinions about abortion, but they fall into several major camps; one argument derives from a maternal perspective and three from a fetal perspective.

Maternal argument – women's rights over their bodies

In this argument, the moral status of the fetus is irrelevant and abortion is justifiable as women have domain over their own bodies. People believing this have to explain whether there are any abortions that would be wrong, such as terminations in the third trimester for very minor abnormalities.

Fetal arguments – full, none or some moral status

Full moral status

A person who believes in the absolute sanctity of life from conception, that can never be intentionally ended, must reject all abortions even in cases of rape or fetal abnormality. It is a shame, but unavoidable, that parents will be caused suffering if abortion is always refused (e.g. families coping for a lifetime with an unwanted handicapped child, or having to watch newborns die from such disorders as pulmonary hypoplasia or anencephaly).

No moral status

A person who believes that abortion is justifiable because the fetus is not a 'person' with rights will also have to accept termination for the most trivial reason. They may need to explain whether there is any distinction from infanticide.

Some moral status

Those who are left with the more pragmatic, and pluralistic view that the fetus develops increasing moral status throughout pregnancy and that a justification must be made for an abortion, as the lesser of two evils (killing a fetus versus harm to an adult human or her other children), have a view that corresponds to the law in most Western countries. If a pregnancy is unwanted because of abnormality, this is often considered justification enough.

Additional considerations for congenital abnormality

The moral status of the fetus is central to the acceptability of abortion when a mother has an unwanted pregnancy that affects her life, health or lifestyle. Prenatal diagnosis is often made in pregnancies that were wanted, but changed to unwanted when an abnormality was found. Additional ethical dilemmas when considering termination of fetuses with congenital malformations are:

- How severe does the malformation have to be for a termination to be justified?

- How late can diagnosis and termination be justified?
- Does the distinction between fetuses reflect into adult life?

These moral questions are not for parents and doctors alone to answer, and society, for example through the UK Abortion Act (1967, amended 1990), has created some difficulties. In England, Scotland and Wales there is no upper time limit for termination if there is 'a substantial risk that if the child were born it would suffer from such physical or mental abnormalities as to be seriously handicapped'. Can an ethical explanation be made by any of the camps that justify having a different gestation rule for abortion of the abnormal fetus? This new distinction between normal and abnormal fetuses might discriminate against the disabled amongst us. If a handicap *in utero* distinguishes fetuses who can be aborted and those who cannot, do adults with the same handicap also have less moral status and protection from harm? Differences in gestation limits between terminations for abnormality and social reasons might indicate changing values about adults, unless a special argument, to do with future suffering, can be made for late abortions.

SPECIAL RELATIONSHIPS

Let us next consider what governs the relationship between the health professional and the pregnant woman regarding prenatal diagnosis. The moral relationship of any two humans to one another would be that which we would expect of two strangers (maybe there is not much of an obligation to help one another out, but each has a right not to be harmed by the other).

In addition to the basic, there are a variety of special moral relationships including parent–child, teacher–pupil, shopkeeper–customer and friends. These may entail greater obligations and rights than those of two strangers. Parents are expected to make financial sacrifices to help their children, whereas shopkeepers are not. Teachers are supposed to educate pupils, whereas friends are not. In prenatal diagnosis, the important special relationships are mother–fetus and doctor–patient. The professional might be a doctor, midwife or genetic counsellor, but the models described apply to all. I have tended to use the term patient throughout (meaning a person attending a doctor for care), although client or customer have also been proposed. All are value-loaded terms implying different ethical camps before we even analyse what the relationship is! Parent applies equally to mother and father, whereas only the woman is pregnant. Client or customer may imply a more contractual and less caring relationship.

Different versions of the doctor–patient relationship

There are two main versions of the doctor–patient relationship:

1. Traditional, beneficence (doing good) approach

The doctor must do his or her best for the patient to prolong life and relieve suffering. Need is assessed objectively by the professional, and not merely accepted as the subjective experience. This approach has been thought to lead to extreme paternalistic 'doctor knows best' behaviour and, although traditional, is being challenged. Paternalism may be modernized (by incorporating more respect for patient empowerment and choices into doing good) or rejected outright for another model.

2. Modern, autonomy (freedom to choose) approach

To replace the beneficence model, the relationship may be described as a professional–client relationship, where the passivity expected of patients is rejected. The professional must maximize life-enhancing potentials, by restoring health and respecting autonomous choices. If an autonomous and informed client really wants a certain treatment or procedure in the belief that it will enhance life, then the doctor should give it.

Both traditionalists and modernists, paternalists and utilitarians, claim that they wish to construct a more equal relationship between partners in care, and to respect *both* beneficence and autonomy. However, when pushed or in direct conflict, one of the principles, beneficence or autonomy, must give way.

Basic components of the doctor–patient relationship

Some of the central components of the doctor–patient relationship and their description in different moralities are shown in Table 1.3 below. The reasons the qualities are central to the special relationship are subtly different depending on the viewpoint. Present professional guidelines are based on a duty-based view of the doctor–patient relationship.

Table 1.3 The components of the doctor–patient relationship

Quality	Duty	Goal	Right
Confidentiality	To keep promises	Useful to protect history and secrets	To have confidences kept
Consent	To respect bodily integrity	Examinations and investigations permitted	Not to be interfered with
Competence	Doctor must do his/her best	Helpful to have high standard of management	To have a good doctor

Taking confidentiality as one example, there are profound implications. A promise of confidentiality given to a patient that was duty-based should not be broken (as it is wrong to break promises, unless a greater wrong is committed such as allowing a patient to commit a serious crime). If respecting confidentiality were right-based, the information belonging to and given by the patient should be absolutely protected (the only exceptions being when the patient agrees or is incompetent). If it were goal-based, the decision whether to respect or breach confidentiality would depend on the balance of harms and goods. Confidentiality is useful to encourage patients to give private information, but sometimes it would be right for doctors to breach confidentiality to give important information to others.

Who is the patient/client?

It may be each person at a time, the mother and father together, a whole family or the fetus. If it is more than one at a time, then conflicts of interest may arise. Fetuses, siblings and parents may have different interests in the results of prenatal diagnosis, which they exert to effect on one another. If a doctor's job is to do the best for each individual, then treating couples or families as whole units means that sometimes one person's interest will be sacrificed for another's. There is no problem when the interests of the different parties coincide or overlap, but this is not always the case. Traditional doctor–patient relationships are based on a one to one promise of care. Genetic counselling has often taken a wider view on families and extended families.

Non-directive counselling and informed consent

These ideological tenets sound irreproachable. After all, who would recommend directive counselling or uninformed consent? Aside from the practical problem of achieving non-directiveness, what is the purpose or virtue of non-directive counselling?

Are we aiming for non-directive counselling because it is the way to do the best for patients, or because it enhances their autonomous reproductive choices? This is not an irrelevant distinction, because in an extreme case where doing best and choice collide the doctor will end up with different decisions. For example, if a woman requested a second chorionic villus sample, and explained rationally, having had non-directive counselling, that she was particularly anxious and needed reassurance that a mistake had not been made in the laboratory, what should the doctor do? She fully understands the higher chance of miscarriage but says it is her body, her risk and her choice. A traditionalist doctor who sees non-directive counselling as a means, but not the end, to doing what is best for the patient can refuse to repeat the chorionic villus sample as it is harmful. A modernist doctor believes that non-directive counselling is an aim in itself, something that is necessary to enhance autonomous choices. This doctor then has two courses of action: either to do the repeat chorionic villus sample as this is this woman's carefully considered personal choice, or declare that she is too irrational and anxious to be autonomous, so the request does not have to be fulfilled.

A similar problem can occur with informed consent. How informed does it have to be? Do we give general details, enough information to make a decision, or full information so that all the implications can be considered? What happens if the information is not understood in fine detail? Can too much information about prenatal diagnosis actually do harm by making people anxious or paralysed by indecision? Again, the question is whether information is a means to doing good (in which case the doctor may judge when enough has been given) or necessary in itself to be autonomous (in which case the patient decides, and articulate patients are entitled to as much time as they require).

Non-directive counselling and informed consent are often described as vital to avoid the manipulation of parents and suggestions that prenatal diagnosis and abortion are being used to improve the human race (reminiscent of Nazi eugenic policies to rid the world of diseased people). However, is there actually anything wrong with the aim of having less genetic disease and suffering in the world (rather than the means to achieve it)? And does non-directive counselling really protect against the charge of eugenics? Imagine that a gene for homosexuality or shortness or needing glasses was discovered, and parents wanted, after very careful non-directive counselling, to abort fetuses that would become homosexual, short or bespectacled; would that make it acceptable? Counsellors give the facts and allow people with beliefs about the value of different humans to act on them. Is that really morally neutral, or could it be eugenics by collusion or default? Does fulfilling non-directive counselling just let health workers off the moral hook, but allow parental prejudice full sway? It might be considered a private matter for parents since they have to bring up the children.

DEALING WITH CONFLICT

Many situations induce a feeling of ethical unease; 'I'm not sure that this is right. I feel very uncomfortable with this decision or course of action. I am being pressurized into something that feels wrong'. The conflicts can be between professionals, between professionals and their individual patients or between professionals and society. There are often many layers to a problem. Some, such as communication problems, inexperienced staff or inadequate resources, may be resolvable. Fundamental ethical conflicts cannot be resolved, but may be clarified.

When an ethical problem arises in real practice, there are many ways to deal with it:

1. Recognize the problem
Ethical unease should be attended to. What is the dilemma? By talking about and analysing a problem, it can usually be broken down into its component parts, medical, social, psychological or ethical.

2. Return to medical facts
Good and accurate information about prognosis or the risk/benefit ratio of a course of action often settles ethical dilemmas, as they prove to be less acute or contentious than at first sight. Whatever the moral framework, there is a strong obligation for professionals in the field to be well trained and updated. It is mistaken to guess, bluff or fail to ask for help when needed.

3. Identify the different parties and the different interests
It may be that someone has a very strong case, but it is nothing to do with professional obligations. Regular sympathy may be all that is required. Health professionals tend to want to help everyone, including future generations, but it is not clear that they have to do so.

4. Examine personal feelings

Sometimes the ethical unease is a personal sensitivity (related to personal experience of disease or fertility problems). Is a course of action being followed whilst ignorant or inexperienced? Fear of failure or stepping out of line can be powerful inhibitors of rational thought. Is there an emotional element whereby this particular patient evokes powerful feelings of concern, anger or helplessness? 'Know thyself' is important for getting out of self-made ethical dilemmas. By contrast, are some insights too uncomfortable or painful such that they are being suppressed by strong beliefs (religious, political or ideological)?

5. Recognize pressures to cut ethical corners

There may be financial pressures from a fee-paying patient or the salary-paying employer, career pressures to coerce patients to take part in research.

6. Ensure good communication

Many conflicts arise from poor communication or understanding of the patient's story, situation or experience. Breakdowns of communication may be avoidable, and when they have occurred can often be remedied.

7. Adhere to professional codes of conduct

In the UK, general guidance is given by the General Medical Council 'Duties of a doctor' (http://www.gmc-uk.org/standards/doad.htm) and by the Royal Colleges of Nurses and Midwives. There are equivalents in other countries. Specific guidance is sometimes offered from specialty organizations.

8. Obtain a second opinion

It is helpful to articulate a problem for clarification. Colleagues may help elucidate the key issues in a complex case, confirm the proposed course of action, or be prepared to take a different course of action.

9. Obtain a legal opinion

The law acts in a practical way to resolve disputes between parties in society. When ethical dilemmas are seemingly insoluble, an opinion from a medical defence society or medical lawyer may help.

10. Respect new law – from the Courts and Parliament

In the highly contentious area of reproduction, and with the advances in technology, the law sometimes frames the limits of acceptable medical behaviour. Parliament may make limiting or enabling law as a reflection of public opinion.

11. Ensure continued ethical education

This can be by reading journals or books, attending courses and listening to patients and their concerns. Ethical case presentations can be brought to multidisciplinary groups for discussion. Everyone involved in prenatal diagnosis should be constantly reassessing their opinions and views, and be prepared to explain the ethical stance they take.

12. Maintain continuing debate in society

A creative debate continues amongst and between professionals and the general public. This occurs through the media, professional journals, ethics groups and special interest groups. Toleration of different views, and respect for the goodwill of opponents are qualities that help mutual understanding, if not agreement. Philosophers, theologians and lawyers may help untangle problems, although it is unlikely that there will ever be an ethical expert who can be called in to solve all the problems raised by prenatal diagnosis!

Key points

- It is impossible to avoid ethical dilemmas in prenatal diagnosis.
- Fetal moral status is contested.
- There are a limited number of arguments as to why any abortion may or may not be permissible.
- Different moral frameworks may give different reasons to support or reject an action, but may also throw up challenging inconsistencies elsewhere.
- Doctors have to justify their attitudes and actions and be prepared to defend them.
- Some practical steps can be taken to improve the quality of thinking about ethical issues.

---

2 LEGAL ISSUES IN PRENATAL DIAGNOSIS IN ENGLAND AND WALES

Jonathan Montgomery

INTRODUCTION

The law serves a number of functions in relation to health care practice. It structures the relationship between professionals and patients/clients, setting the ground rules on which the health professions practice. Thus the law governing consent, access to health records and confidentiality help determine the character of the therapeutic relationship, hopefully as a partnership, rather than one dominated by either a paternalistic professional or a consumerist patient. The law also has a role in setting limits to acceptable practice on behalf of society. Controversial ethical issues, such as those that arise when the termination of pregnancy is being considered, are regulated through a legal framework. This will rarely force a single solution upon unwilling professionals and clients, but it will often rule out some options.

The law also has an important function as a mechanism for enforcing these basic principles. It provides remedies to enable patients/clients to vindicate their rights. Sometimes, this can be done through court orders requiring that things are done, or not done. This ensures that clients receive the services to which they are entitled. Sometimes, the problems only come to light when it is too late, rights have been overridden or proper standards of care were not met. Here, the law can only offer compensation for the victims of problems caused by substandard care.

It would be wrong for health professionals to assume that these functions mean that the law is a threat to their work. In most areas it reinforces professional standards rather than undermines them. While the increase in litigation clearly brings genuine worries, the problems relate more to the financial consequences for health services than to restrictions on practitioners that prevent them exercising their clinical judgment in the best interests of their patients/clients. There are widely expressed worries about the phenomenon of defensive medicine. However, if this term describes health professionals doing things that they believe are against their clients' interests merely because the law requires it, then it is a myth. Such practices will not give health professionals better protection in law, because the law almost invariably requires them to achieve satisfactory standards as judged by their own peers not by judges (Jones and Morris, 1989).

The corollary of the fact that the law reinforces basic professional standards is that staying within the law is not in itself a guarantee of ethical practice. The law marks out boundaries more than it determines what should happen. It tends to leave the professions to establish their own canons of ethics. Thus, awareness of the legal aspects of prenatal diagnosis will help professionals to avoid poor practice, but it cannot absolve them from grappling directly with the ethical issues. This chapter discusses the interaction between the law and clinical practice and outlines the English legal framework within which prenatal diagnosis is carried out. Laws differ considerably between countries, so it is not possible to explore the rules applicable in different countries in any detail. However, the conclusion to this chapter considers briefly the variations that can be found in other legal systems.

THE IMPACT OF THE LAW ON PRENATAL DIAGNOSIS

There are few legal rules designed specifically to solve the difficulties encountered in offering prenatal diagnosis. Instead, the implications of general principles need to be worked out. The law is therefore examined in relation to four stages in the process.

First, there are decisions on whether to offer such testing. These may be taken at a macro level, when commissioners decide how far National Health Service funding will be made available for prenatal diagnosis. There will also be choices to be made about individual patients, choosing which tests (from amongst those that are possible) should be made available to them. The second stage in the process concerns the need for proper counselling if it is decided to offer testing. The third point at which legal standards are relevant concerns the testing itself. Fourthly, it is necessary to consider the law governing the use of the results of prenatal diagnosis. This includes rules on the control of the information and also the termination of pregnancy.

The provision of prenatal diagnosis

Under the National Health Service Act (1977) the Secretary of State for health is obliged to provide a comprehensive health service. However, this does not mean that the National Health Service, or individual health professionals working within it, must provide everything possible; nor does it mean that they must always give patients/clients what they want. Attempts to use the courts to force professionals to offer care when it does not have priority within existing resource constraints have consistently failed. Providing the decision is taken properly, with due care and without discrimination on the basis of the sex or race of the patient/client, it should be safe from legal challenge (Montgomery, 2002). Although these principles have not been tested in relation to services for prenatal diagnosis, they have been established in other contexts.

In 1980 a group of patients tried to use the courts to force a health authority and the Secretary of State to enhance orthopaedic services. It had been accepted that improvement was necessary and the Secretary of State had agreed to the building of a new hospital. However, the plans were then shelved due to lack of funding. The Court of Appeal rejected the patients' claim that the duty to provide a comprehensive health service had been breached. The judges stated that resource allocation was a political issue that was properly addressed through

Parliament, not the courts (*R* v *Secretary of State for Social Services*, ex p. *Hincks*, 1980). Thus, it appears that a purchaser who claimed that there was insufficient money to provide services for prenatal diagnosis would be safe from challenge through the courts.

Where the service is available, patients/clients may feel aggrieved if it is not offered to them. Such matters have also come to court. In 1987 a baby was being cared for in a Birmingham hospital awaiting an operation to repair a hole in his heart. There were insufficient nursing staff to offer the operation to all the babies who would benefit from it. The parents of the baby sought an order from the court instructing the hospital to treat him. The Court of Appeal rejected their application. They said that they could not get involved in the managerial questions of resource allocation, nor could they rearrange waiting lists. They would interfere only if a health authority acted wholly unreasonably (*R* v *Central Birmingham HA*, ex p. *Walker*, 1987).

There is little guidance as to what would be counted as an unreasonable decision. The courts have indicated that it would be improper to select patients on the basis of race (*R* v *Ethical Committee of St Mary's Hospital* {Manchester}, ex p. *Harriott*, 1988). Presumably discrimination on the basis of sex would similarly be unacceptable because, like racial discrimination, sex discrimination is prohibited by statute. It will usually be improper to decide whether to offer prenatal diagnosis to people on the basis of religious affiliation. This appears to happen in Judaism, but this is not due to religious affiliation; rather, it is because Ashkenazi Jews are an ethnic group with an increased risk for some disorders, such as Tay-Sachs disease. Discrimination on the basis of Disability is also unlawful (Disability Discrimination Act 1995) and it would probably be unreasonable to differentiate between the pregnancies of women who themselves have disabilities and those who do not.

These sorts of factors may, of course, be important where a particular group wishes to use prenatal diagnosis as a way of pursuing objectives (such as sex selection) that are unacceptable to health professionals. It would be dangerous to refuse diagnostic testing to patients/clients merely on the basis of their sex, religion or race. This does not mean that there may not be acceptable reasons for refusing to cooperate with such plans. In particular, it may be that in many cases there is no scope within the law for using the information that would be generated. If sex alone could not justify an abortion, then it would be proper to refuse testing on the basis that it could not produce any useable information and would thus be a waste of resources. The relevant aspects of abortion law are discussed below.

These examples illustrate how reluctant the courts have proved to be to interfere with managerial decisions on resource allocation within the National Health Service. They have gone further still in their deference to clinical judgment. While they have reserved the right to override unreasonable decisions about the use of resources, they have stated (in the context of the care of *disabled* newborns) that doctors are entitled to 'refuse to adopt treatment ... on the basis that it is medically contraindicated or for some other reason is a treatment which they could not conscientiously administer' (Re J, 1990, p. 30). Even more explicitly, it has also been held that it would be an abuse of the powers of the courts to force a doctor to treat a patient against his or her clinical judgment (Re J, 1992). This principle would also be applied to cases outside the National Health Service.

The law previously described means that it would be very difficult indeed to obtain an order from a British court requiring that a patient be offered prenatal diagnosis. The implementation of the Human Rights Act 1998, requiring public bodies in the UK to respect citizens' rights under the European Convention on Human Rights has had little impact on the courts' reluctance to intervene in resource allocation decisions. To date, judges have suggested that the Convention cannot be used to create rights to specific services (*R* v *NW Lancashire HA*, ex p. *A*, 2000; *R* v *Secretary of State for the Home Department*, ex p. *Mellor*, 2001).

In practice, most challenges will be made after the event, alleging that the professional acted negligently, that is without reasonable care. That legal doctrine requires proof that the course of action taken would not be accepted as proper by a responsible body of professional people skilled in the area in question (*Bolam* v *Friern* HMC, 1957). This effectively means that where health professionals believe that testing is inappropriate, then the law will allow them to withhold it from patients even when the patients are keen to have it. Where there are differing opinions within the professions, providing that the refusal to offer testing is acceptable to at least one school of thought, it will not be negligent (*Maynard* v *West Midlands RHA*, 1983). The courts will only intervene where there is no logical basis for the view adopted by the health professionals (*Bolitho* v *City and Hackney HA*, 1997).

It should be noted that where patient/clients are offered specialist services, they are entitled to expect that they will be properly carried out, and the standard of care is tailored to responsible professional practice in those specialties. Thus, if prenatal diagnosis is offered it is no excuse for a mistake that some units could not offer such a service at all. Further, on this principle, hospitals as well as individual professionals may be liable if the services they deliver fail to meet the promised standard (*Wilsher* v *Essex AHA*, 1988).

The net effect of these decisions of the English courts is that patients cannot demand prenatal diagnosis when health professionals genuinely and reasonably believe that it should be withheld. From one perspective, this enables health professionals to protect patients from a self-destructive desire for knowledge at all costs. From another, it is paternalistic and permits health professionals to impose their views of the ethics of prenatal diagnosis on their patients/clients. In the private sector, the persuasive power of money may minimize the likelihood of this occurring. In the state-funded National Health Service, it is an example of the general lack of patient power (Montgomery, 1996).

Counselling on testing

If it is decided to offer diagnostic testing, it will be necessary to obtain the consent of the person from whom the material to be tested will be obtained

(Kennedy, 1992). Such consent needs to be real, but in English law (in contrast to the position in many countries) it does not have to be fully informed. English law draws a distinction between the fact of consent to the procedure and the obligation to counsel patients. The former requires the patient to be informed in broad terms of what is to happen to them, to be capable of deciding to agree to it and to be free from coercion in doing so. A health professional may negate an otherwise valid consent by withholding information for improper reasons, but the failure to inform a patient/client of all the risks and alternatives will not usually render the test unlawful.

The extent of the duty to counsel patients/clients is determined by the test for negligence. This means that, providing professional practice is followed, there will be no scope for legal action. The courts have suggested that patients should normally be fully informed, especially if they ask questions, but have declined to set more precise legal standards for the health professions. Some guidance has been offered in the course of judicial discussion. Health professionals should be particularly diligent in informing patients of any special risks involved, that is risks that would (if they materialized) be particularly significant for them. The judges have also accepted that it is permissible to withhold information if it would harm the health of patients to reveal it. The general position is that judges expect that professionals will ask themselves whether information would be regarded as significant by a reasonable person in the patient's position (*Pearce* v *United Bristol Hospitals NHS Trust*, 1998). This guidance is not, however, legally binding. When the crunch comes, the courts have always returned to the professional standards test (Montgomery, 1988), although they have asserted the right to consider whether there is a logical basis for the practice of the professionals (Montgomery, 2002).

In practice, therefore, once again English law basically leaves the health professions to police themselves. It would almost certainly be negligent to fail to counsel a patient fully about the implications of prenatal diagnosis. However, this would be because professional opinion would regard a failure to counsel them as irresponsible, not because a judge has reached that conclusion independently.

Carrying out the test

Where prenatal diagnosis involves carrying out tests on the mother during pregnancy, then her consent will be sufficient to authorize it. However, where it involves preimplantation testing on gametes or embryos, it may need to be done under a licence from the Human Fertilisation and Embryology Authority. The Human Fertilisation and Embryology Act 1990 prohibits the storage of human gametes, and the creation and storage of human embryos, unless such a licence has been granted. The Authority has indicated that it will license pre-implantation genetic diagnosis for severe or life-threatening conditions (HFEA, 2001).

If the diagnostic test goes ahead, and something goes wrong, once again the legal action would be for negligence (Montgomery, 2002). This would be so whether the mishap was an inaccurate result, an injury to the child *in utero*, or the loss of the baby. If there has been a genuine accident, without negligence, the action will fail. Proving that a medical accident during prenatal testing was the result of negligence would involve two stages:

1. Patients/clients would need to show that there had been an unacceptably poor standard of practice.
2. The person suing would have to prove that they had suffered 'damage' as a result of the mistake.

The first stage of the process involves the standard of care outlined above. The patient/client would have to prove that the person carrying out the tests failed to meet the standards expected of them by their own peers. This does not mean that there must be uniform practice, but it means that the way in which the test was carried out must be regarded by experts from the profession as within the range of approaches that are regarded as legitimate. A mistake will constitute negligence if it is an error that would not have been made if responsible practice had been followed.

The courts have elaborated this test in a number of ways. It has already been pointed out that the courts will not prefer one accepted professional approach to another. The test for negligence is not designed to stifle innovation. Nor is it concerned with enforcing the best possible practice. Provided a minimum level of competence is attained, then the professional carrying out the tests has not been negligent.

The courts have also held that the victims of accidents should not lose out because the person caring for them is inexperienced. The hospital has an obligation to provide professional services, and if they fail to do so they will be liable to compensate anybody who suffers injury as a result. Inexperienced hospital staff are expected to be competent to provide the services on offer, but, if they are unsure of their skill, they may escape liability for accidents by recognizing their limitations and calling in more senior staff to confirm their diagnoses or carry out tricky procedures (*Wilsher* v *Essex AHA*, 1988). Thus an individual practitioner may be protected from a negligence action, but the patient will still be compensated.

The second stage of a legal action, showing that damage was caused by the mistake, raises two issues. First, is the damage suffered something that the courts recognize as amenable to compensation through the law? Injury to the baby will qualify and the courts have accepted that the birth of an unwanted baby may also be damage for these purposes, although no compensation will be payable for the birth itself, only for the financial consequences of any disability. Physical injury to the mother would also suffice, and pain and suffering that goes with it would also be compensated. However, distress alone, short of clinically diagnosed mental illness, is not compensated by English law. This would mean that if an abnormality is falsely diagnosed and the woman (or couple) decides to continue with the pregnancy, and a healthy infant is born, then there would probably be little chance of a successful negligence action.

In practice, it will often be the case that the causal link between the injury suffered and the negligence will be unclear. It is for the person suing to prove the causal link, and uncertainty will protect the professional. In essence, the professional's defence would be that their mistake made no difference; any damage that the patient/client suffered would have occurred even without their mistake. The detailed application of this principle will vary according the type of case.

Where there is a failure to diagnose an abnormality, the court would need to consider whether anything could, or would, have been done to avoid the birth if the professionals had acted properly. If no legal abortion would have been available, even if a disabililty had been detected, the chain of causation between mistake and injury would be broken. No action to prevent the birth could have been taken without breaking the law. Thus the birth of the disabled child would not have been a result of the mistake, but of the legal rules (*Rance* v *Mid-Downs HA*, 1991). This makes the grounds for the termination of pregnancy (discussed below) significant in some negligence actions. Similarly, if the parents would not have chosen to terminate had they known the correct position, then the mistake would have made no difference.

Complications arise when the child is suing for errors in prenatal diagnosis. This cannot happen unless the child is born alive and there has been a breach of duty towards the mother (Congenital Disabilities (Liability) Act 1976). Even when this is the case, however, the courts have refused to accept claims for damages based on the claim that the person suing would rather not have been born at all (*Mckay* v *Essex AHA*, 1982). These are sometimes known as 'wrongful life' claims. Thus, a negligent failure to diagnose an abnormality or to counsel about the possibility of termination will not give rise to a legal action by the child. Where, however, a mistake in the diagnostic procedure actually causes an injury to the child, then it may sue once it has been born.

Acting on the result

The first decision that has to be made once the results of prenatal diagnosis come through concerns informing the parents of the results. A distinction needs to be drawn between the obligations of health professionals to inform their patients/clients in response to specific questions and the rights of patients to seek information out. Failing to volunteer information would be legal unless the standard of care in negligence, as outlined above, was breached. It is therefore essentially a matter for the professions. However, it must be questionable whether professional practice would support testing when it was not intended to reveal the results. To fail to pass on the results of the test would thus probably be unlawful in many circumstances. The real problems arise when professionals wish to reveal some of the information obtained from prenatal testing, but not all of it. This raises the second issue.

Patients have rights of access to their records under data protection law (Data Protection Act 1998; Data Protection (Subject Access Modification) (Health) Order 2000). However, these rights are not absolute. Access can be refused where it would cause serious harm to the physical or mental health of the patient or another person to allow it. As a fetus cannot generally constitute a legal person until it is born, it would not be possible to justify withholding the results of a test because they would be used to terminate a pregnancy. In order to avoid problems, health professionals might limit the amount of information recorded after tests to the minimum necessary for their clinical purposes.

This might become an issue where the test had been carried out to screen for an abnormality that the professional would have regarded as a legitimate ground for an abortion and that abnormality was excluded, but the test revealed other information that the patient/client (but not the professionals) regarded as a ground for termination. An obvious example would be the sex of the fetus. No professional could be forced to test for fetal sex against his/her wishes (see above). However, once the information is incorporated into the notes, patients will be entitled to see it on request unless the health professional responsible for their care can show that the patient's health would be at risk from having access to the facts.

A final legal issue in relation to the dissemination of the results of prenatal diagnosis concerns the position of the father of the fetus. Where testing has been carried out on a pregnant woman, technically the results are confidential to her. They should not, therefore, be passed on to her partner without her agreement. It would be safest to establish her views before carrying out the diagnostic tests. There would be no difficulty where tests are carried out on gametes of embryos *in vitro*, because both parents would be involved as patients (because the law requires both their consents).

The next decision to which the law is relevant concerns the possibility of abortion. There is no right to an abortion in English law. Rights imply entitlement, which is not secured by English law. The law establishes when abortions may be legal, and within those limits it makes two doctors the gatekeepers to the procedure (Abortion Act 1967, as amended by the Human Fertilisation and Embryology Act 1990). This means that a woman is never entitled to a termination of pregnancy, just because it would be lawful to carry one out. Professionals who oppose abortions on principle have an express legal right to opt out under the 'conscience clause' (Abortion Act 1967, s 4). However, if a doctor believes that a particular woman's case is insufficiently meritorious she or he may simply decline to offer termination on the basis that the legal grounds have not been established. This point can be seen more clearly from an examination of the grounds set out in the Act.

Two of the four grounds on which terminations of pregnancy are legal may be in issue. They apply to selective reductions of multiple pregnancies as well as the termination of single pregnancies. The first is the so-called 'social ground' that is available up to 24 weeks. This covers cases where two doctors believe in good faith that the continuance of the pregnancy would involve risk, greater than if the pregnancy were terminated, of injury to the physical or mental health of the pregnant woman or any existing children of her family. The second is available until birth itself and covers cases where two doctors believe in good faith that there is a substantial risk that if the child were born it would suffer from such physical or mental abnormalities as to be seriously handicapped.

The precise meaning of each of these two grounds is unclear. It is sometimes argued that statistical evidence shows that it is always safer to terminate a pregnancy in the early stages than to carry the baby to term and deliver it. If this is the case, then there will always be a justification for abortions before the 24th week. No court has ever been asked to consider whether this approach would be legal. It is, however, clear that doctors have filled in the forms citing only 'pregnancy' as the justification for abortions and have not been prosecuted. This 'statistical argument' could be used covertly to permit the abortion of fetuses of the undesired sex. It has also been argued that sex selection through termination of pregnancy may be openly practised on the basis that the woman would suffer ill-health due to the social stigma of having a baby of the 'wrong' sex (Morgan, 1988, 2001). Again, no court has had the opportunity to pronounce on the legality of such a practice.

The 'social grounds' for termination are available only before the end of the 24th week of pregnancy. Unfortunately, there is some doubt as to the way in which pregnancies are to be dated. Some commentators have suggested that the 24 weeks begin to run from the point of conception (Grubb, 1991; Murphy, 1991). However, the best view is probably that the words refer to the usual clinical practice of dating from the first day of the woman's last menstrual period, correcting if necessary after ultrasonic scan (Montgomery, 2002). This is the assumption made by the Abortion Regulations 1991 (although the regulations cannot alter the meaning of the statute).

There is no gestational age limit on terminations on the basis of fetal handicap. That ground is therefore available right up until the time of birth. However, it is unclear what degree of handicap would satisfy the test (Morgan, 1990). One case suggests that in essence the question is whether the child's life would be worth living (*Mckay* v *Essex AHA*, 1982). Some help is given by the cases concerning the selective non-treatment of neonates. The courts have recognized that it is sometimes legitimate to withhold treatment, even though it is known that the result of doing so is likely to be the child's death. They have refused to authorize such a plan of care in relation to Down syndrome (Re B, 1981), but have accepted it where there was no prospect of prolonging the baby's life for any significant time (Re C, 1989). The Court of Appeal has also endorsed the decision of a paediatric team to decline to ventilate a child born very prematurely, severely brain damaged and expected to be quadriplegic, blind, deaf and dumb (Re J, 1990).

The courts have rejected, however, suggestions that they should set out quasi-statutory guidelines on the degree of disability that would justify non-treatment. These decisions cannot really be taken to establish rules that the particular handicaps in issue would always be treated in the same way. The courts have also rejected the suggestion that parents are entitled to decide whether a disability is so serious that treatment should be withheld. The issue is what is in the best interests of the child not whether the parents' views are reasonable (Re C (HIV Test), 1999).

One of the implications of this uncertainty is that there is considerable scope for doctors to interpret the law so that it is line with their own moral views on what grounds provide an ethical justification for the termination of pregnancy. The legality of a termination does not actually depend on the precise meaning of (for example) 'seriously handicapped'. What matters is whether the doctors believed in good faith that this might be the case. Thus, it is medical opinion that ultimately determines whether an abortion can be carried out, and unless it can be shown that the doctors acted in bad faith it would be very difficult to impugn their decision.

CONCLUSION

This chapter has surveyed the main legal issues raised by prenatal diagnosis. It has aimed to state the relevant principles of English law clearly, without becoming embroiled in the ethical problems discussed in the previous chapter. It has shown that in most areas the legal standards are determined by the health professions rather than the courts. The best way to avoid brushes with the law is therefore to pursue good professional practice. However, it is unlikely that the consciences of those practising prenatal diagnosis will be satisfied with merely avoiding legal difficulties. Staying within the boundaries of legally acceptable practice is no guarantee of good ethics. It may be the beginning of good ethical practice, but it is not enough.

The focus on English law has been deliberate because the degree of variation between legal systems is such that a comprehensive survey would have to be of enormous length (see Giesen, 1988, for such a survey). However, in every legal system the same four categories of legal problem will arise. Access to services will be determined largely by the way in which services are organized in the country in question. Where the provision is private, then it will rarely be possible to force a professional to offer tests, although malpractice laws may come close to doing so.

In many countries the legal standards required of health professionals in relation to both counselling and malpractice are more intrusive of clinical judgment than in England. There is, therefore, no guarantee that other legal systems are so supportive of professional ethics as the English system. More commonly, the courts will assess whether professional standards are reasonable when considered in the light of prevailing community standards. This is particularly true in the area of informed consent, where English law is out of line with the predominant global view that patients should be given the information that they would regard as significant, even where professionals are reluctant to convey it.

The regulatory system established by the Human Fertilisation and Embryology Act 1990 is generally regarded as one of the more sophisticated regimes. In some countries there is no regulation and in others the dealing with embryos *in vitro* is banned. There may also be legislative restrictions on what grounds are regarded as legitimate for tests. In relation to the grounds for termination of pregnancy, English law is neither particularly restrictive nor especially liberal (Glendon, 1987). The fundamental point, however, is that each legal system must be considered in its own right.

By focusing on one system, that applied in England and Wales, the issues have been highlighted and the position in those countries explained. This should enable English and Welsh practitioners to avoid legal problems. It should also assist those from other countries to discover their own laws by identifying the questions that they should ask.

Key points

- In all countries, the law structures the relationship between professionals and patients/ clients, setting the ground rules on which the health professions practice. This impacts on the provision of prenatal diagnosis, counselling on testing, carrying out the test and acting on the result.
- The law reinforces professional standards rather than undermining them. Defensive medicine (doing things that are not in their client's interests because the health professional believes the law requires it) does not give health professionals better protection in law, because English law almost invariably requires them to achieve satisfactory standards as judged by their own peers rather than by judges.
- The National Health Service is obliged by law to provide a comprehensive health service, but NHS health professionals are not obliged to provide everything possible, nor must they always give patients/clients what they want.
- A mistake made by a professional will constitute negligence if it is an error that would not have been made if responsible practice had been followed. The test for negligence is not designed to stifle innovation nor to enforce the best possible practice. If an acceptable level of competence is attained, then the professional has not been negligent.
- In England and Wales, patients have the right of access to their records, but health professionals may limit the amount of information recorded to the minimum necessary for their clinical purposes.

REFERENCES

Bolam v *Friern Hospital Management Committee* (1957) 1 Butterworths Medico-Legal Reports 1–13.

Bolitho v *City and Hackney HA* (1997) 4 All England Law Reports 771.

Data Protection (Subject Access Modification) (Health) Order (2000), SI 2000 No 413.

Giesen D (1988) *International Medical Malpractice Law*. Martinus Nijhoff Publications, Dordrecht, Holland.

Glendon MA (1987) *Abortion and Divorce in Western Law*. Harvard University Press, Cambridge, MA.

Grubb A (1991) The new law of abortion: clarification or ambiguity? *Criminal Law Review*, 659–670.

Human Fertilisation and Embryology Authority (2001) Ethical issues in the creation and selection of preimplantation embryos to produce tissue donors (opinion issued 22 November 2001).

Jones MA, Morris AE (1989) Defensive medicine: myths and facts. *Journal of the Medical Defence Union*, 5; 40–43.

Kennedy I (1992) Consent to treatment: the capable person. In *Doctors, Patients and the Law* (ed. Dyer, C). Blackwell Scientific Publications, Oxford.

Maynard v *West Midlands RHA* (1983) 1 Butterworths Medico-Legal Reports 122–131.

Mckay v *Essex AHA* (1982) Law Reports, Queens Bench 1166.

Montgomery J (1988) Power/knowledge/consent: medical decision-making. *Modern Law Review*, 51; 245–255.

Montgomery J (1996) Patients first: the role of rights. In E*ssential Practice in Patient Centred Care* (eds Fulford KWM, Ersser S, Hope T). Blackwell Science, Oxford.

Montgomery J (2002) *Health Care Law*, (2nd edn). Oxford University Press, Oxford.

Morgan D (1988) Foetal sex identification, abortion and the law. *Family Law*, 18; 355–359.

Morgan D (1990) Abortion: the unexamined ground. *Criminal Law* Review, 687–694.

Morgan D (2001) Legal and ethical dilemmas of fetal sex identification and gender selection. In *Issues in Medical Law and Ethics* (Morgan D), Cavendish Publishing, London.

Murphy J (1991) Cosmetics, eugenics and ambivalence: the revision of the Abortion Act 1967. *Journal of Social Welfare & Family Law*, 375–393.

Pearce v *United Bristol Hospitals NHS Trust* (1998) 48 Butterworths Medico-Legal Reports 118.

R v *Central Birmingham HA*, ex p. *Walker*; R *v Secretary of State for Social Services*, ex p. *Walker* (1987) 3 Butterworths Medico-Legal Reports 32–36.

R v *Ethical Committee of St Mary's Hospital* (Manchester), ex p. *Harriott* (1988) 1 Family Law Reports 512.

R v *North West Lancashire HA*, ex p. *A* (2000) 2 Family Court Reports 525.

R v *Secretary of State for the Home Department*, ex p. *Mellor* (2001) 2 Family Court Reports 153.

R v *Secretary of State for Social Services, West Midlands RHA and Birmingham AHA*, ex p. *Hincks* (1980) 1 Butterworths Medico-Legal Reports 93–97.

Rance v *Mid-Downs HA* (1991) 1 All England Law Reports 801–824.

Re B (1981) 1 Weekly Law Reports 1421–1425.

Re C (1989) 2 All England Law Reports 782–790.

Re C (HIV Test) (1999) 2 Family Law Reports 1004.

Re J (1990) 6 Butterworths Medico-Legal Reports 25–43.

Re J (1992) 9 Butterworths Medico-Legal Reports 10–21.

Wilsher v *Essex AHA* (1988) 3 Butterworths Medico-Legal Reports 37–91.

3 LEGAL ISSUES IN PRENATAL DIAGNOSIS IN THE USA

James B. Haddow

INTRODUCTION

Health care professionals in the USA often develop the impression that the most remarkable effect of the law on their work is its interference with the delivery of appropriate care. That perception is driven primarily by the frequently exaggerated risk of malpractice lawsuits that result in damage awards against health care providers. The fear of malpractice lawsuits, in turn, gives rise to the view that treatment and advice must take into account a set of standards imposed by the courts, rather than relying exclusively on informed professional judgment. The idea of basing treatment decisions on legal standards, often called 'defensive medicine', springs from a misapprehension of the relationship between the law and health care delivery.

It is true that even the most skilled and careful practitioners may be required to defend themselves against legal action. The actual relationship between health care and the law is, however, both more complex and less threatening than a narrow focus on large malpractice awards might suggest. A web of state and federal laws affects, among many other things, how health care practitioners secure and document their patients' consent to treatment; how they handle their patients' records and other confidential information; and under what circumstances they offer certain ethically sensitive procedures, like abortion and physician-assisted suicide. In each of these areas, professional standards and legal rules combine forces to provide guidelines intended to serve both the interests of individual patients and the broader goals of civil society. Perhaps most importantly, whatever the context, the law looks first to the judgment of health care professionals themselves in making rules that affect them. Where the law provides remedies to patients who have been denied health care to which they are entitled or who have been injured in the course of receiving care, it provides those remedies only when the challenged care falls below a standard that professionals in the field set for themselves and their peers.

Nor are orders to pay money either the exclusive aim or the inevitable result of successful health-care-related lawsuits. Remedies in these cases can take a variety of forms. For example, when a court is asked to intervene while a desired outcome can still be achieved (as when relatives seek withdrawal of life support from a patient in a persistent vegetative state), the court may provide a remedy in the form of an order directing health care providers to take specific action. In other cases, where irreparable harm has been done (as when a patient has lost a limb due to improper treatment of an infection), there is no practical alternative to an award of money damages.

In every action in which a patient seeks money damages from a health care provider, the standard of practice is the *sine qua non*, and, except in a few extraordinary cases, the patient can prove the standard of practice only by producing a witness with appropriate qualifications to explain what it is. The health care practitioner is not an insurer, and a bad outcome alone is not enough to support a remedy. Unless the patient produces a witness with the training and expertise necessary to describe the standard of care, explain how it was breached in the patient's case, and say how the breach caused the patient's injury, the patient will face dismissal of her legal claim (*Garrison* v *Medical Center of Delaware, Inc.*, 1989). In other words, in deciding whether a patient is entitled to any remedy when she is dissatisfied with her health care, courts place paramount importance on standards of practice health care practitioners establish for themselves in their areas of specialty.

United States courts traditionally determined standards of care on a case-by-case basis, by reference to evidence about how physicians in the same geographic area where the challenged treatment occurred commonly handled similar problems (Restatement (Second) of Torts § 299A, 1965). Now, however, most courts rely on evidence of national standards, when such evidence is available (Prosser *et al.*, § 32 at pp. 187–188, 1984).

The standards of care by which defendants in malpractice lawsuits are judged should not be considered aspirational. A health professional is not required by the law to use more than the degree of care and skill expected of a reasonably competent practitioner in the same class to which they belong, acting in the same or similar circumstances (e.g., *Shilkret* v *Annapolis Emergency Hospital Assoc.*, 1975). The standard 'is not that of the most highly skilled, nor is it that of the average member of the profession or trade, since those who have less than median or average skill may still be competent and qualified. Half of the physicians of America do not automatically become negligent in practicing medicine at all, merely because their skill is less than the professional average' (Restatement (Second) of Torts 299A, 1965). Therein lies the fallacy of 'defensive medicine'.

Just as no legal standard is an appropriate substitute for professional judgment, the law also is not, and does not purport to be, a source of rules of ethics for health care professionals. An understanding of the legal principles that apply to the delivery of health care can help practitioners to distinguish real legal risks from imagined ones, and to avoid the real ones more comfortably. Risk management alone, however, will not produce good, ethical practice. This chapter outlines the legal framework within which prenatal diagnosis is carried out in the United States. Much of the law that affects prenatal diagnosis is imposed at the state level, and may vary from state to state. There are, however, broad legal principles of general application, and the descriptions of the law in this chapter will focus on those principles. For the most part, this chapter will not take into account the law of any individual state.

THE IMPACT OF THE LAW ON PRENATAL DIAGNOSIS

By now, in the arena of medical malpractice litigation, many courts have had the opportunity to develop corollaries to the general rules of professional negligence for specific application to cases involving prenatal diagnosis. At the same time, the United States Congress and a number of state legislatures have enacted laws designed to regulate both laboratory procedures used in prenatal diagnosis and disposition of patient samples and confidential information. The resulting set of legal rules affects health professionals involved in prenatal diagnosis at four stages of the process: offering prenatal diagnosis to the patient, communicating with the patient about the risks and benefits of testing, conducting the test, and providing counselling and care based on the test results.

The discussion that follows considers the specific legal issues that face practitioners during each of the four phases of prenatal diagnosis.

The provision of prenatal diagnosis

Presently, the legal duty of health care professionals to offer prenatal diagnosis to their patients is defined in terms of a woman's constitutional right to terminate pregnancy before a fetus becomes 'viable', recognized by the United States Supreme Court in *Roe* v *Wade*, 410 U.S. 113 (1973). Once a fetus is viable, any state may impose regulations on the right to terminate a pregnancy, but the option of abortion must remain available to the extent necessary to preserve the life or health (including the mental or emotional health) of the mother (*Planned Parenthood of Southeastern Pennsylvania* v *Casey*, 1992). A failure to provide prenatal diagnosis can give rise to a successful claim for damages only if it prevents a patient from having access to a legal abortion (*Garrison* v *Medical Center of Delaware, Inc.*, 1989). If the patient would not have terminated her pregnancy anyway, she will not be entitled to recover damages because she was denied access to prenatal diagnosis (*Provenzano* v *Integrated Genetics*, 1999).

The scope of the legal duty to provide prenatal diagnosis and related services is coextensive with the standards of practice established by health care professionals who provide care and treatment to pregnant women. As a matter of law, a health care professional has a duty to offer to their patient at least all prenatal diagnostic tests that a reasonably competent practitioner in their specialty and in those circumstances would offer to a similarly situated patient (2 Louisell and Williams, 17G.07, 2001). If a health care provider recognizes or should reasonably recognize risk factors in a patient that suggest the possibility that her child may be affected by a disorder that can be detected through prenatal diagnosis, the health care provider has a duty to inform the patient of the risks and the availability of the appropriate tests (*Didato* v *Strehler*, 2001). On the other hand, in the absence of recognized risk factors, prenatal diagnosis need not be offered (*Munro* v *Regents of the University of California*, 1989).

In addition to any expert testimony that could be considered on the issue of the standard of care in offering prenatal diagnosis, courts have also taken into account clinical practice guidelines established by organized groups of health care specialists (e.g. *Didato* v *Strehler*, 2001). Because guidelines are usually developed by medical specialty societies or academic medical centres, however, they may carry little weight in the evaluation of care rendered by practitioners with less training or access to resources. It is important to keep in mind that, for this and other reasons, clinical practice guidelines are not, in themselves, determinative of the standard of care (4 Louisell and Williams, ¶ 29.03[4], 2001).

Although, since Roe v Wade, courts across the country have recognized claims by parents for 'wrongful birth' arising from failed prenatal diagnosis, they have (with very few exceptions) rejected 'wrongful life' claims i.e., claims brought on behalf of infants born with disorders that could have been detected by prenatal diagnosis, but were not (*Garrison* v *Medical Center of Delaware, Inc.*, 1989). In declining to recognize these claims, the courts have relied on the fact that, to date, the only alternative to being born with a disorder detectable through prenatal diagnosis was not being born at all. With that in mind, courts have generally agreed that 'the question of whether it would have been better for an impaired child to never have lived at all is a philosophical one not amenable to judicial resolution' (*Garrison* v *Medical Center of Delaware, Inc.*, 1989).

Advances in two areas of health care practice present the potential for changes in these legal paradigms. First, the availability of preimplantation genetic diagnosis (PGD) in connection with *in vitro* fertilization makes it possible for couples to discard embryos before implantation if genetic testing on embryonic cells reveals abnormalities (Harper, 1996; Lissens *et al.*, 1996). By making it possible to know about genetic disorders before an embryo is implanted, PGD presents the opportunity for a patient considering pregnancy to avoid having an affected embryo implanted in the first place, rather than having to resort to termination of the pregnancy. No decision concerning a legal claim arising from failed PGD has been reported in the United States. On one hand, it is worth noting that, in any such claim, the duty to provide accurate diagnostic information to the prospective parent would be entirely unrelated to the constitutional right to terminate a pregnancy. On the other hand, because of the risks associated with *in vitro* fertilization, it is unlikely that any US court would impose on any health care provider a legal duty to discuss PGD with, or offer PGD to, any patient who was not already involved in *in vitro* fertilization for legitimate clinical reasons.

The second advance in health care technology that is likely to affect the legal relationships between health care providers and patients in the area of prenatal diagnosis, if its potential is realized, is effective *in utero* therapy to treat genetic disorders. The potential for effective treatment of disorders that can be detected through prenatal diagnosis raises the possibility that courts will recognize widely for the first time claims by infants based on the failure to provide prenatal diagnosis. These claims would be distinguishable from the generally disfavoured wrongful life claims, because rather than comparing life to non-life, the courts would be in a position to compare life with an untreated disorder to life with effective treatment. Such a claim would, in other words, be very much like any claim by a patient for failure to offer a diagnostic test or procedure when it would have been appropriate (according to applicable professional standards) to do so.

There are no statutes that say, in so many words, that under a specific set of circumstances a health professional must make a certain prenatal diagnostic test available to a patient. Nevertheless, the standards of care for health professionals who provide prenatal care in the United States include offering at least some prenatal diagnosis to most pregnant women in most clinical settings. By defining civil liability for the same health professionals in terms of the breach of these standards, the law reinforces them, and provides an additional incentive to make prenatal diagnosis widely available.

Securing informed consent

The law requires health care practitioners, before conducting any procedure, to secure their patient's consent, after providing the patient with sufficient information about the risks and benefits of the procedure to allow the patient to make an informed choice about whether to go ahead with it (Prosser *et al.*, § 32, 1984). Precisely what information should be conveyed with respect to any specific treatment or procedure has generally been determined, once again, by reference to professional standards of care, but in recent years some courts have begun shifting the focus in informed consent analysis from what reasonable practitioners do to what reasonable patients need to know in order to make informed decisions about their own care (e.g., *Nickel v Gonzalez*, 1985). Regardless of how the standard is formulated, the obligation to provide information is not absolute or unlimited. The prevailing view of the courts is that it is 'obviously prohibitive and unrealistic to expect physicians to discuss with their patients every risk of proposed treatment – no matter how small or remote – and generally unnecessary from the patient's viewpoint as well' (*Canterbury v Spence*, 1972).

These general principles of the law of informed consent have been applied directly in the field of prenatal diagnosis (e.g. *Munroe v Regents*, 1989; *Bedel v University of Cincinnati Hospital*, 1995). Again, clinical practice guidelines sometimes address this question, but should not be considered as the only source of standards for what information should be disclosed to patients facing prenatal diagnostic testing and related procedures.

Carrying out the test

In order to carry out prenatal diagnostic testing, once the health care professional and the patient have decided to do so, a sample must be taken and analysed. Procedures like amniocentesis and chorionic villus sampling, undertaken for the purpose of collecting samples for prenatal diagnostic testing, must be performed according to standards established by the professionals who regularly conduct them. If such a procedure is performed in a professionally unacceptable manner, and if either the patient or the child *in utero* is injured as a result, then the injured party will be entitled to make a legal claim against the practitioner who performed the procedure. As in any such claim, the burden is on the person making it to prove both that the applicable standard of care was breached, and that the breach caused the injury for which compensation is sought.

Once the sample is properly secured, it must be analysed. Laboratory analysis of samples, like other functions performed by health professionals, must be done according to professional standards (*Harms* v *Laboratory Corporation of America*, 2001). As a consequence, a laboratory faces the risk of liability if it fails to perform tests according to the standard of practice among laboratories performing similar tests (*Curlender* v *Bio-Science Laboratories*, 1980; 2 Louisell and Williams, ¶17G.07[5], 2001) or if it fails to report the results accurately (*Provenzano* v *Integrated Genetics*, 1998).

As is the case in other areas of clinical practice, professional organizations have generated sets of guidelines, recommendations and checklists to which courts are likely to look in order to determine the standard of care for laboratory practice. In addition, the Federal government has proposed regulations on Genetic Testing (Federal Register, 2000; 65: 25928–24934), promulgated under the Federal Clinical Laboratory Improvement Amendments of 1988 ('CLIA'). While the primary purpose of these regulations will be to inform the process of certification of laboratories, they are likely to be treated by the courts as evidence of the applicable standard of care. Although other published guidelines (e.g. the College of American Pathologists' Checklist and the American College of Obstetricians and Gynecologists' Standards and Guidelines for Clinical Genetics Testing (http://www.acog.org) are not directly enforceable, they are also evidence of the standard of care applicable to laboratories conducting testing for the purpose of prenatal diagnosis.

Finally, after prenatal diagnosis is discussed, but before any testing begins, the health care practitioner may decide to refer the patient to a specialist for further evaluation or for testing. Even if the practitioner responsible for providing primary care collects samples for testing instead of referring the patient to a specialist, they may choose to send the samples to an independent laboratory for analysis. In either case, if the specialist or the laboratory is known or suspected to be unqualified or to have engaged in substandard practice, and if an act of malpractice by the specialist or the laboratory causes damage to the patient, the primary care practitioner may be liable for negligent referral (see *Estate of Tranor* v *Bloomberg Hospital*, 1999). The obligation to exercise an appropriate degree of care in making referrals or sending samples out for testing is independent of any separate duty that the specialist or laboratory may have to the patient.

Board Certification or accreditation is available in most health care specialty practice areas. Guidelines for the licensing and certification of testing laboratories are in place at both the state and federal levels. The American College of Medical Genetics and the College of American Pathologists also accredit laboratories with specific emphasis on prenatal diagnosis. At a minimum, a health care professional who refers a patient to an uncertified specialist or causes a screening or diagnostic test to be conducted by a laboratory without the appropriate accreditation, certification or licensure risks direct liability to the patient in the event of an adverse outcome.

Acting on the result

Before the United States Supreme Court articulated a constitutional right to terminate pregnancy, the law recognized no duty to provide information that could be used only in deciding whether a pregnancy should be terminated (see *Gleitman* v *Cosgrove*, 1967). Now, however, applicable standards of care dictate not only that prenatal diagnosis be offered in the appropriate circumstances, but also that the results be communicated to the patient (*Turner* v *Nama*, 1997). The first duty of the health care practitioner upon receiving the results of prenatal diagnostic tests is to communicate the results promptly and accurately to the patient.

Somewhat more complicated legal issues surround the disclosure of test results to family members of a pregnant woman, and particularly the other parent of the child she is carrying. Legal guidelines that find their roots in rules of professional ethics prohibit disclosure of patient information to anyone other than the patient herself without the patient's express consent, unless the information concerns a risk of harm to another (2 Louisell and Williams, ¶17G.07[1], 2001). The most comprehensive set of legal privacy guidelines are those published by the Department of Health and Human Services in July of 2001 (45 CFR parts 160, 164). These federal guidelines (fully applicable throughout the United States beginning in April of 2003) require, generally, that most doctors, hospitals, or other health care providers obtain a patient's written consent before using or disclosing the patient's personal health information. There are exceptions to the general rule, however, for certain uses of patient health information, including reporting to public health authorities and (subject to conditions) use of personal health information for research purposes. Under these guidelines, a health care practitioner who breaches a patient's confidentiality faces not only potential civil liability, but also potential criminal prosecution.

Given the obligation to maintain confidentiality of patient information, even if it means withholding information from spouses, partners, children, and other family members (e.g., *MacDonald* v *Clinger*, 1982), it is wise to establish, before prenatal diagnosis begins, who will have access to test results. It is also prudent to have the patient's written consent in advance if the results are to be reported to anyone other than the patient herself. Whether or not a spouse or partner has access to the results of prenatal diagnostic tests, the pregnant woman alone has the right to choose whether or not to terminate her pregnancy (*Planned Parenthood of Southeastern Pennsylvania* v *Casey*, 1992).

It is in the implementation of the decision to terminate a pregnancy that the law surfaces next, in the form of limits on the availability of abortion. As noted above, 'a state may not prohibit any woman from making the ultimate decision to terminate her pregnancy before viability' (*Planned Parenthood of Southeastern Pennsylvania* v *Casey*, 1992). States have, however, imposed various restrictions on the right to terminate a pregnancy after a fetus has become viable. Many states prohibit abortion of a viable fetus except when, in appropriate medical judgment, it is necessary to preserve the health or life of the mother. Because of the definitions of the terms 'viable' and 'necessary to preserve the health of the mother,' however, that prohibition, where it exists, is not as broad as it may seem.

From a legal perspective, 'the definition of "viability" and the application of the presence of a heartbeat, spontaneous respiration, and/or spontaneous movement on the demarcation of viability, are questions better left to medical experts and ethicists' (*WomanCare of Southfield, P.C.* v *Granholm*, 2000). For this reason, on this subject, courts have consistently relied on the expertise of health care professionals. What they have found quite consistently, based on testimony from these experts, is that a fetus can be non-viable either because it has not reached a gestational age at which the majority of fetuses can survive outside the uterus (generally thought to be between 23 and 26 weeks' gestation) or because it suffers from a lethal abnormality (e.g., *WomanCare of Southfield, P.C.* v *Granholm*, 2000). Although some states retain statutes that purport to limit the availability of abortion after a specific gestational age without regard to viability, those statutes are almost certainly unenforceable (*Planned Parenthood of Central Missouri* v *Danforth*, 1976). At least in cases involving diagnoses of fetal abnormalities that are so profound as to be incompatible with life, the constitutional right to abortion extends through the entire pregnancy.

Even when a fetus is indisputably viable, abortion may be available in states that restrict the termination of late-term pregnancies. To begin with, some state statutes restricting post-viability abortions make specific exceptions for cases in which a serious and untreatable fetal defect has been diagnosed. Even where no such exception exists, however, a pregnant woman has a constitutional right to an abortion at any time if it is necessary, in appropriate medical judgment, to preserve her health (*Stenberg* v *Carhart*, 2000). The United States Supreme Court has made it clear that 'necessary' cannot refer to an absolute necessity or to absolute proof. Medical treatments and procedures are often considered appropriate (or inappropriate) in light of estimated comparative health risks (and health benefits) in particular cases. Neither can that phrase require unanimity of medical opinion. Doctors often differ in their estimation of comparative health risks and appropriate treatment' (Id.). In other words, the reasoned and informed judgment of a qualified health care professional that an abortion is necessary to preserve the health of a pregnant woman will be sufficient, as a matter of law, to establish her right to an abortion, even if other qualified professionals might reach the opposite conclusion. Furthermore, at least some federal courts have said that mental or emotional health is entitled to the same protection as physical health when it comes to access to abortion (e.g., *Planned Parenthood of Central New Jersey* v *Verniero*, 1998; *Richmond Medical Center for Women* v *Gilmore*, 1999).

Here again, as in other areas of intersection between health care and the law, much more is determined by the judgment of health care professionals than by the judgment of lawyers and judges.

CONCLUSION

The foregoing discussion addresses the most prominent current legal issues that regularly arise in the field of prenatal diagnosis in the United States. It is important to keep in mind that there are principles of US law that touch prenatal diagnosis in more attenuated ways and are therefore not part of this discussion. Because of the federal system of government in the United States, there are also, as previously noted, variations in the law from state to state. Finally, the law is not static. Because the rules of legal decision in the health care arena rely so heavily on the expertise of health professionals, advances in treatment and technology will result in constant changes in the law.

Internationally, there is wide variation in the approach of legal systems to health care delivery, and it would be impractical to attempt even to summarize the differences here. While the legal rules that face practitioners outside the USA are likely to be fundamentally different from those described in this chapter, the points at which legal issues arise, and the issues themselves, are likely to be essentially the same everywhere:

- Provision of prenatal diagnosis – under what circumstances can or must a practitioner make it available?
- Communication with the patient about testing – what information, if any, must the practitioner provide to the patient in the process of securing the patient's consent to testing, and what consent is required?
- Carrying out the testing – what are a practitioner's legal obligations in collecting and analysing samples?
- Acting on the results – what results can or must be reported to whom, and what treatment options can or must the practitioner make available to the patient?

In practicing prenatal diagnosis, health care professionals will always be working within a legal framework. By being aware of the legal issues that are likely to arise, they will be better equipped to inform themselves about the legal rules that apply to their work, wherever they may pursue it.

Key points

- Legal rules for judging the professional activities of health care providers are, by and large, based on the standards of practice that providers develop for themselves and their peers.
- Failure to provide prenatal diagnosis can give rise to a successful claim for damages only when the standards of practice established by health care professionals specializing in prenatal care dictate that prenatal diagnosis should be offered, and the failure to offer it prevents a patient from having access to a legal abortion.
- The law requires that, before conducting any prenatal diagnostic procedure, health care practitioners must secure their patient's consent, after providing the patient with sufficient information about risks and benefits to allow the patient to make an informed choice about whether to proceed.
- Health professionals who collect samples for prenatal diagnostic testing must do so according to standards established by the professionals who regularly conduct the same kinds of sample collection procedures.
- Legal guidelines that find their roots in rules of medical ethics prohibit disclosure of patient information to anyone other than the patient herself without the patient's express consent, unless the information concerns a risk of harm to another.
- In the areas of intersection between health care and the law, much more is determined by the judgment of health care professionals than by the judgment of lawyers and judges.

REFERENCES

Bedel v *University of Cincinnati Hospital* (1995) 107 Ohio App. 3d 420, 669 N.E.2d 9.
Canterbury v *Spence* (1972) 464 F.2d 772.
Code of Federal Regulations, 45 CFR parts 160, 164.
Curlender v *Bio-Science Laboratories* (1980) 106 Cal. App. 3d 811, 165 Cal. Rptr. 477.
Didato v *Strehler* (2001) 262 Va. 617, 554 S.E.2d 42.
Estate of Tranor v *Bloomsburg Hospital*, 60 F. Supp. 2d 412.
Federal Register (2000); 65: 25928-24934.
Garrison v *The Medical Center of Delaware, Inc.* (1989) 581 A.2d 288.
Gleitman v *Cosgrove* (1967) 49 N.J. 22, 227 A.2d 689.
Harms v *Laboratory Corporation of America* (2001) 155 F.Supp.2d 891.
Harper JC (1996) Preimplantation Diagnosis of Inherited Disease by Embryo Biopsy: an Update of the World Figures. *Journal of Assisted Reproduction and Genetics*, 13(2); 90–95.
Lissens W, Sermon K, Staessen C *et al.* (1996) Review: Preimplantation diagnosis of inherited disease, *Journal of Inherited and Metabolic Disease*, 19; 709–723.
Louisell DW, Williams H (2001) *Medical Malpractice.* Matthew Bender, Charlottesville, LO.
MacDonald v *Clinger* (1982) 84 A.D.2d 482; 446 N.Y.S.2d 801.

Munro v *Regents of the University of California* (1989) 215 Cal. App. 3d 977, 263 Cal. Rptr. 878.

Nickel v *Gonzalez* (1985) 17 Ohio St. 3d 136, 477 N.E.2d 1145.

Planned Parenthood of Central Missouri v *Danforth* (1976) 428 U.S. 52.

Planned Parenthood of Central New Jersey v *Verniero* (1998) 41 F.Supp. 2d 478.

Planned Parenthood of Southeastern Pennsylvania v *Casey* (1992) 505 U.S. 833.

Prosser W, Keeton W, Dobbs D *et al.* (1984) *The Law of Torts* (5th edn). West Publishing Co., St Paul, MI.

Provenzano v *Integrated Genetics* (1998) 22 F.Supp. 2d 406.

Provenzano v *Integrated Genetics* (1999) 66 F. Supp. 2d 588.

Restatement (Second) of Torts (1965).

Richmond Medical Center for Women v *Gilmore* (1999) 55 F.Supp. 2d 441.

Roe v *Wade* (1973) 410 U.S. 113.

Shilkret v *Annapolis Emergency Hospital Assoc.* (1975) 276 Md. 187, 349 A.2d 245.

Stenberg v *Carhart* (2000) 530 U.S. 914.

Turner v *Nama* (1997) 294 Ill. App. 3d 19; 689 N.E.2d 303.

WomanCare of Southfield, P.C. v *Granholm* (2000) 143 F.Supp. 2d 827.

4 THE HUMAN SIDE OF SCREENING PROGRAMMES

Jean Chapple

INTRODUCTION

The dictionary definition of screening includes 'to sift coarsely' – implying that it is not a precise process. The UK National Screening Committee (2000) defines screening as:

> *a public health service in which members of a defined population, who do not necessarily perceive they are at risk of, or are already affected by a disease or its complications, are asked a question or offered a test, to identify those individuals who are more likely to be helped than harmed by further tests or treatment to reduce the risk of a disease or its complications.*

Public health specialists differ from midwives and doctors involved in clinical medicine in that their 'patients' are whole communities rather than the individuals who make up that community. This creates a potential tension between those making health policy decisions that affect society as a whole and those who have day-to-day contact with individuals and who need resources to deliver that clinical care. In general, what is good for the individual is also good for society. However, UK debates about combined mumps, measles and rubella vaccine and possible associations with autism show that professionals and the public do not always appreciate this. Diagnosing and treating one person may mean that no resources are left to diagnose and treat another. These are the opportunity costs of a programme – Dr Paul may be robbing Dr Peter of his or her chance to treat the patient sitting in front of them (Mooney, 1992).

Screening has important ethical differences from clinical practice as the health service is targeting apparently healthy people in an attempt to help individuals to make better-informed choices about their health. However, there are risks involved and it is important that both professionals and patients have realistic expectations of what a screening programme can deliver (UK National Screening Committee, 2000). This chapter looks at some of the challenges in running prenatal and genetic screening programmes whilst treating individuals as people and not inanimate products on a eugenic production line.

Acheson (1988) defines public health as the science and art of preventing disease, prolonging life and promoting health through the organized efforts of society. Public health has six main roles to play in prenatal diagnosis and screening:

1. assessing when and why malformations occur;
2. assessing the need for screening;
3. evaluating pilot screening projects;

4. teaching professionals and the public about screening;
5. informing public policy decisions about screening;
6. monitoring the results of population screening programmes.

ASSESSING WHEN AND WHY MALFORMATIONS OCCUR

The core science of public health is epidemiology, the study of the distribution and determinants of disease. This means looking at data from large populations to see what malformations occur, how often they occur and who is affected.

Congenital malformations are generally rare, with about 2% of all fetuses having a major malformation. The average family doctor who looks after about 3000 patients will have no more than 60 new babies in the practice each year and would expect to see less than one baby each year with a major genetic problem. If a new health hazard arises which doubles the rate of malformations, it is easy to see that the family doctor would regard two babies with malformations in a year as entirely due to chance clustering of rare events. It is easier to see the effects of a teratogen in a maternity hospital, with between two to six thousand births a year. However, if only a low proportion of women or their partners are exposed to the teratogen, the numbers of babies affected will still be small and again may be ascribed to chance. It is not until figures on malformations from hundreds of thousands of pregnancies are aggregated that effects of health hazards can be shown with any degree of certainty. This can be done using congenital malformation and genetic registers. The power of regional registers can be increased if they cooperate to pool results, as happened in the EURO-HAZCON study to look at the risk of congenital anomalies near hazardous-waste landfill sites in Europe (Dolk *et al.*, 1998).

Registers use information from individuals as part of good epidemiological studies. This use of information vital for public health worries some health professionals who fear that it conflicts with their obligation to preserve confidentiality. In the UK this has resulted in legislation to regulate the use of information (Section 60 of the UK Health and Social Care Act 2001). Epidemiological studies lead to the formation of hypotheses as to the cause of malformations in populations that can be tested scientifically (Fielder *et al.*, 2000). This may suggest ways of detecting the malformation through screening individuals in that population who have the characteristics that make that malformation more likely to happen (the high-risk population).

Epidemiological analysis has found the cause of some malformations, such as the effects of thalidomide on limb formation in fetuses, the effects of maternal rubella (Sullivan *et al.*, 1999), and of some anti-epileptic drugs (Jones *et al.*, 1989) and the increased incidence of malformations in women on insulin who have poorly controlled diabetes at the time of conception (Becerra *et al.*, 1990).

ASSESSING THE NEED FOR SCREENING

There is always a possibility that any plans to implement screening for congenital malformations and disorders may be seen as public health specialists conducting a 'search and destroy mission' sacrificing individuals with a problem for the greater good of society – the utilitarian approach mentioned in Chapter 1.

Resources for health care are finite and so commissioners of health care have a 'portfolio' of services which they buy. In a publicly funded system, this usually means buying a little of everything rather than excellent health care for only one section of society. Commissioners need to buy evidence-based, cost-effective health care that provides good outcomes for the public money spent on them. Cost-effectiveness analysis can cause problems when used for prenatal screening programmes. It seems to imply that terminating an abnormal pregnancy saves the state or insurance company from having to pay for expensive lifelong health care for a disabled person and so money spent on screening is money saved on health care elsewhere. However, this is only true if screening is done only if parents agree to have a termination if there is an abnormality. Naturally, this view disturbs those born with disease or malformations, as it begins to suggest that health care for any particular disorder may not be provided by a state- or insurance-funded health service if that disorder can be detected prenatally.

One of the main values put on prenatal screening and diagnosis is the information that it yields to individuals to enable them to make informed choices about their situation. It is impossible to put a monetary value on this to include in a cost–benefit analysis.

Technology exists to screen and diagnose several hundred genetic disorders and malformations and many of the population will want to take advantage of new tests. Public health can contribute to the debate about what tests should be available by using epidemiology to look at and assess the need for screening services – what are the commonest genetic disorders in the local population; what are the areas where intervention could reduce the burden of disease by preventing future and further disability?

EVALUATING PILOT SCREENING PROJECTS

A screening test is not usually in itself diagnostic; it detects a subgroup of those tested who are at higher risk of having the disease or disorder than the original population screened. This subgroup should be offered further investigation with a diagnostic test that is often more time-consuming, expensive and invasive than the screening test. For example, the questions 'How old are you?' and 'What ethnic group do you belong to?' are both screening tests to determine a subgroup who are at higher risk of having a baby with a problem than the general population – Trisomy 21 in the case of maternal age, and sickle cell anaemia, thalassaemia or Tay–Sachs disease in the case of ethnic group. This information then has to be converted to a risk assessment.

It is rare for a screening test to provide discrete variables where the answer is either 'yes' or 'no' – even ethnic group may be difficult to define precisely. Most screening questions or tests give results in the form of continuous variables and need a decision defining a cut-off point above which the answer or test result is declared 'positive'. For example, if 'How old are you?' is used as a screening test, then at what age is the test positive: if the woman is over 35, 37 or 40, or any other age?

Further investigation (a diagnostic amniocentesis or a maternal blood test to pick up sickle-cell trait) is needed to confirm or refute that the condition is present. Once the diagnosis is confirmed, treatment or preventive advice and action can be offered. This in itself creates conflicts – public health can supply figures on the risks of having a baby with an abnormality on which to base informed consent, but if you have a 1 in 1000 risk, and you are the one, that is 100% of you.

Whilst screening has the potential to save lives or improve quality of life through early diagnosis of serious conditions, it is not a foolproof process. Public health specialists have a duty to the general population to ensure that any screening programme is effective. Screening can reduce the risk of developing a condition or its complications but it cannot offer a guarantee of protection. In any screening programme, there is an irreducible minimum of false positive and false negative results. The UK National Screening Committee is increasingly presenting screening as risk reduction to emphasize this point. Many programmes are abandoning the use of 'positive' or 'negative' results but reporting the risks directly to the person tested (Nicolaides *et al.*, 1994).

A screening test may be read as negative even if the disease is present (a *false negative*), thus giving both the person screened and their carers false reassurance that all is well. It may be read as positive when a disease is not present (a *false positive*), which will lead to further unnecessary investigation before the actual health of the person or fetus screened is confirmed. These errors occur because most screening tests are not discrete and do not measure the absolute presence or absence of disease. Instead, they measure biochemical parameters or other markers of a disorder. For example, serum alpha-fetoprotein is found in maternal serum in all pregnancies; an arbitrary cut-off point for high and low values at different gestational ages is needed to use the value of serum alpha-fetoprotein as a screening test for open neural-tube defects and for chromosomal abnormalities. Biophysical parameters such as nuchal translucency also occur in continuous distributions (Nicolaides *et al.*, 1994). The efficacy of the programme in picking up a high proportion of true cases without subjecting hundreds of pregnancies to the potential dangers of an invasive diagnostic test, such as amniocentesis, needs a careful balance of risks which must be explained to those being screened (Edwards *et al.*, 2002).

To assess the effectiveness of a screening programme, two questions need to be asked:

1. To what extent can the test discriminate between affected and unaffected individuals? There are two measures to assess the discriminatory powers of a screening programme. *Specificity* refers to the proportion of unaffected individuals who have a negative result on screening: for example, the proportion of women with pregnancies unaffected by a neural-tube defect who have AFP values which put them at low risk for a neural-tube defect. The *false positive*

rate is calculated by taking the specificity from 100. *Sensitivity* is the proportion of affected individuals who give a positive result on screening and is the *detection rate* of the programme. For example, how many women who actually have a pregnancy with a fetus with neural-tube defect have a high serum AFP?

2. What is the chance that those who have a positive screening test really have the disease? This is a measure of the proportion of true positive screening tests to all positive screening tests and is known as the *positive predictive value*. The sensitivity and specificity of a screen remains the same however many cases there are in a population. In contrast, the predictive value depends on the prevalence of the disorder in the population screened. If tests are introduced in populations where there is a high prevalence of the disease (for example, relatives of people with inherited disorders), the odds of being affected may be high and a screening test will pick up many cases. However, the screening test will be less impressive in the general population, where the prevalence of the disorder is lower.

Genetic and prenatal screening

We offer antenatal screening programmes routinely to all members of the pregnant population. As this target population consists of people who are healthy, it is extremely important that the advantages of testing for the disorder are not outweighed by the disadvantages. Some screening may be more effective if it is done in two stages: a high-risk group can be identified because of a specified attribute (such as ethnicity), and then the screening test can be offered to that subsection of the population.

People known to be at high risk of genetic disease because a member of their family has developed the illness are usually counselled about their risks and are aware of the possibilities of prenatal diagnosis. They may be very keen to have testing whereas people who are offered a test to pick up a disease that they have never heard of and have never considered might cause problems for them may be less keen. Although carrier status may be common, it is relatively rare for carriers to pair up with other carriers. Even when two carriers have children, there is only a one in four risk of being affected for each of their children, so family history of disease is in fact uncommon, even in families where there are carriers. Individuals may be angry if they are carriers and go on to have an affected child but were not offered a simple screening test which would have detected their carrier status.

The term 'reduce the risk of disease' differentiates genetic from other forms of screening. We usually design screening programmes to benefit directly the individual tested, by offering either early diagnosis and treatment or prevention or by reassurance that there is one less disease that the person tested currently has to worry about. The only direct benefit to individuals tested in a genetic screening programme is to allow them to make choices about their future family. Carrier status does *not* mean that the carrier of a recessive disorder is diseased, as their other 'normal' gene will compensate for the presence of the abnormal one. However, without such screening, definitive prenatal diagnostic tests cannot be offered.

There is a very real danger genetic screening may lead to the perception that carriers are abnormal and diseased. In 1974 in Seattle, Hampton and colleagues showed that hastily introduced screening programmes led to sickle cell 'non disease' with carrier children regarded as 'different' by parents. Current debate in the UK seeks to ensure that insurance companies cannot discriminate against carriers – will a private company insure a couple with a one in four risk of having a child with cystic fibrosis unless they undertake to terminate any affected pregnancy?

As the genes that cause disease are mapped and cloned, it will become more common to perform a screening test that is also diagnostic in that it detects the actual presence of a gene mutation causing a disease rather than a biochemical test that detects and measures the gene product. Genetic screening is therefore starting to differ from most other forms of screening in that it is the final arbiter of whether the person tested is positive or negative for the 'risk of disease' or presence of the gene. The possibility of screening for carriers of cystic fibrosis was raised by the identification in 1990 of the most common cystic fibrosis mutation (a three base pair deletion, delta F508, in the structural gene for cystic fibrosis on the long arm of chromosome seven; Rommens et al., 1990). The realization of the technical feasibility of cystic fibrosis carrier screening by detecting the faulty gene itself has produced strong arguments both for and against its introduction (Modell, 1990; Wilfond and Fost, 1990).

The greatest difference between screening for genetic diseases and for other disorders is that true primary prevention is not currently possible for genetic disorders. There are several options open to carriers of an inherited disease to avoid the birth of an affected child, but many of these are not generally acceptable to individuals or couples:

- to remain childless;
- to select a partner who is not a carrier of the same disease (in the case of recessive disorders);
- to use artificial insemination by donor or ovum donation;
- to ensure that only a non-affected fetus implants (using preimplantation genetic diagnosis on an eight cell embryo; Coutelle et al., 1989; Handyside et al., 1992; Chapter 9 of this book);
- to have prenatal diagnosis and terminate affected pregnancies.

Recent advances in the field of gene and cell transplantation (Editorial, 1990a) may offer true hope of effective long lasting treatment and increase the acceptability of genetic screening programmes. However, the spectre of eugenic control of 'designer baby' future generations hangs over genetic screening programmes. In the UK, the Human Fertilisation and Embryology Authority governs these issues and encourages public debate. Given that primary prevention is not a current possibility, the objectives of genetic screening developed by the Royal College of Physicians of London (1989) are different from those of other screening programmes. They are:

- to allow the widest possible range of informed choice to women and couples at risk of having children with an abnormality;
- to provide reassurance and reduce the level of anxiety associated with reproduction;
- to allow couples to embark on having a family knowing that they may avoid the birth of seriously affected children through selective abortion;
- to ensure optimal treatment of affected infants through early diagnosis.

There are many different screening programmes for many different types of conditions. Various sets of criteria by which to judge whether a screening programme is likely to bring benefits to those screened have been published. (Thorner and Remein, 1961; McKeown, 1968; Wilson and Jungner, 1968; Cochrane and Holland, 1971; Cuckle and Wald, 1984; UK National Screening Committee, 1998).

To summarize the criteria for a successful screening programme, the genetic disorder which is being sought by the programme should be:

- well defined;
- of known natural history;
- an important health problem for the individual and for the community as it is severe, or common or both;
- of known incidence and prevalence;
- preventable by acceptable methods;
- have a beneficial influence on reproductive decision-making by detection of carrier status.

The screening test must:

- be simple, safe, precise and acceptable;
- be valid, that is, both sensitive and specific with a high predictive value;
- be repeatable;
- be relatively inexpensive;
- have a known distribution of test values in affected and unaffected individuals – the extent of overlap must be sufficiently small and a suitable cut off level defined;
- operate in the context of an agreed policy on further diagnostic investigation of individuals with a positive test result and on the choices available to those individuals.

We offer screening tests to people who are well in an attempt to stop future ill-health, so it is vital that tests are acceptable and do not cause iatrogenic disease. Acceptability varies according to culture and perceived seriousness of the disorder. It is accepted in Western countries that women should not mind having a vaginal examination with a speculum for a cervical smear to be taken, because it is perceived that the screening procedure will have a significant benefi-cial effect on mortality from cervical cancer. Rectal examinations in men to screen for prostate cancer are viewed in a different light!

In any screening programme, it is inevitable that certain individuals will be subject to what is later proved to be unnecessary worry and that some will be falsely reassured and thus be even more devastated by the birth of a child with a congenital malformation. Evaluation of screening programmes is therefore essen-tial if individuals in society are to have access to appropriate technology which overall does more good than harm.

TEACHING PROFESSIONALS AND THE PUBLIC ABOUT SCREENING

Public health specialists also have a duty to ensure that services are given to each person efficiently – that is, that the input of resources into screening programmes produces the maximum output in the form of information that can be used by couples to give informed consent to procedures. Screening has been applied to a variety of diseases with no simple genetic origins (for example hypertension and urine dip stick testing for diabetes and proteinuria are all screened for during pregnancy, and there are UK national programmes for cervical and breast cancer screening). There is a wide variety of success in achieving the primary aim of screening – to prevent morbidity and mortality from the disease (Mant and Fowler, 1990). We should learn lessons from screening programmes applied to these diseases. These include how to educate health care professionals and those in the target group about the screen and how to feed back the results of the screen (whether positive or negative) so that diagnostic tests, treatment or preventive measures can be offered. Education of both professionals and public is essential if the screening test is to be offered to the whole target population and accepted or rejected in an informed manner. In multicultural societies, professionals also need to know of different cultural perceptions (see Chapter 7) and how to use interpreters effectively (Adams, 2002). The full potential benefits of a programme can only be realized if a large proportion of the target group voluntarily attends for screening.

There is evidence that good training and support for professionals (see Chapter 18) can result in a significant increase in take-up of screening programmes. Uptake of antenatal HIV screening depends more on the midwife than the method of offering the test (Gibb *et al.*, 1998; Simpson *et al.*, 1998). The availability and performance of well-trained and motivated professionals determines the success of screening programmes (National Electronic Library for Screening, 2002). It is essential that they understand what screening is, and what it can and cannot do.

I have found Figure 4.1 overleaf helpful as a visual aid to show the effects of changing the shape and size of holes in the screening 'sieve' (the screening test) and the shape and size of the cubes and spheres being screened (the screened population). I also came across another teaching aid when buying groceries on-line. I typed in 'ham' and was confronted by a list which included a wide variety of products by Moet et Chandon, Lansom, Vidal Sassoon and Wella – *cham*pagnes and *sham*poos. My on-line search was sensitive – it picked out everything with 'ham' in it – but not specific, as I was tempted by many other products beside the one I was searching for. However, I missed some delicious European offerings such as 'jambon' or 'proscuitto'. I have also asked students to screen each other for gender. Measuring height results in a range of continuous variables and the need for a cut-off point above which a student is at high risk for having XY chromosomes. The question 'Are you wearing trousers?' produces discrete variables and a positive and negative group. This screening test is highly sensitive for men (they all wear trousers) but not specific (in our student population in winter, most women wear trousers too).

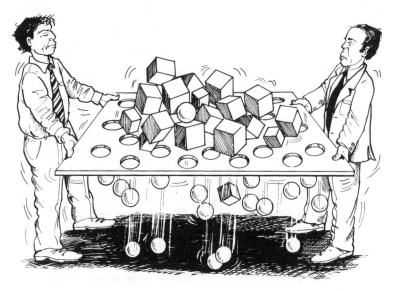

Figure 4.1 Diagnostic or screening tests (from Greenhalgh T [1997], with permission of the British Medical Journal).

INFORMING PUBLIC POLICY DECISIONS ABOUT SCREENING

Costs of medical care are rising worldwide and the premise on which the UK National Health Service was founded – if money is spent on health care, then the need for health care systems to treat disease will reduce over a period of time – has been shown to be wrong time and again. Better health services bring higher expectations in the population that funds the service through taxes or insurance contributions, and an increased demand for care. Steep rises in spending on health care have led to the introduction of cash limits to nationalized health care services and limits as to what insurers will pay in private health care systems. Those funding health care are concerned about value for the money they spend and this has led to the need to show that clinical practice in obstetrics is both safe and effective. Failure of free markets for health care and the need for equal access to care for all citizens are the reasons why in all countries the state has a role in preventive and curative health services.

Such issues are an integral part of the debate between politicians, health professionals, managers and the public before change in maternity services can occur. In reality, this involves an on-going dialogue between parents represented by pressure groups, health care professionals and politicians, none of whom can claim an exclusive right to have the definitive solution. There is a conflict between the personal, family view of giving birth as a tremendously important life event versus the requirements of politicians, taxpayers, insurance companies and professionals for safety and value for money. In our present day egalitarian society, public debate is regarded as entirely acceptable but there are undoubtedly drawbacks in compromise solutions that attempt to satisfy all parties.

The arrival of technology as an established part of care in pregnancy, while solving many problems, has also introduced new ones. The pregnant woman and her obstetrician no longer wait for delivery accepting that whatever happens is 'God's will'. The woman expects that those who care for her have access to the latest technology for the care of her and her baby, and that she will be kept fully informed of the implications of using that technology and of any abnormal findings.

We use screening tests for fetal wellbeing in all maternity units. These range from methods for detecting fetal abnormality, to biophysical and biochemical assessment of the fetus. Clinical decision-making is very dependent on such tests – for example, whether or not to terminate a pregnancy when a fetal anomaly is suspected. Chalmers and colleagues (1989) drew attention to the considerable variation in the validity of some of these tests and interventions.

If care is to be evaluated scientifically, it is important for women and their partners to understand the basis of randomized trials so that they will agree to take part in the studies needed. If women do not agree to be allocated by drawing numbers to specific treatment or non-treatment groups, professionals cannot give future mothers the benefit of proper information on which to base their choices. Many women are altruistic enough to agree to take part in trials where they cannot see any particular advantage or disadvantage to being in one or other group.

However, unless trials take place soon after the introduction of a new technique or technology, women can be as blinded by the perceived but anecdotal and unquantified advantages or disadvantages as their carers. For example, routine ultrasound screening for fetal anomaly has never been subjected to a scientific evaluation in the form of a randomized controlled trial. However, its use in the United Kingdom is now so widespread that it would probably be considered unethical not to offer an anomaly scan to one group in a randomized controlled trial. Provision of scanning as a routine has been driven by clinicians who want to detect abnormality and by parents who want the chance to see and welcome their baby in the womb and confirm their child's normality. Tensions arise because the aims of these two groups are actually at odds with each other.

Health care professionals treat individuals, but treating an individual may produce other consequences which affect third parties – for example, immunizing a person against rubella not only gives that individual protection, it also makes them less likely to pass the disease on to women who may be pregnant (Normand, 1991). Many people pay for their own health care through insurance or directly from their own pockets, but a considerable amount of care is paid for by the state through taxation. The consequence of this is that benefits produced for one section of the community may mean that resources are not available for care that would benefit others (the opportunity costs). Screening programmes that would benefit individuals directly may not be initiated if the results are not important for the community as a whole. An example of this is screening for toxoplasmosis in pregnancy.

The parasite *Toxoplasmosis gondii* can cause fetal infection resulting in severe and lasting neurological damage in the baby when the mother contracts the infection for the first time in pregnancy. The disease in the mother is usually symptomless and not all infections in pregnancy produce disability in the baby. Screening programmes on maternal blood have been running in France and Austria for some time. An initial test is done at booking and, if the mother has not had a previous *Toxoplasma* infection, the tests are repeated monthly to ensure that any new infection is detected and treated *in utero* or a termination of pregnancy offered if necessary. About 20–25% of French women need repeat testing (Editorial, 1990b).

In the UK, about 25 new cases of congenital toxoplasmosis are reported each year to the British Paediatric Surveillance Unit in 680,000 births. This is about half the expected number estimated from data on acute *Toxoplasma* infection in pregnancy and transmission rates (Editorial, 1990b). Only 20% of women tested in London had previously had a toxoplasmosis infection (Fleck, 1969), so a screening programme in the United Kingdom would need to test 680,000 women at the start of their pregnancy and subsequently 80% or 540,000 pregnant women in each month of their pregnancy to detect 25–50 cases each year. The resources required to do this mean that it is highly unlikely that the UK will introduce toxoplasmosis screening. This is in spite of vigorous lobbying by well-informed and highly motivated pressure groups of families who have discovered that their child has been damaged by a potentially detectable and treatable disease. The cost per case discovered, however beneficial to the individual family concerned, is simply too high. Greater benefit to the community as a whole may result in spending the same amount of money on other forms of more cost-beneficial health care. Health education about minimizing the risks of contracting toxoplasmosis during pregnancy through food hygiene in preparing raw meat and in avoiding cat faeces is a more cost-effective way of reducing the incidence (RCOG Multidisciplinary Working Group, 1992).

A similar dilemma arises with triple screening for the chromosomal defect, Trisomy 21 (Down syndrome). Past screening programmes based on offering amniocentesis to older mothers (37 years old or more) subjected about 5% of pregnancies in the United Kingdom to amniocentesis and picked up about one third of fetuses with Trisomy 21. Theoretical research studies using markers found in maternal blood, have been shown retrospectively to pick up between 60 and 85% of all cases for the same or much lower (1%) amniocentesis rate (Wald *et al.*, 1988, 1999). In some parts of the UK, 15% of women are now over 37. If we are to keep relatively low overall amniocentesis rates, older mothers will have to forego their absolute right to a diagnostic test and will only have an amniocentesis if indicated by the blood test, which misses some cases.

There are also real problems in presenting screening results as risks rather than 'positive' or 'negative'. Everybody interprets risk differently and many of us see 'chance' as a more positive statement than 'risk'. We happily bet money on national lotteries with a one in a million 'risk' of winning vast sums of money. We may not interpret a 1 in 100 chance of an affected child the same as a 99% chance that the baby will be normal (Abramsky and Fletcher, 2002). If we cannot estimate what level of risk leads to the request for a diagnostic test, it is difficult to plan for every request to be met.

Screening tests that are complex and/or spread out over time present special problems. For example, some women may not understand why they have to wait several weeks for the results of screening in the first and second trimester to be combined in the integrated test for Down syndrome. Considerable resources will be needed to explain the test fully so that women can give informed consent. Others will simply not be able to attend twice because of the costs of time and travel or being moved to a different city under an asylum seekers programme. Research is needed to look at the uptake and outcome of running a simpler programme with lower detection and higher false positive rates against the outcome and uptake in practice of more complex screening programmes.

Cost–benefit evaluation is needed for all screening programmes, together with surveys on what those who are most affected by the results, the parents, think of what is offered to them. Health care planners also need to consider how to ensure equity of access to screening programmes, including treatment. Every society has its disadvantaged groups – refugees and asylum seekers, those who do not speak the native language, those with disability and disease and those living in poverty. Access for some groups can be improved by relatively simple measures – ensuring that leaflets are translated into appropriate languages and videos, tapes and interpreters provided for those who cannot read, hear or understand. There can be advantages of pooling resources between maternity units and using the same patient information tools across screening programmes, as this reduces the cost of translation into different languages and media considerably.

MONITORING THE RESULTS OF POPULATION SCREENING PROGRAMMES

Screening programmes include not only applying screening tests to populations, but also diagnostic procedures, treatments and interventions. The UK National

Screening Committee (1998) has proposed seven criteria for screening programmes:

1. There should be evidence from high-quality randomized controlled trials that the screening programme is effective in reducing mortality or morbidity.
2. There should be evidence that the complete screening programme is clinically, socially and ethically acceptable to health professionals and the public.
3. The benefit of the screening programme should outweigh the physical and psychological harm caused by the test, diagnostic procedures, treatment or intervention.
4. The opportunity cost of the screening programme (the services that cannot be offered if resources are used instead for another programme) should be economically balanced in relation to expenditure on medical care as a whole.
5. There should be a plan for managing and monitoring the screening programme and an agreed set of quality assurance standards.
6. Adequate staffing and facilities for testing, diagnosis and treatment and programme management should be available prior to the commencement of the screening programme.
7. All other options for managing the condition should have been considered (such as improving treatment, providing other services).

All parts of the programme should be monitored, both locally by professionals assessing their own care and across the entire programme. For example, the Medical Research Council trial of amniocentesis (1978) found that miscarriage directly related to amniocentesis occurred in 1–1.5% of pregnancies tested in this way. This rate is commonly quoted to parents, but the outcome is also related to the experience of the operator: if more than two insertions are made during any one procedure, the fetal loss rate is increased (Simpson *et al.*, 1976; Lowe *et al.*, 1978). What parents really want to know is 'What are the risks of a miscarriage if you or a member of your team do my amniocentesis?'

It is not possible for individual units to do their own randomized clinical trials, but careful use of audit should enable them to compare their performance with other centres. Audit is the systematic review of how a technique proved by research to produce good patient care is applied in practice. In local units, clinicians have a duty to audit their own practice to identify areas where they could improve and to ensure they achieve specified standards of care. Public health specialists and commissioners have a duty to ensure that audit takes place and appropriate changes to improve care are implemented.

Research findings do not translate directly into programmes that produce exactly the health gain predicted from the research. Retrospective analysis of stored serum from pregnancies that resulted in a fetus with Trisomy 21 (Wald *et al.*, 1988) suggested that two thirds of cases could be picked up for a 5% false positive rate. In practice (Wald *et al.*, 1992) just over half the cases were picked up in a demonstration project, largely because take up of screening varied considerably. If the public votes with its feet and does not take up screening programmes, their effectiveness decreases and tough decisions have to be made as to whether to divert more resources into promoting the programme or to stop the programme. Policy is shifting towards taking greater care that people participating in any screening programme do so on the basis of informed consent, and this may affect take-up (Marteau and Kinmouth, 2002).

Starting and stopping screening entails considerable debate and needs good evidence of efficacy and efficiency rather than anecdotes. The practice of good public health can raise the standard of this debate and can address the conflicts engendered in preventing disease, prolonging life and promoting health for the individual through using the efforts and resources produced by society in an effective, open and organized way.

Key points

- Public health specialists differ from other health professionals involved in clinical medicine in that their 'patients' are whole communities rather than the individuals who make up that community.
- It is part of the public health remit to assess the need for screening, inform the public and professionals about it, develop policy and monitor the implementation and results of screening programmes.
- Resources used to screen for a condition are not available for use elsewhere. The public health specialist must assess whether resources are being used wisely.
- Screening tests do not usually detect with certainty the presence or absence of a condition; they estimate level of risk, and it is in their nature that they have false positives and false negatives.
- We offer antenatal screening tests to all members of the pregnant population. It is extremely important that the advantages of testing for the disorder are not outweighed by the disadvantages.

REFERENCES

Abramsky L, Fletcher O (2002) Interpreting information: what is said, what is heard – a questionnaire study of health professionals and members of the public. *Prenatal Diagnosis*, 22(13) 1188–1194.

Acheson D (1988) *Public Health in England* – the report of the committee of enquiry into the future development of the public health function. HO Cm289 1988, London.

Adams K (2002) Making the best use of health advocates and interpreters. *British Medical Journal*. Career focus supplement 325; s9–s10.

Becerra JE, Khoury MJ, Cordero JF *et al.* (1990) Diabetes mellitus during pregnancy and the risks for specific birth defects: a population based case-control study. *Pediatrics*, 85; 1–9.

Chalmers I, Enkin MW, Kierse MJNC (eds) (1989) *Effective Care in Pregnancy and Childbirth*. Oxford University Press, Oxford.

Cochrane AL, Holland WW (1971) Validation of screening procedures. *British Medical Bulletin*, 27; 3.

Coutelle C, Williams C, Handyside A *et al.* (1989) Genetic analysis of DNA from single human oocytes: a model for preimplantation diagnosis of cystic fibrosis. *British Medical Journal*, 299; 22–24.

Cuckle HS, Wald NJ (1984) Principles of screening. In *Antenatal and Neonatal Screening* (ed. Wald NJ) Oxford University Press, Oxford, pp. 1–21.

Dolk H, Vrihied M, Armstrong B *et al.* (1998) Risk of congenital anomalies near hazardous-waste landfill sites in Europe: the EUROHAZCON study. *Lancet*, 352; 423–427.

Editorial (1990a) Myoblast transfer in Duchenne's muscular dystrophy. *British Medical Journal*, 301; 77–78.

Editorial (1990b) Antenatal screening for toxoplasmosis in the United Kingdom. *Lancet*, ii; 346–347.

Edwards A, Elwyn G, Mulley A (2002) Explaining risks: turning numerical data into meaningful pictures. *British Medical Journal*, 324; 827–830.

Fielder HMP, Poon-King CM, Palmer SR *et al.* (2000) Assessment of impact on health of residents living near the Nant-y-Gwyddon landfill site: retrospective analysis. *British Medical Journal*, 320; 19–23.

Fleck DG (1969) Toxoplasmosis. *Public Health*, 83; 131–135.

Gibb DM, MacDonagh SE, Gupta R *et al.* (1998) Factors affecting uptake of antenatal HIV testing in London: results of a multi-centre study. *British Medical Journal, 316; 259–261.*

Greenhalgh T (1997) How to read a paper: Papers that report diagnostic or screening tests. *British Medical Journal*, 315; 540–543.

Hampton ML, Anderson J, Lavizzo BS *et al.* (1974) Sickle cell 'nondisease', a potentially serious public health problem. *American Journal of Diseases of Childhood*, 128; 58–61.

Handyside AH, Lesko JG, Tarin JJ *et al.* (1992) Birth of a normal girl after in vitro fertilisation and preimplantation diagnostic testing for cystic fibrosis. *New England Journal of Medicine*, 327; 905–909.

Jones KL, Lacro RV, Johnson KA *et al.* (1989). Pattern of malformations in the children of women treated with carbamazepine during pregnancy. *New England Journal of Medicine*, 320; 1661–1666.

Lowe CU, Alexander D, Bryla D *et al.* (1978) *The safety and accuracy of mid-trimester amniocentesis.* US Department of Health, Education and Welfare DHEW Publication number (NIH) 78–190.

Mant D, Fowler G (1990) Mass screening: theory and ethics. *British Medical Journal*, 300; 916–918.

Marteau TM, Kinmouth AL (2002) Screening for cardiovascular risk: public health imperative or matter for individual informed choice? *British Medical Journal*, 325; 78–80 .

McKeown T (1968) Validation of screening procedures. In *Screening in Medical Care. Reviewing the evidence.* The Nuffield Provincial Hospital Trust, Oxford University Press, Oxford.

Medical Research Council (1978) An assessment of the hazards of amniocentesis. *British Journal of Obstetrics and Gynaecology*, 85 (Suppl 2); 1–41.

Modell B. (1990) Cystic fibrosis screening and community genetics. *Journal of Medical Genetics*, 27; 475–479.

Mooney G (1992) *Economics, Medicine and Health Care* (2nd edn). Harvester Wheatsheaf. Hemel Hempstead, Herts.

National Electronic Library for Screening (2002) www.nelh.nhs.uk/screening

Nicolaides KH, Brizot ML, Snijers JM (1994) Fetal nuchal translucency: ultrasound screening for fetal Trisomy in the first trimester of pregnancy. *British Journal of Obstetrics and Gynaecology*, 101; 783–786.

Normand C. (1991) Economics, health, and the economics of health. *British Medical Journal*, 303; 1572–1577.

RCOG Multidisciplinary Working Group (1992) *Prenatal Screening for Toxoplasmosis in the United Kingdom*. Royal College of Obstetricians and Gynaecologists, London.

Rommens JM, Ianuzzi MC, Kerem B-S *et al.* (1990) Identification of the cystic fibrosis gene: chromosome walking and jumping. *Science,* 245; 1059–1065.

Royal College of Physicians of London (1989) *Prenatal Diagnosis and Screening – Community and Service Implications*. Royal College of Physicians, London.

Simpson NE, Dallaire, L Miller JR *et al.* (1976) Prenatal diagnosis of genetic disease in Canada: report of a collaborative study. *Canadian Medical Association Journal,* 115; 739–746.

Simpson WM, Johnstone FD, Boyd FM *et al.* (1998) Uptake and acceptability of antenatal HIV testing: randomised controlled trial of different methods of offering the test. *British Medical Journal*, 316; 262–267.

Sullivan EM, Burgess MA, Forrest JM (1999) The epidemiology of rubella and congenital rubella in Australia, 1992–1997. *Communicable Disease Intelligence*, 23; 209–214.

Thorner RM, Remein QR. (1961) *Principles and Procedures in the Evaluation of Screening for Disease*. Public Health Monograph No 67, US Department of Health Education and Welfare.

UK National Screening Committee (1998) *Handbook of Population Screening Programmes*. Department of Health, London. (www.doh.gov.uk/nsc/pdfs/nsc_handbookfirstdraft.pdf)

UK National Screening Committee (2000) (www.doh.gov.uk/nsc/whatscreening/whatscreen_ind.htm)

Wald NJ, Cuckle HS, Densem JW (1988) Maternal serum screening for Down syndrome in early pregnancy. *British Medical Journal*, 297; 883–887.

Wald NJ, Kennard A, Densem JW *et al.* (1992) Antenatal maternal serum screening for Down's syndrome: results of a demonstration project. *British Medical Journal*, 305; 391–394.

Wald NJ, Watt HC, Hackshaw AK (1999) Integrated screening for Down's syndrome based on tests performed during the first and second trimesters. *New England Journal of Medicine*, 7(341); 461–467.

Wilfond BS, Fost N (1990) The cystic fibrosis gene; medical and social implications for heterozygote detection. *Journal of the American Medical Association*, 263; 2777–2783.

Wilson JMC, Jungner G (1968) *Principles and practice of screening for disease*. Public Health Papers, WHO No 34.

5 WOMEN'S EXPERIENCES OF PRENATAL SCREENING AND DIAGNOSIS

Josephine M. Green

INTRODUCTION

Although most pregnant women worry about the possibility that there might be something wrong with their baby, few have any specific grounds for this. Statham *et al.* (1997) found 'the possibility of something being wrong with the baby' to be one of the highest scoring worries in a sample of over 1800 women in early pregnancy, with only 11% being not at all worried. However, when asked 'Have you any reason to think that your baby might be more likely than any other to have some sort of a problem?' only 13% said 'yes', and these were primarily on grounds of age. Most women take part in screening programmes in order to be reassured that their babies are healthy, rather than with any expectation that they are not (Farrant, 1985; Green *et al.*, 1993a; Weinans *et al.*, 2000), and it is important for service providers to appreciate the implications of this.

In this chapter I shall give an overview of what is known about women's experiences of prenatal screening and diagnosis. I shall conclude with some observations about the context of prenatal screening and, in particular, serum screening for Down syndrome. Earlier reviews of the literature on the psychological effects of fetal diagnosis on pregnant women can be found in Green (1990) and Green and Statham (1996). A systematic review entitled 'Psychosocial aspects of genetic screening of pregnant women and newborns' is due to be published by the NHS R and D Health Technology Assessment programme in the UK in 2003 (http://www.hta.nhsweb.nhs.uk/).

DIAGNOSIS VERSUS SCREENING

In discussing diagnostic tests and screening tests different issues arise, so it is best to clarify the distinction before we start. Diagnostic tests are those that can give a (fairly) definitive answer to the question 'Does the baby have . . . (a particular disorder e.g. spina bifida or Down syndrome)?' If we had diagnostic tests for common disorders that were cheap and risk free, then we could apply them to everybody, and we would not need screening tests. However, the reality is that the available diagnostic techniques for genetic and chromosomal anomalies (principally amniocentesis and chorionic villus sampling) are not cheap and they do carry a risk of miscarriage. It is therefore not considered appropriate for everybody to have them. Rather, we screen pregnant women to identify a subgroup who have a higher than average chance of having a baby with the disorder in question and for whom the costs and risks are therefore thought to be justified. The screening may be done on the basis of a woman's age, ethnic group or family history, or it may involve a screening test (e.g. measuring maternal serum alpha-fetoprotein). Either way, screening *per se* can not tell us that the baby definitely does or does not have the disorder, only that there is a relatively high or low likelihood of that being the case. It is therefore in the nature of screening tests that they 'get it wrong', i.e. some people with a 'high risk' screening result (or 'screen positive') have babies that are fine ('false positive') and some with a 'low risk' ('screen negative') do in fact have affected babies ('false negative'). Cut-offs are usually chosen to minimize the number of false negatives, but that often means a high proportion of false positives.

WOMEN'S EXPERIENCES OF DIAGNOSTIC TESTS

Women who have diagnostic tests fall into four groups: women who have had a previous disabled child; women with a family history of a genetic disorder; women of 'advanced maternal age' (usually 35 plus); and women who have had positive screening tests. The two tests that we will consider in this chapter are amniocentesis, which is generally performed in the second trimester at 15–16 weeks, and chorionic villus sampling (CVS), which is performed at 11–12 weeks. Because it is done so early, CVS has mainly been used for risks that are known at the start of pregnancy, such as age and family history. Women whose risk is determined as a result of screening tests carried out during the second trimester of pregnancy generally do not have this option. However, the development of first trimester screening techniques means that CVS is now sometimes an option following a positive result of a screening test.

Despite considerable methodological variation (Green, 1990), some consistent findings about women's experiences of amniocentesis emerge from the literature. These concern worries about potential miscarriage and the stressful nature of the period waiting for results, followed (usually) by a drop in anxiety once normal results are given. Although the waiting time for results has now been reduced somewhat, this period continues to be a time of stress. An ongoing randomized controlled trial is investigating whether decreasing the uncertainty about when and how results will be given can help with this. Apart from this, it appears that little attention has been given to ways of reducing anxiety in this context.

After receiving reassuring results, are tested women less anxious than those who are not tested? The first controlled study (Fava *et al.*, 1982, 1983) found no differences between the groups by mid-pregnancy and therefore concluded that amniocentesis does not allay anxiety. Three subsequent studies (Phipps and Zinn, 1986; Marteau, 1991; Statham *et al.*, 1993) have also failed to find significantly lower anxiety scores for women who have had negative amniocentesis results compared to untested controls. The latter two studies have concluded that differences between groups are likely to relate to pre-existing characteristics, which is a recurring theme in this area (Green, 1990).

Comparison of women aged less than 35 who were allocated to having amniocentesis without any particular indication for the procedure, with those having amniocentesis on the grounds of their age (Tabor and Jonsson, 1987), showed a decline in anxiety immediately after the procedure for the younger women while for older women it did not drop until normal results had been given. Another Scandinavian study (Sjogren and Uddenberg, 1990) found that younger women who were having prenatal diagnosis because of self-reported anxiety, were actually not particularly anxious once their request for the test had been granted. As one said: 'Now, when I am allowed to have the test, I don't worry about what will follow'. These findings underline the other main message that emerges from the literature, which is that the main determinant of women's reactions to the process of prenatal diagnosis is the reason for having it.

As early as 1975, Robinson *et al.*, reporting on women having amniocentesis on the grounds of their age, stated that they 'saw the test as an appropriate part of intelligent prenatal care and expected a benign outcome'. Evers-Kiebooms *et al.* (1988) compared women having amniocentesis for maternal age with those who had had a previous child with Down syndrome or a neural tube defect. Mothers of children with Down syndrome were most anxious while waiting for the results, while those who had previous experience of a neural tube defect were the ones least likely to be reassured by a negative result. Other studies have also generally shown that women who have had previous affected children are more anxious and less likely to be reassured, while women being tested simply on grounds of age are the least anxious (e.g. Chervin *et al.*, 1977; Beeson and Golbus, 1979). However, the literature also shows very clearly another group for whom amniocentesis is particularly stressful: those having amniocentesis because of a high-risk serum screening result (see below). Farrant (1980) showed that, in contrast to the situation described for older women, amniocentesis was not viewed as a routine component of antenatal care, rather it was seen as part of a relentless process challenging what was previously believed to be a normal pregnancy.

It is often assumed that CVS is less stressful for women than amniocentesis for three reasons:

1. They do not have to wait so long to have the test done (11 weeks after their last period instead of 16 weeks).
2. They do not have to wait so long for results (1 week versus 2 or 3 weeks for conventional karyotyping).
3. Termination of pregnancy, if requested, can be carried out in the first trimester and thus by dilatation and curettage rather than by inducing labour at 20 weeks or more.

The first two assumptions are, on the whole, supported by the literature. McCormack *et al.* (1990), for example, in a retrospective study of 152 women who had had CVS, found high acceptability and willingness to accept higher miscarriage rates as a trade off for the benefits of earlier and quicker results. This was especially true for women at known risk of passing on a genetic disorder. Data have, until recently, been lacking with respect to the third assumption: that earlier terminations are less distressing. However, a recent study (Statham *et al.*, 2001) which followed up 148 sets of parents who had terminated a pregnancy following diagnosis of a fetal abnormality found that gestation was *not* a significant predictor of emotional wellbeing in either the short or the longer term. (See also Chapter 13 in this book.)

The first study comparing experiences of CVS and amniocentesis involved 61 women enrolled in the Canadian randomized control trial (Spencer and Cox, 1987, 1988). Robinson *et al.* (1988) published a separate study, based on another 54 women from the same trial. Both studies indicated that CVS evoked less anxiety over a shorter period of time than amniocentesis. Spencer and Cox reported that women having amniocentesis were suppressing their attachment to their fetus until after they had had a negative result. Robinson *et al.* did not measure attachment until 22 weeks, at which point there was no difference between the groups. However, they subsequently investigated a different set of women, not part of the trial (Caccia *et al.*, 1991), and did find that attachment scores rose after a reassuring test result, whether this was at 15 weeks (for the CVS group) or at 21 weeks (for the amniocentesis group). This finding may be taken as support for Barbara Katz Rothman's idea of the 'tentative pregnancy' (Rothman, 1986). Kolker (1989) suggests that these 'positive' feelings after negative test results are a function of the anxiety created by the test itself: had the test not raised anxieties, there would be no need for reassurance. This interpretation is consistent with the findings from the amniocentesis studies quoted above that found no net benefit to tested women compared to those who were not tested.

In evaluating the data in this area, it is important to know whether women are undergoing a procedure that they have chosen or whether they have been randomized. Verjaal *et al.* (1982) showed that women who actively sought amniocentesis started from a position of greater commitment to the procedure and were likely to be loyal to their choice. The irony of randomized trials is that they can create differences between groups: those that get what they want versus those that do not. In Britain, for example, the trial comparing amniocentesis and CVS got off to a very slow start because most women did not want to be randomized (MacKenzie *et al.*, 1986). Having been counselled as to the two methods, they had formed a preference and did not want their fate decided by the toss of a coin. To tolerate the delays and anxieties of amniocentesis when everyone else is in the same boat is one thing; to tolerate them in the knowledge that you could have had your results 2 months sooner, had you been otherwise randomized, is quite different. That women did have more negative feelings about amniocentesis in this context is clear from the Spencer and Cox study where 100% of the 31 women planning further pregnancies said that they would want CVS next time. In contrast, another study looking at women who had chosen which technique to have (Tunis *et al.*, 1990) compared 30 women who had opted for amniocentesis with 151 who had chosen CVS, and found virtually no differences between the groups on a range of psychological indices.

There is one other important point to be made about CVS versus amniocentesis, which is raised by Robinson *et al.* (1991) concerning miscarriage after

CVS. Compared with amniocentesis, a relatively large number of women will miscarry after CVS, partly because it does actually cause more miscarriages than amniocentesis and partly because there is a higher rate of spontaneous loss at this earlier stage of pregnancy. However, no one can know whether their particular miscarriage was a consequence of the procedure or was one that would have happened anyway. Robinson *et al.* found that women who miscarried after CVS experienced a great deal of guilt and blamed their loss on their selfish desire for an earlier test result. They, in fact, had even less reason for feeling this way than might be supposed because they were part of the randomized trial and had not actually chosen to have CVS. This is an important point that should be taken into account when counselling women for prenatal diagnosis. Related to it is the higher rate of terminations of pregnancy for fetal chromosomal anomaly following CVS, compared with amniocentesis (Medical Research Council Working Party on the Evaluation of Chorionic Villus Sampling, 1991). The working party was, unfortunately, not able to say how many of these were false positives because post-termination karyotyping was not always carried out. Neither, of course, were they able to say how many true positives would have aborted spontaneously before the sixteenth week. Either way, the higher termination rate is another risk of the procedure that women should be aware of.

WOMEN'S EXPERIENCES OF SERUM SCREENING

Maternal serum alpha-fetoprotein screening for neural-tube defects has been in common use in the United Kingdom since the late 1970s. In the late 1980s and early 1990s the same test started to be used to screen for Down syndrome, and, since then it has been refined in various ways to improve its efficacy as a screen for Down syndrome (e.g. the 'triple' test). The test is usually carried out at 16 weeks. As a screening test (see above), it necessarily has false positives and false negatives. The test's sensitivity and specificity depend critically on gestational age being correctly known, since the level of alpha-fetoprotein increases by about 19% per week in the second trimester (Wald and Cuckle, 1984), while the level of hCG (human chorionic gonadotrophin) declines with gestational age.

Research has looked at psychological effects on women who have a false positive screening result. The effects of false positive alpha-fetoprotein results were first reported by Farrant (1980) and Fearn *et al.* (1982), who both found exceedingly high levels of anxiety. Fearn *et al.* found that the anxiety persisted even when they were told that there was not a problem after all. The most severe levels of anxiety were found in women who, having gone on to have amniocentesis, were not told the results. They were just told to assume that all was well if they did not hear to the contrary. It is to be hoped that this practice no longer occurs. The finding that abnormal serum screening results are associated with anxiety has been confirmed in all subsequent studies, both when screening for neural-tube defects (Berne-Fromell *et al.*, 1983a; Burton *et al.*, 1985b; Marteau *et al.*, 1992b; Green *et al.*, 1993b) and for Down syndrome

(Evans *et al.*, 1988; Marteau *et al.*, 1988; Abuelo *et al.*, 1991; Keenan *et al.*, 1991; Roelofsen *et al.*, 1993; Statham and Green, 1993; Santalahti *et al.*, 1996; Fairgrieve, 1997; Robinson, 2001).

There has been less research looking at the effect of screening on women whose screening result is normal. Early large scale studies comparing anxiety in screened and unscreened women in Sweden (Berne-Fromell *et al.*, 1983b; Berne-Fromell and Kjessler, 1984), and the USA (Burton *et al.*, 1985a) concluded that any differences between screened and unscreened women were minor, favoured the screened women and did not suggest long-term harm resulting from participation in the screening programme. Two large British studies (Marteau *et al.*, 1992a; and the Cambridge Prenatal Screening Study [Green *et al.*, 1993b; Statham *et al.*, 1993]) also concluded that serum screening for neural-tube defects was not causing higher anxiety, but was being accepted by those who were more anxious initially. This interpretation was supported by the further finding from the Cambridge study that tested women were neither more nor less worried than women in hospitals where the test was not offered. In other words, while the test was not generating worries, neither did it seem to be allaying them, although both studies do suggest the possibility of lower anxiety in tested women in late pregnancy.

Another group of women who have received little attention are those with false negative results, i.e. the screening test does not indicate a problem, but the baby does in fact have an abnormality. The paucity of research here is in part due to the major ethical and methodological challenges presented. Approaching such women clearly requires particular sensitivity. Furthermore, if our question is 'Is it worse to give birth to a child with Down syndrome after a negative screening test than it would have been without the screening test?' then there are real difficulties in finding appropriate comparisons because there are likely to be some pre-existing differences between women who had screening and those who did not. For example, we might expect that parents who decline screening are more willing to cope with a child with Down syndrome than those who accept.

Hall and colleagues (2000) interviewed 261 sets of parents of children with Down syndrome with different screening histories. Eighty-two (31%) were excluded because their account of the screening history differed from the medical records. This is in itself an interesting and worrying finding. None of the parents who had declined screening blamed others for the birth of their child with Down syndrome, whereas 28% of those in the false negative group and 13% who were not offered screening did blame others. Blaming others was associated with poorer scores on a number of measures. Thus, a clear message is that parents should not be encouraged to attribute blame, since blaming others is clearly not a helpful way of coping. We should bear in mind that blaming others may be a personality characteristic associated with accepting or declining the test. For example, those who decline tests may be more willing to take responsibility for what happens to them. Thus, the conclusion that a false negative result is the *cause* of slightly poorer adjustment, is not justified.

WOMEN'S EXPERIENCES OF ULTRASOUND SCANNING

Ultrasound scanning is in a different category from other techniques for investigating fetal well-being. First, it gives instant results, the process is happening there and then. Second, it does not fit easily into a classification of 'screening' versus 'diagnosis'. In the sense that it is used on everybody (in the United Kingdom), irrespective of risk status 'just to make sure that the baby is alright', it is being used as a screening technique. It may reveal findings that are of limited significance in their own right but are known to be associated with certain syndromes. In these cases the scan findings will be the cue for further diagnostic investigations. This is increasingly happening for chromosomal disorders (Nicolaides *et al.*, 1992). However, scans may also give definitive information, e.g. about structural abnormalities, number of fetuses, and fetal death, so in this sense they are diagnostic. The NHS R and D Health Technology Assessment programme has recently published a systematic review of ultrasound in pregnancy (Bricker *et al.*, 2000). This includes a very useful chapter on women's experiences. Two other recent publications also review this topic (Clement *et al.*, 1998; Baillie *et al.*, 1999).

Considering how widespread ultrasound scanning is, we know surprisingly little about women's experiences. Only a handful of studies, for example, have looked at women who have an actual or potential problem detected via a scan (Jöergensen *et al.*, 1985; Green *et al.*, 1992; Baillie, 1997; Statham *et al.*, 2001). There has been no randomized controlled trial that has compared psychological outcomes for scanned and unscanned women. Women's experiences of nuchal translucency scanning as a specific screen for Down syndrome and other chromosome disorders is also largely unexplored. We know rather more about attitudes: women are generally very enthusiastic about scanning; they do not, on the whole, regard it as a 'test'. Women who decline other forms of screening because they do not want information about fetal abnormalities, often still want scans (e.g. Esen and Olajide, 1997; Santalahti *et al.*, 1998). A number of studies have shown, however, that women are not well-informed about the purpose of scans and it has been suggested that women should be giving 'informed consent' for scans as they would for any other investigative procedure.

Early studies on women's experiences date from the early 1980s, e.g. Milne and Rich (1981) and the Kings College Hospital study (Campbell *et al.*, 1982; Reading *et al.*, 1982; Reading and Cox, 1982). These showed that what women liked about scans was a moving image that was interpreted for them. Nowadays that is what women expect. For most British women, 'seeing' the baby on scan is a high spot of the pregnancy, an event to be shared with the baby's father and siblings. We asked the women in the Cambridge Prenatal Screening Study if they felt that they could have said 'no' to the scan. Many clearly found this an extraordinary question: why should they wish to say no? Roberts (1986) found that the scan operator was the single most important determinant of women's satisfaction with the scan. However, to quote from Campbell *et al.* 'In busy clinics, insufficient attention may be given to providing feedback and in some cases reassurance'. We see the evidence of this, not from studies that are focused on ultra-sound, but on those which have retrospectively sampled (and thus not altered) everyday practice. Jacoby (1988), for example, quotes one woman's experience of ultrasound: 'I was not spoken to. The scan was not explained and my questions were totally ignored. I felt I was just a nuisance, and was sure something was wrong with the child as the comments written were placed in a large firmly sealed envelope ...'.

Similar comments were given by some mothers in Hyde's (1986) study. 'I've seen it on television, and I was led to believe it would be explained.' 'You build yourself up, then they don't say anything'. Hyde's study is of considerable interest because it was carried out in the United Kingdom during the very small time window when ultrasound scanning was becoming common but was not yet the norm. She found that unscanned women in hospitals where ultrasound was not used routinely were less likely to see scans as a source of reassurance. This would seem to be a classic example of the belief that 'what is must be best' as observed by Porter and Macintyre (1984).

When Hyde was carrying out her survey in 1982, many women were still very suspicious of this new technology. Nowadays, women's main complaint about ultrasound in pregnancy – as we found in the Cambridge Prenatal Screening Study – is that they do not get enough of it. However, concerns about ultrasound may not in fact be so far below the surface. Thorpe et al. (1993) asked mothers of newborn children about their views of ultrasound scanning in a non-routine context: cerebral scanning of neonates. Many mothers had misgivings about this, which they then had to accommodate within their framework of acceptance of antenatal scanning, for example: 'I know it's not harmful through me – it is just the thought of doing it on him.' 'She is only a baby, she's not old enough to have one whereas I am.'

One of the most telling comments from Thorpe's respondents was 'This [cerebral] scan looks for things that are wrong whereas the scan in pregnancy checks to see that the baby is OK'. This distinction between 'checking that everything is OK' and 'looking for abnormalities' is probably one of the keys to women's enthusiasm for scans: they do not view them as a threat that might give them bad news (like amniocentesis), but as a benign procedure which allows them to see their baby and confirm that it is healthy. Their assumption that the procedure is benign is, of course, encouraged by the fact that scans are routine and given to everyone. Thus, to quote another of Thorpe's participants: 'If it was necessary I would have [consented] – if it was routine – no problem.'

CONCLUSIONS

Prenatal screening and diagnosis do not happen in a vacuum, and a woman's experiences are related to both the broad societal context (Green et al., 1992) and the more specific circumstances that have led her to be having this test at this time. Perhaps the most neglected of these circumstances has been the historical context. One thing that is clear from the literature is that women react differently to tests that are new, or to tests that they have actively sought, compared to those that are accepted as routine procedures (Richards and Green, 1993). When the first edition of this book was being written in 1993, the 'hot topic' was the introduction of serum screening for Down syndrome. This caused a lot of difficulties to both women and health professionals (Statham and Green, 1993; Green 1994). To understand these difficulties we have to consider context. Firstly, the test was being introduced at a time when the ethos of health-care in general and maternity care in particular was shifting towards one in which women were to be told much more about what was happening to them. This was in contrast to the situation which had pertained for serum screening for neural-tube defects, where a large proportion of women did not know whether they had had the test or not. Serum screening for Down syndrome was also replacing (at least in theory) another method of screening – age – which is not actually recognized by most people as being a screening test at all. The message that older women are at risk for chromosomal abnormalities has been so effective that the fact that two thirds of Down syndrome babies are born to younger women has been buried.

The concept of a screening test which necessarily has false positives and false negatives is poorly understood. Screening tests for all manner of ills are now such a major aspect of health care that the population as a whole needs to be better educated about the underlying principles and key concepts. One such concept is that of the 'positive predictive value' which refers to the proportion of people with a screen positive result who do actually have the condition in question. The positive predictive value of the triple test is approximately 1 in 68, in other words 67 out of every 68 women who screen positive will not have an affected baby. (This compares with figures for neural-tube defect serum screening varying from 1 in 15 to 1 in 66, depending on incidence). Using age alone as the screening method for Down syndrome has considerably poorer positive predictive value. Even at age 40, when the risk is 1 in 110, that still means that 109 out of 110 40-year-olds have been selected for amniocentesis but do not have an affected baby. It may be that the poor predictive value of age is one of the factors which makes it a less threatening screening method: a woman selected for amniocentesis on the basis of her age is, on average, only half as likely to have a Down syndrome baby as one selected by the triple test. However, it is likely that the other factor that makes serum screening so much more alarming to women is the fact that it is based on specific information about this particular pregnancy, not just membership of an impersonal risk group.

Until now, the provision of serum screening for Down syndrome in the UK within the NHS has been idiosyncratic. In a number of centres it has been offered only to older women, which negates the underlying assumptions and purpose of the test. The UK National Screening Committee has now recommended that serum screening for Down syndrome be made available to all women irrespective of age (www.nsc.nhs.uk/antenatal_screen/antenatal_screen _ind.htm). They held back from making such a recommendation until a suitable support infrastructure could be in place. The findings of a recent survey of community health professionals (Statham *et al.*, 2002) give cause for concern in this regard since it appears that in many places GPs and community midwives are not being informed of positive screening results and are thus ill-placed to offer support. The prenatal detection rate of Down syndrome in England and Wales has been around 45% in women under 35 years and 70% in women older than 35 (Mutton *et al.*, 1998). The availability of second-trimester serum screening to all may well mean that the detection rate in the younger age group rises to around 60%. The number of false positive results in this group will, of course, also increase. This means that health professionals must anticipate an increased workload in dealing with the anxieties raised which may be particularly high in younger women (Bryant *et al.*, 2001).

Key points

- Women experience considerable anxiety while waiting for the results of diagnostic tests, particularly if they believed themselves to be 'low risk' at the start of pregnancy.
- Earlier diagnosis is welcomed but the grief of parents terminating early is no less than that of those terminating later.
- Positive screening test results cause a great deal of anxiety, which may not be fully resolved by a negative diagnostic test result.
- Ultrasound scanning is not seen primarily as a test of fetal abnormality; what women like about scans is a moving image that is interpreted for them and the social aspects that allow other family members to see the baby.
- Women's feelings about screening and diagnostic tests depend very much on the context; for example, whether the procedure is new or routine and whether they have actively chosen it.
- Screening tests are now such a major aspect of health care that the population as a whole needs to be better educated about the underlying principles and key concepts.

REFERENCES

Abuelo DN, Hopmann MR, Barsel-Bowers G *et al.* (1991) Anxiety in women with low maternal serum alpha-fetoprotein screening results. *Prenatal Diagnosis*, 11; 381–385.
Baillie C (1997) PhD thesis: Lay explanations of positive screening test results and their psychological consequences. Leeds University, Leeds.
Baillie C, Hewison J, Mason G (1999) Should ultrasound scanning in pregnancy be routine? *Journal of Reproductive and Infant Psychology*, 17; 149–157.
Beeson D, Golbus MS (1979) Anxiety engendered by amniocentesis. *Birth Defects Original Articles Series*, 15; 191–197.
Berne-Fromell K, Kjessler B (1984) Anxiety concerning fetal malformations in pregnant women exposed or not exposed to an antenatal serum alpha-fetoprotein screening program. *Gynecologic and Obstetric Investigation*, 7; 36–39.

Berne-Fromell K, Uddenberg N, Kjessler B (1983a) Psychological reactions experienced by pregnant women with an elevated serum alpha-fetoprotein level. *Journal of Psychosomatic Obstetrics and Gynaecology*, 2; 233-237.

Berne-Fromell K, Kjessler B, Josefson G (1983b) Anxiety concerning fetal malformation in women who accept or refuse alpha-fetoprotein screening in pregnancy. *Journal of Psychosomatic Obstetrics and Gynaecology*, 2; 94–97.

Bricker L, Garcia J, Henderson J *et al.* (2000) Ultrasound screening in pregnancy: a systematic review of the clinical effectiveness, cost-effectiveness and women's views. *Health Technology Assessment*, 4(16); 41–62.

Bryant L, Green M, Hewison J (2001) Prenatal screening for Down's syndrome: some psychosocial implications of a 'screening for all' policy. *Public Health*, 115; 356–358.

Burton BK, Dillard RG, Clark EN (1985a) Maternal serum alpha-fetoprotein screening: the effect of participation on anxiety and attitude toward pregnancy in women with normal results. *American Journal of Obstetrics and Gynecology*, 152; 540–543.

Burton BK, Dillard RG, Clark EN (1985b) The psychological impact of false positive elevations of maternal serum alpha-fetoprotein. *American Journal of Obstetrics and Gynecology*, 151; 77–82.

Caccia N, Johnson JM, Robinson GE *et al.* (1991) Impact of prenatal testing on maternal-fetal bonding: chorionic villus sampling versus amniocentesis. *American Journal of Obstetrics and Gynecology*, 165(4); 1122–1125.

Campbell S, Reading AE, Cox DN *et al.* (1982) Ultrasound scanning in pregnancy. *Journal of Psychosomatic Obstetrics and Gynaecology*, 1; 57–61.

Chervin A, Farnsworth PB, FreedmanWL *et al.* (1977) Amniocentesis for prenatal diagnosis. *New York State Journal of Medicine*, August, 1406–1408.

Clement S, Wilson J, Sikorski J (1998) Women's experiences of antenatal ultrasound scans. In *Psychological Perspectives on Pregnancy and Childbirth* (ed. Clement S). Churchill Livingstone, Edingburgh, pp.7–24.

Evans MI, Bottoms SF, Carlucci T *et al.* (1988) Determinants of altered anxiety after abnormal maternal serum alpha-fetoprotein screening. *American Journal of Obstetrics and Gynecology*, 159; 1501–1504.

Esen UI, Olajide F (1997) Expectations and fears of women regarding two methods of prenatal screening. *International Journal of Gynaecologic Obstetrics*, 57(2); 193–194.

Evers-Kiebooms G, Swerts A, van den Berghe H (1988) Psychological aspects of amniocentesis: anxiety feelings in three different risk groups. *Clinical Genetics*, 33; 196–206.

Fairgrieve S (1997) Screening for Down's syndrome: what the women think. *British Journal of Midwifery*, 5(3); 148–151.

Farrant W (1980) Stress after amniocentesis for high serum alpha-feto-protein concentrations. *British Medical Journal*, 281; 452.

Farrant W (1985) 'Who's for amniocentesis?' The politics of prenatal screening In: *The Sexual Politics of Reproduction* (ed. Homans H). Gower, London.

Fava GA, Kellner R, Michelacci L *et al.* (1982) Psychological reactions to amniocentesis: a controlled study. *American Journal of Obstetrics and Gynecology*, 143; 509–513.

Fava GA, Trombini G, Michelacci L *et al.* (1983) Hostility in women before and after amniocentesis. *Journal of Reproductive Medicine*, 28; 29–34.

Fearn J, Hibbard BM, Laurence KM *et al.* (1982) Screening for neural-tube defects and maternal anxiety. *British Journal of Obstetrics and Gynaecology*, 89; 218–221.

Green JM (1990) Calming or harming? a critical review of psychological effects of fetal diagnosis on pregnant women. *Galton Institute Occasional Papers*, Second series, No 2.

Green JM (1994) Serum screening for Down's syndrome: the experiences of obstetricians in England and Wales. *British Medical Journal*, 309; 769–772.

Green JM, Statham H (1996) Psychosocial aspects of prenatal screening and diagnosis. In *The Troubled Helix: Social and Psychological Implications of the New Human Genetics* (eds Marteau TM and Richards MPM). Cambridge University Press, Cambridge.

Green JM, Statham H, Snowdon C (1992) Screening for fetal abnormalities: attitudes and experiences. In: *Obstetrics in the 1990s: Current Controversies* (eds Chard T and Richards MPM). McKeith Press, London, pp. 65–89.

Green JM, Snowdon C, Statham H (1993a) Pregnant women's attitudes to abortion and prenatal screening. *Journal of Reproductive and Infant Psychology*, 11; 31–39.

Green JM, Statham H, Snowdon C (1993b) Pregnancy: A Testing Time. Unpublished Report of the Cambridge Prenatal Screening Study, Centre for Family Research, University of Cambridge, Cambridge.

Hall S, Bobrow M, Marteau TM (2000) Psychological consequences for parents of false negative results on prenatal screening for Down's syndrome: retrospective interview study. *British Medical Journal*, Feb 12, 320(7232); 407–412.

Hyde B (1986) An interview study of pregnant women's attitudes to ultrasound scanning. *Social Science and Medicine*, 22; 587–592.

Jacoby A (1988) Mothers' views about information and advice in pregnancy and childbirth: findings from a national study. *Midwifery*, 4; 103–110.

Jöergensen C, Uddenberg N, Ursing I (1985) Ultrasound diagnosis of fetal malformation in the second trimester: the psychological reactions of the women. *Journal of Psychosomatic Obstetrics and Gynaecology*, 4; 31–40.

Keenan KL, Basso D, Goldkrand J et al. (1991) Low level of maternal serum alpha-fetoprotein: its associated anxiety and the effects of genetic counselling. *American Journal of Obstetrics and Gynecology*, 164; 54–56.

Kolker A (1989) Advances in prenatal diagnosis: social-psychological and policy issues. *International Journal of Technology Assessment in Health Care*, 5; 601–617.

McCormack MJ, Rylance ME, Newton J et al. (1990) Patients' attitudes following chorionic villus sampling. *Prenatal Diagnosis*, 10; 253–255.

MacKenzie IZ, Boyd P, Ferguson J (1986) Chorion villus sampling and randomization. *Lancet*, i (8487); 969–970.

Marteau TM (1991) Psychological aspects of prenatal testing for fetal abnormalities. *Irish Journal of Psychology*, 12; 21–132

Marteau TM, Kidd J, Cook R et al. (1988) Screening for Down Syndrome. *British Medical Journal*, 297; 1469.

Marteau TM, Johnston M, Kidd J et al. (1992a) Psychological models in predicting uptake of prenatal screening. *Psychology and Health*, 6; 13–22.

Marteau TM, Cook R, Kidd J et al. (1992b) The psychological effects of false positive results in prenatal screening for fetal abnormality: a prospective study. *Prenatal Diagnosis*, 12; 205–214.

Medical Research Council Working Party on the Evaluation of Chorion Villus Sampling (1991) MRC European Trial of chorion villus sampling. *Lancet*, 337; 1491–1499.

Milne LS, Rich UJ (1981) Cognitive and affective aspects of the responses of pregnant women to sonography. *Maternal–Child Nursing Journal* (Pittsburg), 10; 15–39.

Mutton D, Ide RG, Alberman E (1998) Trends in prenatal screening for and diagnosis of Down's syndrome: England and Wales, 1989–1997. *British Medical Journal*, 317; 922–923.

Nicolaides KH, Snijders RJM, Gosden CM *et al.* (1992) Ultrasonographically detectable markers of fetal chromosomal abnormalities. *Lancet*, 340; 704–707.

Phipps S, Zinn AB (1986) Psychological response to amniocentesis: I. Mood state and adaptation to pregnancy. *American Journal of Medical Genetics*, 25; 131–142.

Porter M, Macintyre S (1984) What is, must be best: a research note on conservative or deferential responses to antenatal care provision. *Social Science and Medicine*, 19(11); 1197–1200.

Reading AE, Cox DN (1982) The effects of ultrasound examination on maternal anxiety levels. *Journal of Behavioral Medicine*, 5; 237–247.

Reading AE, Campbell S, Cox DN *et al.* (1982) Health beliefs and health care behaviour in pregnancy. *Psychological Medicine*, 12; 379–383.

Richards MPM, Green JM (1993) Attitudes toward prenatal screening for fetal abnormality and detection of carriers of genetic disease: a discussion paper. *Journal of Reproductive and Infant Psychology*, 11; 49–56.

Roberts J (1986) The consumer's viewpoint on ultrasound in pregnancy. *Bulletin of the British Medical Ultrasound Society*, Feb/Mar; 18–19.

Robinson GE, Garner DM, Olmstead MP *et al.* (1988) Anxiety reduction after chorionic villus sampling and genetic amniocentesis. *American Journal of Obstetrics and Gynecology,* 159; 953–956.

Robinson GE, Carr ML, Olmsted MP *et al.* (1991) Psychological reactions to pregnancy loss after prenatal diagnostic testing: preliminary results. *Journal of Psychosomatic Obstetrics and Gynaecology*, 12; 181–192.

Robinson J (2001) Prenatal screening: a retrospective study. *British Journal of Midwifery*, 9(7); 412–417.

Robinson J, Tennes K, Robinson A (1975) Amniocentesis: its impact on mothers and infants. A 1-year follow-up study. *Clinical Genetics*, 8; 97–106.

Roelofsen EEC, Kamerbeek LI, Tymstra TJ (1993) Chances and choices. Psycho-social consequences of maternal serum screening. A report from The Netherlands. *Journal of Reproductive and Infant Psychology*, 11; 41–47.

Rothman BK (1986) *The Tentative Pregnancy: Prenatal Diagnosis and the Future of Motherhood.* Viking, New York.

Santalahti P, Aro AR, Hemminki E *et al.* (1998) On what grounds do women participate in prenatal screening? *Prenatal Diagnosis*, 18(2); 153–165.

Santalahti P, Latikka AM, Ryynanen M *et al.* (1996) Women's experiences of prenatal serum screening. *Birth*, 23(2); 101–107.

Sjogren B, Uddenberg N (1990) Prenatal diagnosis for psychological reasons: comparison with other indications, advanced maternal age and known genetic risk. *Prenatal Diagnosis*, 10; 111–120.

Spence W, Cox DN (1987) Emotional responses of pregnant women to chorionic villi sampling or amniocentesis. *American Journal of Obstetrics and Gynecology,* 157; 1155–1160.

Spencer JW, Cox DN (1988) A comparison of chorionic villi sampling and amniocentesis: acceptability of procedure and maternal attachment to pregnancy. *Obstetrics and Gynecology*, 72; 714–718.

Statham H, Green JM (1993) Serum screening for Down syndrome: some women's experiences. *British Medical Journal*, 307; 174–176.

Statham H, Green J, Snowdon C (1993) Psychological and social aspects of screening for fetal abnormality during routine antenatal care. In: *Proceedings of the 1992 Research and the Midwife Conference* (eds Robinson S, Thomson A, Tickner V), Manchester School of Nursing, University of Manchester.

Statham H, Green JM, Kafetsios K (1997) Who worries that something might be wrong with the baby? A prospective study of 1072 pregnant women. *Birth*, 24(4); 223–233.

Statham H, Solomou W, Green JM (2001) When a baby has an abnormality: a study of parents' experiences. *Part 1 of the Final report to the NHS Executive (Mother and Child Health Initiative)* of Grant no. MCH 4–12.

Statham H, Solomou W, Green JM (2002) When a baby has an abnormality: a study of health professionals' experiences. *Part 2 of the Final report to the NHS Executive (Mother and Child Health Initiative)* of Grant no. MCH 4–12.

Tabor A, Jonsson M (1987) Psychological impact of amniocentesis in low risk women. *Prenatal Diagnosis*, 7; 443–449.

Thorpe K, Harker L, Pike A *et al.* (1993) Women's views of ultrasonography: a comparison of women's experiences of antenatal ultrasound screening with cerebral ultrasound of their newborn infant. *Social Science and Medicine*, 36; 311–315.

Tunis SL, Golbus MS, Copeland KL *et al.* (1990) Patterns of mood states in pregnant women undergoing chorionic villus sampling or amniocentesis. *American Journal of Medical Genetics*, 37; 191–199.

Verjaal M, Leschot NJ, Treffers PE (1982) Women's experiences with second trimester prenatal diagnosis. *Prenatal Diagnosis*, 2; 195–209.

Wald NJ, Cuckle HS (1984) Open neural-tube defects. In: *Antenatal and Neonatal Screening* (ed. Wald NJ), Oxford University Press, Oxford.

Weinans MJ, Huijssoon AM, Tymstra T *et al.* (2000) How women deal with the results of serum screening for Down syndrome in the second trimester of pregnancy. *Prenatal Diagnosis*. 20(9); 705–708.

6 COUNSELLING AROUND PRENATAL TESTING

Lenore Abramsky

INTRODUCTION

What constitutes a prenatal diagnostic test? Why do women need to be counselled prior to having prenatal diagnostic tests? Who should do the counselling and how should it be done? How, when, where and by whom should results of tests be given to women? This chapter will consider all these issues and explore some of the dilemmas created by new genetic and obstetric technology. My first dilemma is how to refer to the counsellor who because of the constraints of the English language must be assigned a gender. I have decided to give her my own. The term 'counsellor' will be used to refer to anyone doing counselling, whatever the actual training or qualifications of that person may be. The term 'prenatal tests' will be reserved for investigations done to identify fetal abnormality.

WHY COUNSEL BEFORE A PRENATAL SCREENING OR DIAGNOSTIC TEST?

Why is more in-depth counselling of a woman required before taking her blood for serum screening for Down syndrome than is required prior to taking blood to see if she is anaemic? The essential difference between these two tests lies in the purpose for which the tests are done.

We take a mother's blood to see if she is anaemic to safeguard the health of the mother and therefore of the baby. If the mother is anaemic, she can take iron supplementation, which is an acceptable intervention for most women. The implied value judgement expressed in doing this test and acting upon it is that it is a 'good thing' if both mother and baby are kept as healthy as possible. Most women concur with this value judgement unless it involves what for them is an unacceptable amount of interference in their lives or in the pregnancy. By contrast, the purpose of prenatal screening and diagnostic tests is, for the most part, quite different. They are done so that if the baby is affected with a serious disability the parents can choose to have the pregnancy terminated if they wish (Crawfurd, 1983). The implied value judgement expressed in doing these tests is that if the quality of life will not be good enough (which is open to interpretation) then it is preferable that there be no life.

Many people, but by no means everyone, would agree with this statement. The counsellor who says 'We recommend an amniocentesis for all women with your screening result' rather than 'we offer an amniocentesis for all woman with your screening result' is assuming that the woman agrees that in the case of the disability in question, it is preferable that there be no life. She is putting subtle pressure on the woman to have the test. For those who do not agree that having no life is preferable to having life with a serious disability, it is far from clear that it is always beneficial for them to know early in pregnancy that the baby will be born with a serious disability (Statham *et al.*, 2001). I have certainly been told by some people that they would rather not have known about the condition before the baby was born while others are very grateful that they did know.

An analogous situation that does not involve pregnancy illustrates the qualitative difference between the purpose of prenatal screening and diagnostic tests and most other medical tests. If a person suffering from fatigue goes to their family doctor for a check-up, the doctor is probably safe in assuming that the patient would like to have a blood test to check for anaemia, so that treatment can be initiated if the patient is anaemic. By virtue of being there, the patient has expressed an interest in maintaining their health. It would be a very different story if the doctor were doing the blood test not in order to treat any abnormality found, but with a view to offering the patient euthanasia if the result were abnormal. If this were the purpose of the test, the doctor would not be correct in assuming that the patient wanted the test just because she presented for care. It would be necessary to counsel the patient and to obtain informed consent before doing any tests. In the same way, the doctor or midwife in the antenatal clinic or the genetics clinic cannot assume that just because a woman is there she wants prenatal diagnostic tests, with a possible consequence of being offered a termination of pregnancy.

Another consideration is that some prenatal diagnostic tests are invasive and carry with them a risk to the pregnancy (Rodeck and Nicolaides, 1983; Turnbull and MacKenzie, 1983; Canadian Collaborative CVS-amniocentesis Clinical Trial Group, 1989; Medical Research Council Working Party on Chorion Villus Sampling, 1991; Johnson *et al.*, 1999; Roper *et al.*, 1999; Papantonio *et al.*, 2001). No parents should be asked to take that risk unless they fully understand it and are entirely sure that the information obtainable from the test is worth the risk.

WHAT CONSTITUTES A PRENATAL SCREENING OR DIAGNOSTIC TEST?

If it is accepted that counselling is appropriate before prenatal screening and diagnostic tests are done, the next issue is identifying which investigations are prenatal screening or diagnostic tests. We would probably all agree that amniocentesis, chorionic villus sampling, and fetal blood sampling are prenatal diagnostic tests and that nuchal translucency scanning and serum screening for Down syndrome are part of the process leading to prenatal diagnosis. Many people are not however fully aware that ultrasound scanning is our most powerful tool in the field of prenatal screening and diagnosis. It is a screening procedure offered more than once in pregnancy to most women and it is the investigation that most often detects or raises suspicion of a fetal abnormality (Chitty *et al.*, 1991; Levi *et al.*, 1991; Shirley *et al.*, 1992; Chitty, 1995).

PRE-TEST COUNSELLING

The more physically invasive the test is, the more risk it poses to the pregnancy and the more counselling the woman is likely to have prior to the test. So a woman may have considerable and lengthy counselling prior to fetal blood sampling and absolutely no counselling prior to an ultrasound scan. This takes into account the woman's right to decide whether or not to expose the pregnancy to risk but ignores her right to decide whether or not she wants to have certain information about her baby.

It is important to consider the purposes of the counselling and what constitutes adequate counselling. These questions have been considered by a number of authors. A good review of the literature in this area up to 1990 was prepared by Green (1990), while a recent discussion on the subject can be found in Marteau and Dormandy (2001).

Providing information

First, pre-test counselling must ensure that the woman is adequately informed about the condition(s) being tested for and knows as much as possible about the test being offered so that she and her partner can make a fully informed decision about whether or not to have it (RCOG and RCPCH Report, 1997).

This means she needs to know:

- what sorts of conditions can be screened for or diagnosed and what sorts of conditions cannot be screened for or diagnosed by the test in question;
- the effects and the long-term outlook of the condition(s) which the test may detect; this cannot be done so specifically if a single test (such as ultrasound) looks for many anomalies;
- what her prior risk (without the benefit of the test results) is for the condition to be tested and how this compares to other people's risk;
- whether it is a screening test or a diagnostic test and how accurate (both sensitively and specifically) it is for a person in her situation;
- how, when, and where the test would be done;
- what the test would feel like;
- what preparations and aftercare might be needed;
- what risks it poses to the pregnancy;
- the possible consequences of receiving the information the test provides;
- how, when and where she would get the results of the test;
- what alternative tests are available to look for the same condition.

Clearly, a lot of information must be provided if the woman is to be fully informed. This amount of information cannot be imparted without a good deal of time being spent. Staff who are not fully informed themselves cannot inform others. Most people cannot remember a large amount of verbal information accurately, so it is important to back it up with clear written or taped material in a language in which the couple are fluent.

It is worth noting here that some women change their minds when they become better informed about the tests, even if they have stated at the outset of counselling that they have already made up their minds about what they will do (Abramsky and Rodeck, 1991). Three pieces of information which women cited in that study as reasons for changing their minds about tests were:

- the level of risk they had for the condition in question;
- the miscarriage risk of the test being considered;
- the method of termination that would be offered if they chose to terminate the pregnancy following an abnormal result from the test in question.

Facilitating decision-making

The second purpose of pre-test counselling is to help those women or couples who are having trouble making a decision, to reach a decision which is suitable for them, given their values, situation, hopes and fears (Marteau and Dormandy, 2001). Essentially, the role of the counsellor is to help people to see what all the possible consequences of having or not having the tests in question would be, and to determine which set of consequences is the most acceptable (or the least unacceptable) to them.

This requires time, skill, and sensitivity on the part of the counsellor. It very definitely does not involve counsellors giving advice that is essentially what they think they would do in the situation. What the counsellors would do is entirely irrelevant. It is not their baby and they will not have to live with the consequences of any decisions that are made. It is important to help the woman and her partner to explore the pros and cons of having the test in question, a different test, or no test. Many people are helped in this by a 'worst scenario exercise' (Lippman-Hand and Fraser, 1979). They may, for example, want to consider whether, to them, the miscarriage of a healthy baby would be more, less, or equally bad as the birth of a disabled child. With the 'worst case scenario' it is necessary for the couple to keep in mind the relative likelihood of the various end results. If handled well, this exercise can help a lot of people to come to a decision that is right for them. A number of strategies for helping people make decisions appropriate for them are discussed in Egan (1998).

CAN PRE-TEST COUNSELLING BE NON-DIRECTIVE?

I have argued that pre-test counselling should be non-directive, since it is the couple and not the counsellor whose entire future life may be affected by decisions made at the session. However, we must ask whether non-directive pre-test counselling is achievable. Powerful arguments have been made that it is not possible (Clarke, 1991; Anderson, 1999; Williams et al., 2002). Those present at the third European meeting on psychosocial aspects of genetics (1992), voted by a narrow majority that non-directive genetic counselling was not achievable in practice.

This is partly because the counsellor comes to the session with her own cultural background, personality, and life experiences. She may have her own views about what she thinks she would do in the situation or what she thinks a responsible person should do. These views may be conscious or unconscious, but they will influence her choice of words in describing conditions, tests and probabilities. They will influence her facial expression, body language, the order in which things are explained and the amount of time spent on different topics. The good counsellor will do her best to understand her own feelings and to try to keep them out of the counselling situation, but this may not always be entirely successful.

The second stumbling block to non-directive counselling in the antenatal context is the fact that many women having prenatal tests do not approach someone asking for them. They are offered such tests as 'routine' anomaly scanning, carrier testing for thalassaemia, sickle cell disease, Tay–Sachs disease or cystic fibrosis, and amniocentesis for a high risk of Down syndrome. When we offer such tests, surely we are implying that the condition being tested for is undesirable and that we are offering them the opportunity of knowing about it in time to end the pregnancy if the baby is affected (Hildt, 2002). We therefore start many counselling sessions in a manner that suggests a possible direction; many women find it difficult to refuse a test that has been offered (Sjogren and Uddenberg, 1988). We have a genuine problem, however. If we do not offer the tests, then the only people to have access to prenatal diagnosis will be well-informed women who ask for it, and this is clearly unjust. It seems that we cannot offer tests without being somewhat directive, but we must therefore be extremely careful with both verbal and written information to explain to people the optional nature of these tests and the fact that it is entirely acceptable to decline the offer. We must be certain to say that we 'offer' all women (or all those in a given category) the test but not to say that we 'advise' them to have it.

WE COMMUNICATE WITH WORDS

However careful the counsellor is, it is not possible to be entirely neutral. It is not feasible to say absolutely everything about a condition or about all the possible courses of action. The counsellor must decide what is important enough to be said and what is unimportant enough to leave unsaid. The information cannot all be given at the identical moment, so the counsellor must choose the order in which it is presented. The words used will rarely be value-free; words have connotations other than their dictionary definitions.

In a recent forced-choice questionnaire study (Abramsky and Fletcher, 2002) significantly more respondents found:

- 'an abnormality' more worrying than 'a variation from the usual';
- 'a rare abnormality' more worrying than a 'common abnormality';
- a condition that had the word syndrome or disorder attached to it more worrying than one without;
- a technical word (for example, trisomy) more worrying than its less-technical counterpart (for example, an extra chromosome);

- a proportion (1 in X) level of risk more worrying than the equivalent percentage (%);
- the chance of a desired outcome happening (99%) more reassuring than the corresponding chance for the undesired outcome happening (1%).

Counsellors need to bear in mind what connotations (both positive and negative) words have and to use them in such a way as to give the intended message. They should also take great care when communicating risk figures (Tversky and Kahneman, 1981; McNeil *et al.*, 1982; Marteau, 1989; Shiloh and Sagi, 1989; Shaw and Dear, 1990; Calman and Royston, 1997; Hallowell *et al.*, 1997; Campbell, 1998; Jasper *et al.*, 2001; Lloyd, 2001, Schapira *et al.*, 2001; Edwards *et al.*, 2002).

HOW IS PRE-TEST COUNSELLING DONE IN PRACTICE?

Pre-test counselling probably comes closest to the ideal in the context of the genetics services. In such services couples are counselled by clinical geneticists and specialist genetic counsellors who are likely to have up-to-date information, to understand what it means, to be skilled in explaining it and to have the necessary aids such as pictures and diagrams. They are also experienced at this particular type of counselling. In addition, the time allowed for such discussion in the genetics services is far greater than that allowed in most antenatal clinics and there is often a greater degree of privacy. Perhaps most importantly, the ethos of genetic counselling has traditionally been such that the counsellor provides information so that the patient or relative can make informed choices (Fraser, 1974; Harper, 1981; Marteau *et al.*, 1994; Brunger and Lippman, 1995; Michie *et al.*, 1997; Emery, 2001).

This contrasts sharply with the practice in most other fields of medicine in which both doctors and nurses may be used to telling patients what they should do: 'you should lose weight, stop smoking, take exercise, take antibiotics'. It is extremely difficult for someone who has offered directive counselling for years to become non-directive for particular occasions. So it is not surprising that in the context of ordinary antenatal care, tests are often presented as routine rather than as one possible course of action. In one study (Marteau *et al.*, 1992) looking at counselling prior to serum alpha-fetoprotein tests, it was found that over half the doctors presented it as routine saying things such as 'And also we do a routine blood test for spina bifida' and did not invite the woman to make a decision. This is even truer of anomaly scanning which in the UK tends to be presented as routine care, often with no discussion about the possibility of finding abnormalities or about whether the woman would like to have it done. Literature given to women may say that the scan is 'to make sure that the baby is developing normally'. One leaflet, when referring to urine and blood tests and scans, said of them '... tests are the routine ones carried out on all pregnant women'.

It is not possible or desirable for all pregnant women to have full scale genetic counselling, so the vast majority of women will continue to receive what pre-test counselling they get from those looking after them in the course of their routine antenatal care. The challenge facing maternity services is to ensure that obstetric and midwifery staff who counsel women about prenatal tests have the training and time which will enable them to reach and practice at a high standard. It is also vital that they be supplied with high quality written information and is desirable that genetic counsellors are involved in the preparation of this material. It is essential to avoid inaccurate, unclear and directive statements such as the following extracts from actual hospital leaflets being incorporated in information for patients:

> *The only treatment for babies with a serious congenital abnormality is termination of pregnancy.*

> *This [the 19-week anomaly scan] is done to check that the baby has no abnormalities that cannot be detected by the ultrasound at fifteen to sixteen weeks, as it was too early to do this.*

WHAT DO WOMEN SAY THEY WANT FROM PRE-TEST COUNSELLING?

A series of women attending counselling because of advanced maternal age at one obstetric hospital in the early 1990s were asked to write about what they hoped to learn from the session (Abramsky, unpublished). The majority indicated merely that they wanted to know what tests were available and what the risks of these tests were. Nearly half of them said they wanted reassurance about something. Few responses contained specific points for which clarification was wanted: for example, they asked about risks of tests, but did not specifically ask about miscarriage risk, risks of damaging the fetus or risks of damaging the mother. Very few women mentioned the accuracy of the test, and those who did mention this did not distinguish between false positives and false negatives. In short, the questions these women wanted answered were stated in a very general way, and an overburdened or unconscientious counsellor might feel that she had done her job by naming the tests, giving their respective miscarriage risks and reassuring a woman that she could have a test.

So why don't women mention specifics when asked what they want to learn at the session? The answer may be for the same reason as most of us ask few very specific questions about the technicalities of a car repair or a rewiring job. One has to know a lot about a subject in order to know what to ask. People are unlikely to ask about the rate of culture failure if they do not know that the sample is cultured or that cultures sometimes fail. It is the responsibility of the counsellor to answer all the questions that probably would be asked if the pregnant woman knew more about the technology.

Only a tiny number of women said they would like to know what conditions the tests could or could not identify and what their risks were for these conditions. Perhaps they thought, as Sally did, that an amniocentesis or chorionic villus sampling could detect all abnormalities. Sally said '...I want to be sure that the baby that I have is completely healthy and normal, otherwise I am not keeping it...'. It is the job of the counsellor to ensure that the woman does not leave the counselling session with this misapprehension, as Caroline did. Caroline had an amniocentesis for advanced maternal age. The results were normal, but after she received the results an anomaly scan showed that her baby had cystic lungs and that the prognosis was very poor. She was extremely angry and repeatedly said that this could not be so, as the amniocentesis result was normal. It is not always easy to convince women that normal amniocentesis results only rule out specified abnormalities. As many women said, they came to get reassurance, and they may not easily take on board the fact that the reassurance is only partial. However, this problem is greatly compounded if the counsellor is loathe to mention the limitations of the test. Collusion can occur between counsellor and client. More than one woman has been told that the tests are 'just to make sure your baby is normal'.

At the same time, and in complete contrast, women are often told that amniocentesis is a test to look for Down syndrome, with no mention that about half the abnormal results from amniocentesis are not Down syndrome (Ferguson-Smith, 1983; Benn *et al.*, 1995). If the result is an abnormality such as Klinefelter syndrome, the parents who are not aware of such a possibility may close their minds to any information about the condition because they 'know that they want a termination if the baby is abnormal'.

SOME CASES FOR WHICH COUNSELLING HAS BEEN INEFFECTIVE

None of us is a perfect counsellor; we could all improve, and looking at our own and other people's shortcomings is often a way of working towards that improvement. With this in mind, the reader is invited to consider the following cases gathered over many years from many sources.

CASE STUDY I   REBECCA

Rebecca was a Jehovah's Witness expecting her first child. She refused the offer of an alpha-fetoprotein test because she said that she would not contemplate terminating a pregnancy for any reason and therefore did not wish to know if there was a fetal abnormality. She did, however, have an ultrasound scan at about 18 weeks of pregnancy, when anencephaly was diagnosed. Like most women, she did not have counselling prior to the scan and was unaware that one of the main reasons for the scan was to look for fetal anomalies. She and her partner felt very angry about the diagnosis having been made. Her right not to know had not been honoured. She had not been given the necessary information with which to decide whether or not to have a scan. She carried her baby to term in what was a terribly stressful pregnancy.

CASE STUDY 2   BEVERLY

Beverly was a 39-year-old woman who had been trying unsuccessfully for many years to become pregnant. She finally became pregnant as a result of *in vitro* fertilization. At 16 weeks she had an amniocentesis, which revealed that her fetus had Down syndrome. Beverly and her partner requested genetic counselling so that they could find out more about Down syndrome. After hearing what the geneticist had to say, they said that 'it wasn't so bad' and that they had thought the amniocentesis was being done to test for serious abnormalities. They said that they would rather have a Down syndrome baby than no baby, and they decided to carry on with the pregnancy. It appeared that although the pregnancy had been very hard to achieve, Beverly had received only cursory pre-test counselling. It is questionable whether she would have decided to have an amniocentesis with the attendant risk of pregnancy loss if she had fully understood the purpose of it.

CASE STUDY 3   EVELYN

Perhaps the saddest case of all is Evelyn. She was a 24-year-old woman with two healthy children. In her third pregnancy she had biochemical screening and was told she was at increased risk for Down syndrome. The risk was not very high but was about four times higher than her age risk alone. She was offered an amniocentesis but became so upset about the possibility of Down syndrome that she had the pregnancy terminated. Later she became very distressed when she realized that in all likelihood she had aborted a normal baby. She said that she had not been aware that the blood test could provide any information about the chance of the baby having Down syndrome and that this contributed to her sense of shock and anxiety when she was suddenly told that she had a raised risk for Down syndrome. It would appear either that she was not given the relevant information about the screening test or that she did not take in the information. In either case, counselling before screening had been ineffective.

These cases are examples of counselling gone wrong at many different levels. Perhaps one of the main problems that they all had in common was that the counsellor was not really listening to what the woman said or was not responding to non-verbal cues. For example, Rebecca said that she did not want to know if the baby had an abnormality. She may have said that in reply to an invitation to have an alpha-fetoprotein test, but it remained equally true for other tests. If the purpose of the scan had been explained to her, she might have opted to have it, but she might have decided against it. If she had decided to have the scan and then received unwanted information, she might at least have felt less as if she had been assaulted.

Beverly must have made it obvious during the course of her *in vitro* fertilization treatment how desperate she was to have a child. If a counsellor had explained the purpose of amniocentesis to her and had asked her how she felt about taking a risk with the pregnancy, she might well have declined the test.

It is very likely that Evelyn gave some indication (verbal or non-verbal) of her extreme anxiety when she was offered the amniocentesis because of her screening result. Perhaps if this anxiety had been acknowledged and she had been encouraged to talk about it, she would have decided to carry on with the pregnancy. On the other hand, perhaps she was looking for an excuse to terminate it and latched on to that one. In that case, it would have been better if she could have been gently led to explore why she really wanted to end the pregnancy.

THE IMPORTANCE OF LISTENING

Listening is a skill that some people seem to have in abundance and other people seem to lack in equal abundance! To some extent the skill or lack of it may be due to the individual's personality, life experiences and so on. However, it is also a skill that can be learned. It is an unfortunate fact, however, that many health workers finish their training without acquiring the ability to really listen and it is this inability that so often causes problems in the counselling situation.

GIVING THE RESULTS

Once the results of a test are available, clinical staff have the job of imparting them to parents. Staff usually feel that it is important to pass on bad news right away. However, established protocols often give a much lower priority to passing on good news quickly. In fact, it could be argued that it is more important to pass on good news as soon as it becomes available. Anyone who has waited anxiously for news about a loved one, about their own health, about important exam results or a job application will know how agonizing the wait can be. It is entirely inhumane to make someone wait extra hours, days or even weeks to be relieved of this misery.

If an anomaly is detected, it is essential that parents are informed in a sensitive manner, by someone who knows what the diagnosis is and who understands broadly what the implications are. It is vitally important that arrangements are in place for them to be seen promptly by someone who can give them more information, answer their questions and help them consider what the next step should be.

In a recent study on how parents were told their unborn baby had a sex chromosome anomaly (Abramsky *et al.*, 2001) it was found that all too often it was a matter of chance who told the parents and that sometimes the person who made the initial disclosure was, herself, uninformed about the significance of the anomaly. This meant that sometimes the first thing the parents heard was unclear or misleading, which may have coloured how they perceived what they were told later. Although most of the parents in the study went on to get high quality information, this was not universally true.

CONCLUSION

Informative, non-directive counselling before and after prenatal screening and diagnostic tests is essential. The counsellor can only provide this if she has knowledge, skill, sensitivity and time.

Key points

- Prenatal screening and diagnostic tests should only be done with informed consent.
- Informed consent can only be given if accurate, understandable information is given in a non-directive manner.
- The counsellor must be well informed, a good communicator, fluent in the same language as the pregnant woman, and a skilled, sensitive listener.
- Counselling takes time and requires a comfortable and private setting.
- Results should be given to women as soon as they become available and, in the case of positive results, prompt arrangements should be made for parents to be seen for a full consultation with the appropriate expert(s).

REFERENCES

Abramsky L, Fletcher O (2002) Interpreting information: what is said, what is heard – a questionnaire study of health professionals and members of the public. *Prenatal Diagnosis*, 22(13); 1188–1194.

Abramsky L, Rodeck CH (1991) Women's choices for fetal chromosome analysis. *Prenatal Diagnosis*, 11; 23–28.

Abramsky L, Hall S, Levitan J *et al.* (2001) Telling parents about a prenatally detected chromosome anomaly: a telephone interview study. *British Medical Journal*, 322; 463–466.

Anderson G (1999) Nondirectiveness in prenatal genetics: patients read between the lines. *Nursing Ethics* 2; 126–136.

Benn PA, Horne D, Briganti S *et al.* (1995) Prenatal diagnosis of diverse chromosome abnormalities in a population of patients identified by triple-marker testing as screen positive for Down syndrome. *American Journal of Obstetrics and Gynecology*, 173(2); 496–501.

Brunger F, Lippman A (1995) Resistance and adherence to the norms of genetic counselling. *Journal of Genetic Counselling*, 3; 151–167.

Calman KC, Royston GH (1997) Risk language and dialects. *British Medical Journal*; 315; 939–942.

Campbell DM (1998) Risk language and dialects: expressing risk in relative rather than absolute terms is important. *British Medical Journal*, 316; 1242–1243.

Canadian Collaborative CVS-amniocentesis Clinical Trial Group (1989) Multicentre randomized clinical trial of chorionic villus sampling and amniocentesis. *Lancet*, i; 1–6.

Chitty LS (1995) Ultrasound screening for fetal abnormalities. *Prenatal Diagnosis*, 15(13); 1241–1257.

Chitty LS, Hunt GH, Moore J *et al.* (1991) Effectiveness of routine ultrasonography in detecting fetal structural abnormalities in a low risk population. *British Medical Journal*, 303; 1165–1169.

Clarke A (1991) Is non–directive genetic counselling possible? *Lancet*, 338; 998–1001.

Crawfurd M (1983) Ethical and legal aspects of early prenatal diagnosis, *British Medical Bulletin*, 39 (4); 310–314.

Edwards A, Elwyn G, Mulley A (2002) Explaining risks: turning numerical data into meaningful pictures. *British Medical Journal*, 324; 827–830.

Egan G (1998) *The Skilled Helper: A Problem-Management Approach to Helping*. Brooks/Cole Publishing, London.

Emery J (2001) Is informed choice in genetic testing a different breed of informed decision-making? A discussion paper. *Health Expectations*, 2; 81–86.

Ferguson-Smith MA (1983) Prenatal chromosome analysis and its impact on the birth incidence of chromosome disorders. *British Medical Bulletin*, 39(4); 355–364.

Fraser FC (1974) Genetic counselling. *American Journal of Human Genetics*, 26; 636–659.

Green JM (1990) Calming or harming: a critical review of psychological effects of fetal diagnosis on pregnant women. *Galton Institute Occasional Papers*, Second series, no. 2.

Hallowell N, Statham H, Murton F *et al.* (1997) Talking about chance: the presentation of risk information during genetic counselling for breast and ovarian cancer. *Journal of Genetic Counselling*, 6; 269–286.

Harper PS (1981) *Practical Genetic Counselling*, Wright, Bristol.

Hildt E (2002). Autonomy and freedom of choice in prenatal genetic diagnosis. *Medical Health Care Philosophy*, 5(1); 65–71.

Jasper JD, Goel R, Einarson A, Gallo M, Koren G (2001) Effects of framing on teratogenic risk perception in pregnant women. *Lancet*, 358; 1237–1238.

Johnson JM, Wilson RD, Singer J *et al.* (1999) Technical factors in early amniocentesis predict adverse outcome. Results of the Canadian Early (EA) versus Mid–trimester (MA) Amniocentesis Trial. *Prenatal Diagnosis* 19(8); 732–738.

Levi S, Hyjazi Y, Schaaps JP *et al.* (1991) Sensitivity and specificity of routine antenatal screening for congenital anomalies by ultrasound: The Belgian Multicentric Study. *Ultrasound in Obstetrics and Gynaecology*, 1; 102–110.

Lippman-Hand JA, Fraser FC (1979) Genetic counselling – the post counselling period: parents' perceptions of uncertainty. *American Journal of Medical Genetics*, 4; 51–71.

Lloyd AJ (2001) The extent of patients' understanding of the risk of treatments. *Quality in Health Care*, 10; 114–118.

McNeil BJ, Pauker SG, Sox HC *et al.* (1982) On the elicitation of preferences for alternative therapies. *New England Journal of Medicine*, 306; 1259–1262.

Marteau T (1989) Framing of information: its influence upon decisions of doctors and patients. *British Journal of Social Psychology*, 28; 89–94.

Marteau TM, Dormandy E (2001) Facilitating informed choice in prenatal testing: how well are we doing? *American Journal of Medical Genetics*, 106(3); 185–190.

Marteau TM, Slack DMH, Kidd J *et al.* (1992) Presenting a routine screening test in antenatal care: practice observed. *Public Health* 106; 131–141.

Marteau T, Drake H, Bobrow M (1994) Counselling following diagnosis of a fetal abnormality: the differing approaches of obstetricians, clinical geneticists, and genetic nurses. *Journal of Medical Genetics*, 31(11); 864–867.

Medical Research Council Working Party on the Evaluation of Chorion Villus Sampling (1991) Medical Research Council European Trial of Chorion Villus Sampling. *Lancet*, 337; 1491–1499.

Michie S, Bron F, Bobrow M *et al.* (1997) Nondirectiveness in genetic counselling: an empirical study. *American Journal of Human Genetics*, 60(1); 40–47.

Papantoniou NE, Daskalakis GJ, Tziotis JG *et al.* (2001) Risk factors predisposing to fetal loss following a second trimester amniocentesis. *British Journal of Obstetrics and Gynaecology*, 1088(10); 1053–1056.

Rodeck CH, Nicolaides KH (1983) Fetoscopy and fetal tissue sampling. *British Medical Bulletin*, 39(4); 332–337.

Roper EC, Konje JC, De Chazal RC *et al.* (1999) Genetic amniocentesis: gestation-specific pregnancy outcome and comparison of outcome following early and traditional amniocentesis. *Prenatal Diagnosis*, 19(9); 803–807.

Royal College of Obstetricians and Gynaecologists (RCOG) and Royal College of Paediatrics and Child Health (RCPCH) (1997) *Report of a Joint Working Party on Fetal Abnormalities – Guidelines for Screening, Diagnosis and Management.* www.doh.gov.uk/genetics/pgt_ch5.htm

Schapira MM, Nattinger AB, McHorney CA (2001) Frequency or probability? A qualitative study of risk communication formats used in health care. *Medical Decision Making*, 21; 459–467.

Shaw NJ, Dear PRF (1990) How do parents of babies interpret qualitative expressions of probability? *Archives of Disease in Childhood*, 65; 520–523.

Shiloh S, Sagi M (1989) Effect of framing on the perception of genetic recurrence risks. *American Journal of Medical Genetics*, 33; 130–135.

Shirley IM, Bottomley F, Robinson VP (1992) Routine radiographer screening for fetal abnormalities by ultrasound in an unselected low risk population. *British Journal of Radiology*, 65 (775); 564–569.

Sjogren B, Uddenberg N (1988) Decision making during the prenatal diagnostic procedure. A questionnaire and interview study of 211 women participating in prenatal diagnosis. *Prenatal Diagnosis*, 8; 263–273.

Statham H, Solomou W, Green JM (2001), When a baby has an abnormality: a study of parents' experiences. *Report of NHS R and D Study 'Detection of fetal abnormality at different gestations: impact on parents and service implications'.* Centre for Family Research, Cambridge.

Turnbull AC, Mackenzie IZ (1983) Second–trimester amniocentesis and termination of pregnancy. *British Medical Bulletin*, 39(4); 315–321.

Tversky A, Kahneman D (1981) The framing of decisions and the psychology of choice. *Science*, 211; 453–458.

Williams C, Alderson P, Farsides B (2002) Is nondirectiveness possible within the context of antenatal screening and testing? *Social Science in Medicine*, 54; 339–347.

7 PRENATAL SCREENING AND DIAGNOSIS IN A MULTICULTURAL, MULTI-ETHNIC SOCIETY

Jane Sandall, Rachel Grellier, Shamoly Ahmed

INTRODUCTION

In the last decade, there has been increasing discussion about the experiences of women from different ethnic groups using maternity and reproductive health services in the UK. Ethnic minorities now make up over 5% of the UK population (Modood *et al.*, 1997). In 1998, around 635,000 women gave birth in the UK, and of these 86% of mothers were born in the UK, 7% were born in the New Commonwealth, and the remainder were born in other parts of the world (Macfarlane and Mugford, 2000). These figures are based on country of birth of the mother and do not reflect the origins of women from ethnic minorities who were themselves born in the UK.

Recognition of the different norms and values of communities is an important part of providing culturally sensitive maternity care. Many hospitals in the UK serve ethnically diverse areas, and research shows that women's experiences of maternity care often vary according to their ethnicity, religion and culture. Some women and their families have difficulty in communicating with health professionals and may experience insensitive and discriminatory treatment from clinical and administrative staff (Schott and Henley, 1996; Katbamna, 2000). These services need to be offered in a way that is both informative and culturally sensitive. The ongoing development of reproductive genetic technologies and first trimester screening techniques may render acceptable to some women options which were previously unacceptable. Thus, a greater understanding of the implications of offering such services in a society composed of diverse ethnic communities is essential.

DEFINING RACE, ETHNICITY AND CULTURE

The assignment of ethnic identity is complex, and the understanding of the relationship between ethnicity, health and culture correspondingly so. Ethnicity is a multi-dimensional concept that contains notions of shared origins, identity, culture, and tradition and allows us to move away from biological determinism present in the concept of race. The nearest we have to an agreed classification in the UK are the categories used by the Office for National Statistics in the 2001 census which is based on self-assigned ethnic group. This is a pragmatic classification that balances ease of collection against a need to produce data on the population. However, it is of limited use as a measure of socio-cultural differences (McKenzie and Crowcroft, 1996). Other researchers have asked about country of family origin, which is highly correlated with perceived ethnicity (Nazroo, 1997). However, this leaves the status of 'white' as being treated as a relatively homogenous group, which is also problematic (Bradby, 1995).

One of the difficulties with research and policy-making in this area has been that the volume of research on health and 'race' has not produced dividends, either by explaining differences in health experience or in improving provision to ethnic minority communities. Some researchers have focused on the exotic and marginal rather than the central experiences of ethnic minority groups, which often resemble those of the majority. This results in explanations that locate causes of variations in cultural or biological pathology, and ignore the socio-political context (Ahmad, 1996).

For example, congenital malformations make a major contribution to the higher stillbirth and mortality rates in babies born to Pakistani women. The reasons for this are contested, along with how differences between subgroups of ethnic minority populations have been masked in global statistics. Associations have been found between higher rates of congenital malformations and consanguineous marriages (usually first cousins), however, consanguinity may not be the main factor (Bittles *et al.*, 2001). Consanguineous marriage is still the preferred form of marital union for a large proportion of the world population, and our understanding of the effect is still incomplete. Some studies may overestimate the adverse genetic effects, partly due to flawed design in early studies (Ahmad, 1994; Grant and Bittles, 1997).

It is possible that the material, social and psychological disadvantages faced by ethnic minorities are related to geographical location. Aspects of the physical environment can also influence health behaviour by affecting attitudes, access to health facilities and employment opportunities, and increasing exposure to environmental hazards and toxins both at work and home (Shaw *et al.*, 2002), the latter being increasingly important as a factor related to fetal abnormalities.

Interactions between environmental and genetic factors along with the effects of socio-economic deprivation also need to be considered. There is a clearly documented relationship between socio-economic disadvantage and health (Acheson, 1998). A recent survey of the health of ethnic groups in Britain found that across three dimensions of socio-economic status, both Chinese and African Asian groups compared favourably with Whites; Indians were similar to, but slightly worse off than Whites and Caribbeans; Pakistanis and Bangladeshis were clearly worse off, with Bangladeshis the most disadvantaged (Nazroo, 1997). However, the interaction between health, deprivation and ethnicity is complex, and relative rather than absolute deprivation may play a role. Thus, inequality in social position can itself damage health, perhaps because of psychological processes that operate when social comparisons are made (Wilkinson, 1996). However, there is also some evidence that the concentration of ethnic minority groups in particular locations may be protective of health. This may allow the development of a community with a strong ethnic identity, thus enhancing social support, reducing alienation, increasing the group's access to political power, and protecting against the direct effects of racism (Smaje, 1995).

There is some evidence that racial discrimination and harassment have a direct effect on health. The Fourth National Survey (Modood *et al.*, 1997) shows that Bangladeshis were much less likely than African, Asian and Chinese respondents to report racial harassment when they experienced it. Poorer access to some services may explain poorer health. For example, ethnic minority groups reported using primary health services more than other groups, but there is some evidence that they were less likely to be referred for tertiary treatment after controlling for their reported level of health (Cooper *et al.*, 1998). The latest Confidential Enquiry into Maternal Deaths found that women from minority ethnic groups are twice as likely as white women to die in pregnancy and childbirth, and that more ethnic minority women received substandard care, with language barriers a major contributing factor (Lewis, 2001).

ANTENATAL SCREENING POLICY AND PROVISION

Currently, there are variations in the provision of prenatal screening and diagnostic services in the UK (Wald *et al.*, 1998; Lane *et al.*, 2001) and there has been limited national guidance (Royal College of Obstetricians and Gynaecologists, 1993). Recently, the Antenatal Screening Sub-group of the National Screening Committee (National Screening Committee, 2002) announced that all pregnant women in the UK should be offered prenatal screening for fetal anomalies. The aim is to establish an antenatal screening programme for Down syndrome that will ensure equity of access to all pregnant women.

Services previously offered only to women considered to be at a higher risk of Down syndrome due to age or family history are now routinely offered to all pregnant women in many places. However, it can be a 'postcode lottery'. Private screening services are growing and, due to technological developments, an increasing number of genetic, chromosomal and structural anomalies can be prenatally detected. What specific issues do these developments hold for people from different ethnic groups, in addition to issues that are universal concerns for all women?

The rolling-out of prenatal screening services to all pregnant women raises various issues at the heart of the 'new genetics' (Dyson, 1999). Such issues have already been discussed in relation to sickle cell disorders and thalassaemia (Anionwu and Atkin, 2001), and are relevant for all prenatal screening services. First, practical problems include poor practitioner knowledge, late referral for screening and diagnostic testing, and lack of a systematic, properly funded policy (Modell *et al.*, 2000). Second, screening and counselling provision raise concerns about underlying assumptions driving policy (Atkin and Ahmed, 1997). One of the most contested of these is the degree to which informed choice is available against a background of tension between policies of disease prevention and informed decision-making. Such distinctions are crucial as new genetic services disassociate themselves from eugenic thinking and assumptions. Symbolic associations between genetic screening programmes and eugenics have had an impact on haemoglobinopathy screening programmes in the USA. These programmes have been described as racist (Bradby, 1996). There is a need for great care in ensuring voluntary participation and informed decision-making in these programmes.

The 'routinization' of clinical interventions such as prenatal screening brings with it the inherent hazard of assumed consent (Nuffield Council on Bioethics, 1993). This is likely to be exacerbated in the UK by the structure of midwifery care in which midwives have to provide women with large quantities of information about a wide range of issues, including prenatal screening services, during one appointment. In general, the lack of provision of high quality written information to aid informed decision-making in maternity care has resulted in 'informed compliance' (O'Cathain et al., 2002; Stapleton et al., 2002). The pressure of time, differing perceptions of the priority of information, and individual attitudes to prenatal testing impact on the provision of information (Sandall and Grellier, 1999), in spite of attempts to provide non-directive counselling (Williams et al., 2002). As a result, many pregnant women experience mixed levels of care and have expressed differing levels of satisfaction about the screening process (Royal College of Obstetricians and Gynaecologists & Royal College of Paediatrics and Child, Health, 1997; Wald et al., 1998). The sum of such findings undermines the notion that women are giving informed consent when they take part in screening programmes (Marteau et al., 2001). Prenatal screening is often offered within an antenatal care package and information is often about the process rather than informing the decision to participate or not (Marteau et al., 1992). In addition to such general issues, these are overlaid with specific areas of misunderstanding, assumptions and stereotyping due to culture, ethnicity and language.

ETHNIC MINORITY WOMEN'S EXPERIENCES OF PRENATAL SCREENING AND TESTING

A great deal of research has been undertaken to explore women's understanding and experience of prenatal screening and diagnostic tests (for example: Green, 1990; Marteau et al., 1992; Green et al., 1993; Marteau, 1995; Grewal et al., 1997; Helm et al., 1998; Moyer et al., 1999; Hall et al., 2000), however, the majority of this research in the UK has focused on English-speaking women. A few studies have looked at other ethnic groups, but they have tended to emphasise variations in the uptake, specificity and sensitivity of the test in specific ethnic groups (Holloway and Bulusu, 1996), and measure cost-effectiveness by uptake of abortion (Ford et al., 1998). Less consideration has been given to equity of provision, accessibility and appropriateness of the programme to all women. This is compounded by the conflation of offer and uptake in many discussions. There is evidence from national audits of haemoglobin disorders that Pakistani and Bangladeshi women are less likely to be offered screening by health staff (Modell et al., 1997). Some studies (Begum et al., 1993; Bowler, 1993; Bowes and Meehan Domokos, 1996) have explored the views of single ethnic groups, but as they don't compare the views and experiences of a wide range of women receiving prenatal care in the same area, we need to be cautious about attributing views solely to ethnicity, culture or religion (Shaw, 2001). It is also difficult to know if the conclusions drawn from these studies are relevant to women from ethnic or religious backgrounds other than those studied.

Although cultural sensitivity is an important feature of good maternity care, it is difficult for health professionals to provide individualized care without exploring each woman's needs and concerns. Culture is not a static concept, as inter-generational differences exist, geographical variations occur and individual views change and adapt over a lifetime. In addition, ethnicity and religion are not likely to be the only issues to influence women deciding whether or not to have prenatal screening and diagnostic testing. Much of the evidence on women's responses to prenatal screening and diagnosis comes from white populations and the sparse literature illustrates similarities and differences in response. For example, people are generally positive about genetic screening and only about 1 in 50 say they would not want to be screened for genetic conditions (Green and Statham, 1996). However, the uptake of screening in pregnancy varies widely between different ethnic groups. Little is known about the attitudes, health beliefs and experiences of women from a range of ethnic groups with regard to prenatal screening, apart from some largely quantitative studies which allude to difficulties in communication and to cultural issues influencing the uptake of prenatal screening (Gilbert *et al.*, 1996). However, problems have been identified among clients with a limited English vocabulary, which prevents them fully understanding the process of antenatal care due to communication problems and to a lack of sensitivity among health professionals to cultural differences and requirements (Duff *et al.*, 1996).

Understanding some basic assumptions underpinning ethnic and religious identity can help to give health professionals insight into the way in which certain women may contextualize decisions about participation or non-participation in prenatal screening and diagnosis. In a comparative study of Asian and non-Asian women in East London, Woollett *et al.* (1995) found that parity rather than religion was the major variable relating to women's experiences of maternity care, and pointed out the need to go beyond stereotypical views based on ethnicity or religion. Other factors may include:

- previous experience of prenatal screening/diagnosis;
- the views of partner, family and friends;
- views of disability;
- views on abortion;
- economic and social support;
- parity;
- maternal age;
- relationship with health professionals;
- information about the test;
- reproductive history.

Each of these issues, and many more, may have a greater or lesser influence on individual women, and Rapp's work with women in the United States shows the importance of contextualizing the decisions women make within their own cultural and personal identities (Rapp, 2000).

A small, unpublished study found that a significant minority of Bangladeshi women receiving maternity care at one hospital in East London did not understand or know about the existing programme of prenatal screening. Among the women who knew they had been offered screening, 54% refused the test mainly due to religious and 'moral' reasons (Begum et al., 1993). Research that is more recent also suggests that awareness and uptake of prenatal screening is low among ethnically diverse populations in East London (Saridogan et al., 1996; Huttly and Dormandy, 1999).

We will use our own research with women in the ethnically diverse East-end of London to illustrate the ways in which ethnicity and religion affected women's access to, and uptake of prenatal screening and diagnosis (Sandall et al., 2001). The women's descriptions of their experiences also show the ways in which these beliefs can be incorporated into, create conflict with, or be subsumed by other issues influencing their decision-making about prenatal testing.

The hospital where our research was carried out provides maternity care for a diverse range of women from varying ethnic groups, but the three main ethnic groups are Bangladeshi, African-Caribbean and White. We carried out a small-scale comparative study of the factors affecting women's access to serum screening; their understanding and knowledge of the issues involved in antenatal screening and diagnostic tests; their involvement in informed decision-making and their perceptions of the service. Although the small sample size limits the generalizability of the findings, the results give some indication of the commonalities and differences experienced by the women. Ethnicity or religion directly affected some of these, but others reflected individual concerns such as personal circumstance, fear of invasive procedures, or previous reproductive history.

Over a 3-month period (August–October 2000), all women attending the antenatal clinic for their booking session who met the study criteria (over 18 years of age and able to communicate in English, Bengali or Sylheti) were invited to participate in the study (N =169). Participation involved completing a telephone or face-to-face structured questionnaire containing previously piloted and validated questions from the National Audit Commission Survey (Garcia et al., 1998) and an unpublished prenatal screening questionnaire (Begum et al., 1993). One hundred women completed the questionnaire and a subsample of 15 women from a range of ethnic groups, religion and cultures also agreed to take part in a semi-structured in-depth interview held in Sylheti, Bengali, or English according to their individual preference. With the women's permission, the interviews were tape-recorded, translated into English when necessary, and transcribed. The translations were independently assessed for accuracy and appropriateness of interpretation.

Results from the survey gave an overall picture of women's access to and experience of prenatal testing. The interviews provided more detailed information on why and how women decided whether to participate in the screening programme, and their perceptions of the service.

ACCESS TO PRENATAL SCREENING AND DIAGNOSIS

Despite recommendations that prenatal screening should be offered to all pregnant women in the UK, religious and cultural codes of behaviour mean that access to maternity care may be difficult for some women. For example, prenatal screening often needs to be carried out at a specific stage in pregnancy, but it can be difficult for a Muslim woman to attend a hospital appointment at that time if it coincides with Ramadan when a woman's domestic and religious commitments increase considerably and can make it difficult for her to leave the house. In addition, the social norm within the Muslim community is for a female relative or friend to accompany women attending an antenatal appointment and this can compound the problem of accessing routine maternity care.

In the UK, midwives usually offer prenatal screening, and many find it difficult to discuss these tests during their first meeting with a client, because it involves difficult and complex subject matter, such as fetal anomalies. These problems are further exacerbated if midwife and client do not share the same first language or if the client is unfamiliar with the vocabulary used in prenatal screening or does not fully understand the purpose of prenatal screening. Health advocates and interpreters can help but many UK hospitals are understaffed and not all women have access to this service.

Despite suggestions that ethnic minority groups have low levels of awareness about prenatal tests, we found that contrary to previous research, overall awareness was high among all women (82%). However, only 78% of eligible women were given an opportunity to decide whether or not to participate in prenatal screening, and this was associated with ethnicity. Thus, only 7% of White women were not offered screening, compared to 26% of Bangladeshi women and 33% of Afro-Caribbean women. Although all the Muslim women we interviewed refused prenatal screening, they said that they should be given information about the test and have the option to make an informed decision:

> *I think it should be offered. The midwife they are doing their jobs. It didn't seem bad to me, the test. The fact that it's being offered to women I don't think it's a bad thing. The fact that they do all this check-up and everything, to me I think it's good.* (Bangladeshi Muslim)

REFUSING PRENATAL SCREENING

Several studies have found that about 30% of women, irrespective of ethnicity, would not consider termination (Green and Statham, 1996). Refusal of prenatal screening in our study appeared to be clearly associated with ethnicity and, in a reflection of previous research (Begum *et al.*, 1993; Sarodigan *et al.*, 1996; Huttly and Dormandy, 1999; Chilaka *et al.*, 2001) was lowest among Bangladeshi women (31%) compared to acceptance rates of 67% in Afro-Caribbean women and 85% in White women. Responses to our survey indicated the most frequent reason for refusing prenatal screening among all women was that termination of pregnancy would not be considered for any reason. Some women attributed this to religious beliefs, while other women described it more as an individual decision related to whether the pregnancy was planned or not.

> *... We did have a few days when we considered would we keep the baby or not, but we decided that we would in the end ... then at 16 weeks having decided that we're going to have a baby and getting excited about it, the fact of finding that something's wrong and then maybe having to decide to have a termination or something, was something that I didn't want to have to do.*
>
> (White, no religion)

Some women from all ethnic groups described unease at tests that actively looked for fetal anomalies. White women with these concerns tended to accept screening tests but emphasise that they would refuse diagnostic tests and would not have a termination of pregnancy even if fetal anomalies were discovered. Bangladeshi women were more likely to view it as intrinsically wrong to try to look ahead in pregnancy or pre-empt the outcome of delivery and attributed this to their religious beliefs:

> *... If you know about these things in advance it's kind of frightening. I don't know, you just feel frightened about it, because you know religiously you are not really allowed to know beforehand. You just kind of feel frightened and you are separated from your religion.* (Bangladeshi Muslim)

Despite refusing prenatal screening for this reason, two Bangladeshi Muslim women had a series of ultrasound scans because of suspected fetal anomalies. This may be because ultrasound scans are not associated so directly with possible termination of pregnancy by either health professionals or women, even though they can reveal a greater range of fetal anomalies than maternal serum screening does. According to the Shariah (Islamic law) there is nothing wrong with a pregnant woman undergoing medical tests, as these can contribute to the health of the child as well as the mother. It is important, however, that prenatal testing does not turn into a selection process where decisions about termination of pregnancy are made because of disability. Other Islamic scholars, however, present prenatal testing as a temptation, which weakens belief and transgresses the boundaries of their spiritual teachings.

Associating refusal of prenatal screening too strongly with either ethnicity or religion runs the risk of health professionals anticipating women's decisions and becoming selective about what and how much information to give women. Although some women said religion influenced their decision to a certain extent, they also described a number of other reasons that were important to them, although they had not been able to, or had chosen not to, reveal these to a health professional. These included distress at the mention of termination of pregnancy, refusal to have a termination of pregnancy, fear of needles, concern about anxiety while waiting for the results, not wanting to know if the fetus was affected, and having no reason to assume that the fetus might have an anomaly.

Muslim women who refused screening expressed understanding for women who might decide to have a termination if fetal anomalies were discovered and pointed out that social terminations occurred within their communities although this contradicts general Islamic teaching:

> *Once a baby is in your stomach it's been given life, because our religion says for me to kill you it's the same as for me to kill a baby in my stomach ... I can't really terminate, but then you have a lot of Muslim people who do. Accidentally they are pregnant and they don't want a child, I am sure they go and do it, terminate the child. Because in this country you have mixed culture, how many people actually obey the religion or do things according to religion.*
>
> (Bangladeshi Muslim)

In her last sentence this women also recognizes the dynamic nature of cultural and religious beliefs and their impact on the norms of Bangladeshi Muslim behaviour. The basic principle concerning abortion in Islam is that it is unlawful (Haram) (Sheikh and Gatrad, 2000), and only permitted if the mother's life is at risk or if she has been raped. Social values can sometimes override spiritual belief, however, and social values can apply to different generations in different ways. Second generation Bangladeshi Muslims reported that they may be more likely to resort to termination of pregnancy rather than face the shame associated with pregnancy outside marriage, regardless of their religious belief.

Cultural beliefs and values can often be misinterpreted and wrongly held within the group itself to be the preaching of a religion. This can easily happen with a group or community, such as the Bangladeshi Muslim communities in the UK, in which their own special secular and spiritual values are practised. Islam teaches that disability is not associated with punishment for previous wrongdoing, nor should it be seen as a burden or problem and that every individual has a duty to accept a responsibility of care. However, some Muslims view disability as a form of punishment for wrong doings by people close to or related to the afflicted person. The family of a disabled child can be stigmatized and the marriage opportunities for other members of the family substantially reduced.

MAKING THE DECISION ABOUT PRENATAL SCREENING

There were wide variations in acceptance of prenatal screening among women from all ethnic and religious groups. One Bangladeshi woman described the way in which acceptance of divine control over the outcome of childbirth did not negate medical intervention during pregnancy:

I will accept the baby in any way he came ... but to know is OK ... Now I think it's OK to know everything, to do everything, every test to, I don't know, just to stop diseases. We don't know yet whether it's going to stop because it's in God's hands.

(Mixed race Muslim)

In Islam, life is seen as a gift from Allah, and if a person is deprived of certain ability, that individual will have many other abilities to compensate for their inability. According to Islamic belief everyone's fate and provision is predestined. If one is disadvantaged, that disadvantage may be compensated for in many other ways.

Several women, including Muslim clients, said they were initially interested in having serum screening until termination was mentioned as a potential endpoint:

In the beginning I said OK, I am going to do all the things to make sure everything is OK, and then the midwife explained like this one is for this, this one is for this. And when it came down to Down's syndrome, I said OK. This one will you have? You are going to have like another test, have choices to make, having a termination. When she said 'termination' I said 'what'. OK it was an awful decision, to do it .... I think that's the one thing I am scared of.

(African-Caribbean Muslim)

Mention of termination often had sufficient impact for women to immediately refuse prenatal screening. Although termination of pregnancy is not a necessary outcome if fetal anomalies are discovered, many women appeared to understand prenatal screening as resulting in a dichotomized choice – whether to continue or terminate the pregnancy:

They tell you what your options are: you can terminate your pregnancy or you can carry on, but it's not really options.

(White, Church of England)

Few women from any ethnic group described diagnostic tests as potentially advantageous in terms of enabling preparation for delivery at specialist medical centres, planning appropriate clinical treatment, or preparing to care for a child with physical or learning disabilities.

CONCLUSION

In summary, all women gave complex reasons for accepting or refusing screening. Many of these reasons were similar for women from all ethnic and religious groups, particularly the importance of accepting their child whether disabled or not, and opposition to termination of their own pregnancy. However, Muslim women were more likely to describe religion as impacting on their decision. There is a fine line between cultural sensitivity and cultural stereotyping and our own research has shown that although ethnicity and religion may influence decisions about prenatal screening and diagnosis, women from similar backgrounds also express very different opinions about the benefits and disadvantages of discovering fetal anomalies. Conversely, women from very varied backgrounds also describe common views and experiences that cross ethnic and religious boundaries. Health professionals' initial perceptions of their clients may focus on obvious and easily visible aspects of their appearance or health and fail to consider the needs, concerns and requirements of each individual woman (Bowler, 1993).

In one of the few comparative studies of Asian and non-Asian women in East London, Woollett *et al.* (1995) found that parity rather than religion was the major variable relating to women's experiences of maternity care and highlighted a need to go beyond stereotypical views based on ethnicity or religion. The findings from our study echo this need for health professionals to treat their clients as individuals, since women who share ethnic and cultural characteristics may have different beliefs, concerns and requirements in their maternity care. Some women may actively seek out prenatal screening due to personal experience of caring for a disabled child, while others may not consider prenatal testing to have any salience for them, but instead be concerned about other aspects of prenatal care. Health professionals need to try to explore in a culturally sensitive way their clients' knowledge and perceptions of screening and enable each woman to make an individually appropriate decision about whether to accept or refuse prenatal screening and testing.

Race, ethnicity and religion are important factors in the formation of social and individual identities. They also influence the culture of the communities to which we belong and in which we live. Recognition of the different norms and values of communities is an important part of providing culturally sensitive maternity care. Understanding certain basic assumptions underpinning ethnic and religious identity can help to give health professionals insight into the way in which certain women may contextualize decisions about participation or non-participation in prenatal screening and diagnosis. For example, the acceptability of termination of pregnancy at a particular gestation for a Bangladeshi Muslim woman depends upon which Islamic school of thought she follows, as there are differences of opinion amongst Muslim scholars regarding when the spirit is breathed into the embryo (within 40 days of pregnancy or within 120 days of pregnancy). All scholars agree that it is absolutely forbidden to abort the fetus after the spirit has been breathed into it (unless certain conditions justifying abortion apply). The Greek Orthodox Church is also strongly opposed to termination of pregnancy, although the tradition of screening for thalassaemia has led to the Church's acceptance of termination for genetic and chromosomal fetal anomalies. Gendered cultural perceptions about the stigma of, and blame for, disability also influence uptake of prenatal screening and diagnostic services (Dragonas, 2001), as having a disabled child may affect the way women are perceived by their family or the wider community.

Britain is a multi-ethnic society and national and local screening policies face the challenge of providing an equitable service that is sensitive and appropriate to people in different religions, cultures and ethnic communities. The commitment to meeting the health needs of all ethnic groups in the UK has been highlighted in both general health policy (Department of Health, 1997) and that relating specifically to maternity care. The challenges faced are around language difficulties, poor administrative arrangements, equitable allocation of resources, training and education, eliminating discriminatory practices and increasing user involvement.

Key points

- Around 635,000 women gave birth in the UK in 1998; of these, 86% of mothers were born in the UK, 7% were born in the New Commonwealth, and the remainder born in other parts of the world.
- Pakistani and Bangladeshi women are less likely to be offered screening. Inadequate consideration has been given to equity of provision, accessibility and appropriateness of the programme for all women. This is compounded by the failure to distinguish between offer and uptake.
- The take up of prenatal screening between different ethnic groups varies widely, and very little is known about the attitudes, health beliefs and experiences of women from a range of ethnic groups with regard to prenatal screening.
- The routinization of prenatal screening introduces an inherent hazard of assumed consent and/or assumed refusal based on perceptions of culture, religion and ethnicity. It is important to contextualize the decisions women make about prenatal screening within their own cultural and personal identities, their family and community, and to recognize the complexity underlying such decisions.
- In general, more women from ethnic minority groups receive substandard maternity care, with language barriers a major contributing factor. The lack of impact of even high quality written information in maternity care has resulted in 'informed compliance', thus an appropriate format and language that best meets the needs of the local population is crucial.

ACKNOWLEDGEMENT

This research was funded by a local NHS R and D grant.

REFERENCES

Acheson D (1998) *Department of Health Independent Inquiry into Inequalities in Health.* HMSO, London.

Ahmad WIU (1994) Reflections on the consanguinity and birth outcome debate. *Journal of Public Health Medicine,* 16; 423–428.

Ahmad WIU (1996) The trouble with culture. In: *Researching Cultural Differences in Health* (eds Kelleher D, Hillier S). Routledge, London.

Anionwu EN, Atkin K (2001) *The Politics of Sickle Cell and Thalassaemia.* Open University Press, Buckingham.

Atkin K, Ahmed WIU (1997) Genetic screening and haemoglobinopathies: ethics, politics and practice. *Social Science and Medicine,* 46(3); 445–458.

Begum S, Parsons L, Savage W (1993) What do non-English speaking women understand about antenatal screening for Down's syndrome? Academic Dept. Obstetrics and Gynaecology, St. Bartholomew's and the Royal London School of Medicine & Dentistry (unpublished).

Bittles AH, Savithri HS,Venkatesha Murthy G *et al.* (2001) Human inbreeding: a familiar story full of surprises. In *Health and Ethnicity* (eds Macbeth H, Shetty P). Taylor and Francis, London.

Bowes AM, Meehan Domokos T (1996) Pakistani women and maternity care: raising muted voices. *Sociology of Health and Illness,* 8(1); 45–65.

Bowler I (1993). 'They're not the same as us': midwives' stereotypes of south Asian descent maternity patients. *Sociology of Health and Illness,* 15(2); 157–158.

Bradby H (1995) Ethnicity: not a black and white issue. A research note. *Sociology of Health and Illness,* 17(3); 405–417.

Bradby H (1996) Genetics and racism. In: *The Troubled Helix: Social and Psychological Implications of the New Human Genetics* (eds Marteau T, Richards M) Cambridge University Press, Cambridge.

Chilaka VN, Konje JC, Stewart CR *et al.* (2001) Knowledge of Down Syndrome in pregnant women from different ethnic groups. *Prenatal Diagnosis,* 21; 159–164.

Cooper H, Smaje C, Arber S (1998) Use of health services by children and young people according to ethnicity and social class: secondary analysis of a national survey. *British Medical Journal,* 317(17); 1047–1051.

Department of Health (1997) *The New NHS: Modern and Dependable.* Stationery Office, London.

Dragonas T (2001) Whose fault is it? Shame and guilt for the genetic defect. In: *Before Birth: Understanding Prenatal Screening* (ed. Ettorre E). Ashgate Press, Aldershot.

Duff L, Lamping D, Ahmed L (1996) *Maternity services in West and Central London: The Views of Women from the Bangladeshi Community.* Kensington and Chelsea & Westminster Health Commissioning Agency, London.

Dyson S (1999) Genetic screening and ethnic minorities. *Critical Social Policy,* 19(2); 195–215.

Ford C, Moore AJ, Jordan PA *et al.* (1998) The value of screening for Down's syndrome in a socio-economically deprived area with a high ethnic population. *British Journal of Obstetrics and Gynaecology,* 105(8); 855–859.

Garcia J, Redshaw M, Fitzsimons M, *et al.* (1998) *First Class Delivery: A National Survey of Women's Views of Maternity Care.* Audit Commission and National Perinatal Epidemiology Unit, London.

Gilbert L, Nichol J, Alex S *et al.* (1996) Ethnic differences in the outcome of serum screening for Down's syndrome. *British Medical Journal,* 312; 94–95.

Grant JC, Bittles AH (1997) The comparative role of consanguinity in infant and child mortality in Pakistan. *Annals of Human Genetics,* (61); 143–149.

Green JM. (1990) *Calming or harming? A Critical Review of Psychological Effects of Fetal Diagnosis on Pregnant Women.* Occasional papers, Second Series No.2, Galton Institute, London.

Green J, Statham H (1996) Psychological aspects of prenatal screening and diagnosis. In: *The Troubled Helix: Social and Psychological Implications of the New Human Genetics* (eds Marteau T, Richards M). Cambridge University Press, Cambridge.

Green J, Statham H, Snowdon C (1993) Women's knowledge of prenatal screening tests: Relationships with hospital screening policy and demographic factors. *Journal of Reproductive and Infant Psychology*, 11; 11–20.

Grewal GK, Moss HJ, Aitken DA et al. (1997) Factors affecting women's knowledge of antenatal serum screening. *Scottish Medical Journal*, 42; 111–113.

Hall S, Bobrow M, Marteau TM (2000) Psychological consequences for parents of false negative results on prenatal screening for Down's syndrome: retrospective interview study. *British Medical Journal*, 320; 407–412.

Helm DT, Miranda S, Chedd NA (1998) Prenatal diagnosis of Down syndrome: mothers reflections on support needed from diagnosis to birth. *Mental Retardation*, 361; 55–61.

Holloway PJ, Bulusu S (1996) For appreciable ethnic differences in false positive rates, use different cut off points. *British Medical Journal*, 312; 1041.

Huttly W, Dormandy E (1999) *Audit of Maternal Serum Screening for Down's Syndrome in North London, Essex, Hertfordshire & Bedfordshire Regions: April 1997–March 1998*. Wolfson Institute of Preventive Medicine, London.

Katbamna S (2000) *'Race' and Childbirth*. Open University Press, Buckingham.

Lane B, Challen K, Harris HJ et al. (2001) Existence and quality of written antenatal screening policies in the United Kingdom: postal survey. *British Medical Journal*, 322(6); 22–23.

Lewis G (2001) *Why Mothers Die 1997–1999, The Fifth Report of the Confidential Enquiries into Maternal Deaths in the United Kingdom*. RCOG Press, London.

Macfarlane A, Mugford M (2000) *Birth Counts, Statistics of Pregnancy and Childbirth*, Volume 2. The Stationery Office, London.

McKenzie K, Crowcroft NS (1996) Describing race, ethnicity and culture in medical research. *British Medical Journal*, 312; 1054.

Marteau TM (1995) Towards informed decisions about prenatal testing: a review. *Prenatal Diagnosis*, 15; 1215–1226.

Marteau TM, Slack J, Kidd J et al. (1992) Presenting a routine screening test in antenatal care: practice observed. *Public Health* 106 (2); 131–141.

Marteau TM, Dormandy E, Michie S (2001) A measure of informed choice. *Health Expectations*, 4; 99–108.

Modell B, Petrou M, Layton M et al. (1997) Audit of prenatal diagnosis for haemoglobin disorders in the United Kingdom: the first 20 years. *British Medical Journal*, 315; 779–784.

Modell B, Harris R, Lane B et al. (2000) Informed choice in genetic screening for thalassaemia during pregnancy: audit from a national confidential inquiry. *British Medical Journal*, 320; 337–340.

Modood T, Berthoud R, Lakey J et al. (1997) *Ethnic Minorities in Britain: Diversity and Disadvantage*. Policy Studies Institute, London.

Moyer A, Brown B, Gates E et al. (1999) Decisions about prenatal testing for chromosomal disorders: perceptions of a diverse group of pregnant women. *Journal of Women's Health and Gender-Based Medicine*, 8; 521–531.

National Screening Committee (2002) Consultation on draft standards for antenatal screening including specific aspects for Down syndrome screening. www.doh.gov.uk/nsc.

Nazroo JY (1997) *The Health of Britain's Ethnic Minorities*. Policy Studies Institute, London.

Nuffield Council on Bioethics (1993) *Genetic Screening: Ethical Issues*. Nuffield Council on Bioethics, London.

O'Cathain A, Walters SJ, Nicholl JP *et al*. (2002) Use of evidence based leaflets to promote informed choice in maternity care: randomised controlled trial in everyday practice. *British Medical Journal*, 324; 643–646.

Rapp R (2000) *Testing Women, Testing the Fetus: The Social Impact of Amniocentesis in America*. Routledge, London.

Royal College of Obstetricians and Gynaecologists (1993) *Working Party on Biochemical Markers and the Detection of Down's Syndrome*. Royal College of Obstetricians and Gynaecologists, London.

Royal College of Obstetricians and Gynaecologists and Royal College of Paediatrics and Child Health (1997) *Fetal Abnormalities, Guidelines for Screening, Diagnosis and Management: Report of a Joint Working Party of the RCOG and RCPCH*. RCOG, London, www.doh.gov.uk/genetics/pgt_ch5.htm

Sandall J, Grellier, R (1999) *UK Midwives and Prenatal Screening: Results of a National Survey*. Department of Midwifery, City University, London.

Sandall J, Grellier R, Ahmed S *et al*. (2001) *Women's Access, Knowledge And Beliefs Around Prenatal Screening In East London*. Department of Midwifery, City University, London.

Saridogan E, Djahanbakhch O, Naftalin AA (1996) Screening for Down's syndrome: experience in an inner city health district. *British Journal of Obstetrics and Gynaecology*, 108; 1025–1211.

Schott J, Henley A. (1996) *Culture, Religion and Childbearing in a Multiracial Society*. Butterworth Heinemann, Oxford.

Shaw A (2001) Conflicting models of risk: clinical genetics and British Pakistanis. In: *Risk Revisited* (ed. Caplan P). Pluto Press, London.

Shaw M, Dorling D, Mitchell R (2002) *Health, Place and Society*. Prentice Hall, Harlow.

Sheikh A, Gatrad AR (2000) *Caring for Muslim Patients*. Radcliffe Medical Press, Oxford.

Smaje C (1995) Ethnic residential concentration and health: evidence for a positive effect? *Policy and Politics*, 23(3); 251–269.

Stapleton H, Kirkham M, Thomas G (2002) Qualitative study of evidence based leaflets in maternity care. *British Medical Journal*, 324; 639–643.

Wald NJ, Kennard A, Hackshaw A *et al*. (1998) Antenatal screening for Down's Syndrome, *Health Technology Assessment*, 2(1) i—iv; 1–112.

Wilkinson R. (1996) *Unhealthy Societies*. Routledge, London.

Williams C, Alderson P, Farsides B (2002) Is non–directiveness possible within the context of antenatal screening and testing? *Social Science and Medicine*, 54; 17–25.

Woollett A, Dosanjh N, Nicholson P *et al*. (1995) The ideas and experiences of pregnancy and childbirth of Asian and non-Asian women in East London. *British Journal of Medical Psychology*, 68; 65–84.

8 THE SONOGRAPHER'S DILEMMA

Jean Hollingsworth and Elizabeth Daly-Jones

INTRODUCTION

Modern obstetric practice includes ultrasound scans as part of the antenatal care offered to pregnant women. When this facility was introduced into the obstetric care plan it was soon realized that there were insufficient numbers of obstetricians to undertake the volume of work required to satisfy the demand. This role was extended to non-medically qualified staff and soon this group were providing the majority of the obstetric ultrasound service in the UK. It was during these formative years that a number of constraints were placed upon the non-medically qualified practitioners, particularly relating to the communication by the radiographer of the result of the scan to the pregnant woman if a problem was identified.

Today the culture of the relationship between patients and professionals has altered; pregnant women now have access to a wide range of information related to their pregnancies. This information can be explicit when dealing with ultrasound scans. As the technology improves and the public's knowledge about scans increases, expectations about this aspect of care can be extremely high. However, differences in working practices of the various professional groups now involved in obstetric ultrasound may affect direct communication of the scan result when an abnormality is suspected. This chapter considers these constraints, together with other factors that affect communication between sonographer and woman.

Groups giving support to women who have experienced pregnancy loss or fetal abnormalities report that there is often a problem with communication related to the initial scan (Stillbirth and Neonatal Death Society, 1995). They say that many women report being unhappy with what was or was not said, how the information was given and when. There is a perceived lack of awareness of the needs of pregnant women when confronted with distressing news.

These patient indictments do not rest easily with the sonographers who seek to carry out their duties to the best of their abilities within the framework of constraints they encounter daily. What can be done to alleviate this situation so that the sonographers are able to practice in a less restrictive environment and women faced with a problem can be assured that information will be offered honestly and openly?

THE CONSTRAINTS OF PROFESSIONAL DOGMA

Many different groups of people provide obstetric ultrasound services: obstetricians, midwives, cardiac technicians, physics technicians, radiographers, radiologists, sonographers, general practitioners, and other people with a scientific or health care qualification. Some of these groups undertake a formal period of ultrasound training related to general or speciality subjects and may or may not obtain a formal qualification as a result. Others only attend *ad hoc* courses or rely on variable in-service training programmes to be able to conduct, interpret and assess ultrasound examinations. Specific professional groups are regulated in their working practices by their professional codes of conduct and practice and by regulations in the setting in which they work.

In the UK, the largest group is the radiographers, most of whom have had a recognized formal training and have an ultrasound qualification. This group of sonographers, however, are governed not only by their own professional body's rules and regulations, but also by what individual clinical heads of departments perceive to be correct in terms of giving information to women. This leads to wide variation in practice; while many enlightened clinicians give support to non-medical practitioners divulging ultrasound results, others still insist on more formal and dated methods of communication. They argue that non-medical sonographers do not have the necessary background in terms of medical training and that this might result in incorrect information being given to the patient that could have medico-legal consequences. This constraint has the effect of devaluing the sonographer within the professional community when, in fact, sonographers are often more highly qualified and better able to analyse the ultrasound images than members of the other professional bodies.

The role of sonographers in many clinical settings is to provide technical information to the appropriate clinician who then interprets it. This is an archaic system, associated with the radiographer's original role in providing hard copy so that radiologists may diagnose, prognose and report the findings. Sonographers today conduct ultrasound examinations in real time and it is the person who carries out the scan who is best placed to judge whether a problem is present or not. Hard copy ultrasound images do not always reflect what has been identified in real time. Final diagnosis and management must, of course, remain with the medical staff.

Efforts have been made by professional bodies to address this problem. Discussions between sonographers and medical staff have resulted in guidelines tailored to individual departments. The College of Radiographers (1998), in consultation with a multi-professional team, has produced detailed occupational standards for the sonographer. The United Kingdom Association of Sonographers (2001) has also published guidelines that seek to ensure that the highest standards are maintained within the profession. Medical practitioners in the UK are not required to comply with similar codes. Where these guidelines are implemented, a suitable framework will exist for the communication of results to women.

COMMUNICATION ABOUT THE SCAN

Communication skills

An understanding of the ultrasound image is necessary for an explanation to be offered to a woman, but by itself is not sufficient. Interpersonal skills as well as professional constraints affect the ability of the sonographer to communicate with the woman. Some people are naturally able to deal effectively with emotionally difficult situations, while others are unable to cope.

The attitude of the sonographer towards the woman is very important, particularly if the prognosis for the pregnancy is poor. This attitude may depend on the sonographer's underlying personality, but this can be influenced temporarily or permanently by her own life experiences. Many sonographers will have had personal or indirect experiences similar to the woman being scanned, and this may influence their reactions to the situation. A sonographer who is pregnant or trying unsuccessfully to become pregnant or who has recently lost a pregnancy may be particularly vulnerable. Regardless of these factors, most sonographers will conduct their duties with the professionalism expected of them.

The first meeting

Establishing trust between sonographer and patient is part of the professional duty of every sonographer undertaking a scan. Normal courtesies of introduction are important. It is essential that a good relationship is achieved before the scan is commenced, as it is likely that the operator and woman will be meeting for the first time, at what is (for the woman) a very personal and emotional occasion. Good rapport will help to avoid potential difficulties.

Informing women about the purpose of the scan

Clinical staff must make women aware of the purpose of the ultrasound scan. Many women accept the scan as part of routine antenatal care and may not be aware of possible implications. Information leaflets available in many departments describe what ultrasound service is offered in that particular unit, when the scan or scans will be scheduled, how long the average scan may take, what will be looked for on the scan, and any preparation that may be necessary. A verbal explanation by the sonographer should ensure that the woman understands the purpose of the examination and is aware that, although in the majority of cases all will be well, a problem could be detected. If this happens, she should be reassured that the problem will be explained and that further investigations may be offered.

Communicating results

So what are the difficulties surrounding telling women the results of their scans? It would appear quite a straightforward task to explain ultrasound scan results, and this is indeed usually the case when the outcome is good. When there is a problem, however, professional constraints and personal attributes will affect the way in which the sonographer can handle this delicate and sensitive issue.

Initially all appears well, then a subtle change in facial expression, body attitude, and an intense concentration on the monitor is the first indication to the woman that this scan is not as 'routine' as she expected. It might be nothing at all, just a particular image giving rise to extra concentration for a second or two. The sonographer is actually re-evaluating the situation, perhaps to reach a decision as to whether there is a problem or not, before offering an explanation. These non-verbal signals are received well in advance of any verbal communications and are impossible to hide.

The interaction between sonographer and woman may be affected by the presence of other people (Simpson and Bor, 2001). The woman may be accompanied by husband/partner, children, mother, sister, other relatives or friends. Each of these combinations of people will present the sonographer with a different situation in which to establish a suitable communication system and deal with not only the woman but also her companions.

The type of abnormality discovered may also determine the way a particular sonographer will react. The following list is by no means comprehensive but serves to highlight the more common problems that are met during a routine obstetric scan:

- fetal death;
- 'soft' markers that could be associated with a chromosomal abnormality;
- suspicion of an abnormality requiring further investigations;
- unexpected structural abnormalities;
- confirmation of a problem in a high-risk woman;
- multiple pregnancy, either expected or unexpected, with abnormality in one or more babies;
- dating for termination of pregnancy.

If fetal death is unequivocal, then the news conveyed to the prospective parents will be devastating. The sonographer will be thinking about how to reveal this information while still scanning to obtain as much detail as possible to assist clinical management.

When an anomaly is identified, the findings will usually require further evaluation to confirm the diagnosis and prognosis. The practitioner will constantly appraise the situation while scanning, and will endeavour to relay the result to the woman and her companions in the best possible way.

Multiple pregnancies are by their nature special, but each baby has to be scanned as an individual. There are problems in terms of technique alone and these are compounded by the possible permutations of normal and abnormal in a multiple pregnancy.

Soft markers such as choroid plexus cysts, or mild renal pelvic dilatation may be seen on the scan. These can be particularly problematic for the sonographer since the significance of many markers is uncertain and each ultrasound department has its own policy about whether and how these markers are reported to women. In addition, women who have a fetus with these markers may not have given informed consent to screening for chromosome anomalies and may even have declined serum screening or nuchal translucency screening. Thus, whether the ultrasound finding is equivocal or unequivocal, it can present the sonographer with a dilemma.

An important variable is the time gap the woman experiences from the initial scan to actually receiving the result, and this applies to all women, not just those with suspected abnormalities. This may be partially determined by the location of the obstetric ultrasound service in relation to the rest of the antenatal care team.

Women from ethnic minorities may have attitudes towards pregnancy that differ from those of the indigenous population. Language may be a barrier to effective communication and this certainly complicates the interaction between woman and sonographer. In the absence of adequate support such as translation, this group of women will be disadvantaged. Even when support is on hand at the time of the scan, it may be difficult to judge what has been conveyed to the woman, especially if family or friends do the translating. In these situations, non-verbal communication may have great value but care must be taken not to send out inappropriate messages.

No two situations will be identical in all respects. The problem, the sonographer and other conditions may be the same, but the pregnant woman and her family will be different, creating a multitude of different levels of interaction dependent upon the expectations of all taking part. When an abnormality is detected, the relationship between sonographer and patient will be most vulnerable, especially when constraints are introduced into the equation. In this case both the patient and the sonographer who has discovered the problem may find the exchange unsatisfactory. Some sonographers may cope admirably in most situations while others will have more problems, and some sonographers are poor communicators even in the absence of any abnormality.

Withholding information

The sonographer faced with constraints limiting what can be said to the woman may feel compromised, lacking control and frustrated. He or she may be able to avert a potentially difficult situation from developing at that particular time, but this usually involves giving the woman unclear information. Subsequently, when she has a follow-up examination, it will become apparent to the woman that the initial scan must have detected something. It may be argued that this is a damage limitation approach if the follow up scan does not confirm the presence of an anomaly, and so it might be! However, what happens when the woman attends for her next scan without her partner and possibly with young children and is confronted with devastating news without adequate preparation?

If the sonographer has withheld information from the mother, guilt is added to the tally of pressures on him or her. This will affect the interaction between sonographer and patient. Women want, as far as possible, to be told the truth at the time of the scan and are confused as to why this may not happen. Most women would like sonographers to be honest with them about what they see, but some sonographers are not allowed to be honest and others are not personally capable of giving bad news.

Support groups helping women come to terms with what has happened highlight this situation as one of the most difficult to understand. Both the support groups and the women themselves are at a loss as to why this problem occurs (SATFA, 1992).

Referral for a follow-up scan

Different situations will generate different communication problems. The skill mix of staff deployed to various locations will have a direct influence on how communication with women is managed, especially if women are required to attend for another scan if a second opinion is needed. Staff do not set out to create obstacles deliberately, but delays may occur because of the availability of the appropriate person to perform the follow-up scan. The sonographer may be in the unenviable position of having to develop a language that will inform the woman that another scan will be necessary without revealing the nature of the problem to the woman. How well this method of communication works depends very much on the individual sonographer. If the follow-up scan is delayed and the sonographer is prevented from disclosing results of the initial scan, the woman may be lulled into a false sense of security about the outcome of her follow-up scan.

Communication skills training

Obstetric sonographers do not need to become counsellors, but all practitioners must optimize their own communication skills. The hopes and expectations of the prospective parents create a very emotional atmosphere, and the sonographer's ability to communicate well in times of stress is vitally important.

Sonographers welcome the recognition of the value of communication skills training in recent years. The ability to communicate well is as important in the sonographer's repertoire as their ability to scan. Research has found that sonographers feel better able to communicate with women when given clear guidelines within which to work (Simpson and Bor, 2001). Such guidelines functioning within a supportive open environment benefit both the sonographer and the woman.

There has been a huge advance in the training of sonographers in the area of communication in the UK during the last decade. Perhaps now more obstetricians will be willing to remove the constraints imposed on many sonographers.

THE SONOGRAPHER IS HUMAN TOO

In obstetric scanning, the expectations of an accurate result are incredibly high. However, it is not easy to identify some structural defects in the baby. For some sonographers who are newly qualified, lack of confidence in their ability to detect abnormalities means they are likely to suffer a high degree of emotional stress (Smith and Smith, 1995).

The sonographer is in the front line when an abnormality is first detected. Events happening at this interface may be destructive to the sonographer as well as to the person being scanned. It is impossible to standardize codes of behaviour when dealing with human distress, as the whole spectrum of human emotions – from extreme devastation to quiet acceptance – may be displayed upon receipt of less than optimum news. This will have a profound effect on the sonographer who will then be expected to erase this incident instantaneously as if nothing untoward had taken place, in order to proceed with the next scan. The next woman's expectations of her scan will be as high as those of the previous woman. In a busy clinic the sonographer will be like a chameleon, changing styles according to the current situation. This is very stressful.

CURRENT ETHICAL ISSUES FACING THE SONOGRAPHER

There has been rapid technological advancement in the field of obstetric ultrasound. One relatively new development is the nuchal translucency scan. This has been introduced into a number of ultrasound departments as one of a range of screening options. A dilemma can occur when a woman comes for her dating scan having declined serum screening, or even having rejected the offer of a nuchal scan (Venn-Treloar, 1998). What should the sonographer do if the baby has an obviously thickened nuchal translucency? Is the sonographer in breach of the woman's trust if he or she comments on this? Conversely, is there a breach of the sonographer's professional integrity if no comment is made? Should women be encouraged to decline the scan if they do not wish to be told all the findings (Royal College of Obstetricians and Gynaecologists, 2000)?

Ultrasound departments are now able offer fetal sexing at the detailed anomaly scan but this development also creates dilemmas, particularly where it is obvious that the woman or her companions have a strong preference for a particular gender. In a recent study of 92 sonographers, 84% stated that they would not disclose the sex if they suspected the woman might opt for termination on that basis (Simpson and Bor, 2001). The woman might of course argue that to withhold such information on the basis of a suspicion is to breach her right to information.

The typical obstetric sonographer is highly skilled. There are concerns, however, that many are restricted in their practice within individual departments by issues such as quality of equipment and the length of time available for the scan. In the UK, the Royal College of Obstetricians has made recommendations to achieve a more systematic and standardized approach to anatomical examination by the sonographer at the detailed scan (Royal College of Obstetricians and Gynaecologists, 2000, http://www.rcog.org.uk/mainpages.asp?PageID= 439). It could be argued, however, that these recommendations have not been fully implemented, as different departments still offer different services to women.

Conclusion

There has been progressive change over the years in what is required from the obstetric scan by both the clinicians caring for pregnant women and the women themselves. Both the first and second trimester scans are part of the prenatal diagnostic chain and the first link in this chain will probably be the sonographer. While many of the dilemmas discussed in this chapter are an integral part of the job itself, some are the result of too slow a response to rapidly changing circumstances. Radical changes in terms of professional dogma and a greater patient awareness of the implications of the scans they are undertaking are essential to address the expectations of today's obstetric patient. Sonographers, at the sharp end, must come to terms with the dilemmas they face to encourage a more human side to their relationships with their patients in the future.

Key points

- Sonographers are professionally trained and should be permitted to convey information to women regarding their obstetric scan results.
- Every sonographer should be encouraged to attend regular courses to update their counselling skills.
- All ultrasound departments should have clear guidelines in place for imparting obstetric scan results to women.
- Women need to be clearly informed as to the implications of the scans they are undertaking and given a choice as to whether or not they want to be scanned.
- Women will always remember the interaction that occurred between the sonographer and themselves when a problem was detected.

References

College of Radiographers (1998) *Occupational Standards for Diagnostic Ultrasound*. College of Radiographers, London.

Royal College of Obstetricians and Gynaecologists (2000) *Routine Ultrasound Screening in Pregnancy: Protocol, Standards and Training*. Royal College of Obstetricians and Gynaecologists – Report of the RCOG working party July 2000 http://www.rcog.org.uk/mainpages.asp?PageID=439.

SATFA (1992) *Guidelines for Ultrasonographers*. Support After Termination for Abnormality (now called ARC – Antenatal Results and Choices), London.

Simpson R, Bor R (2001) 'I'm not picking up a heart-beat': experiences of sonographers giving bad news to women during ultrasound scans. *British Journal of Medical Psychology*, 74; 255–272.

Smith J, Smith A (1995) Obstetric ultrasound: psychological dimensions. *British Medical Ultrasound Society Bulletin*, 3(4); 25–26.

Stillbirth and Neonatal Death Society. (1995) *Pregnancy Loss and the Death of a Baby. Guidelines for Professionals*. Stillbirth and Neonatal Death Society, London.

United Kingdom Association of Sonographers (2001) *Guidelines for Professional Working Standards – Ultrasound Practice*. United Kingdom Association of Sonographers, London.

Venn-Treloar J (1998) Nuchal translucency – screening without consent. *British Medical Journal*, 316; 1027.

9 PREIMPLANTATION GENETIC DIAGNOSIS

Alison Lashwood

INTRODUCTION

Preimplantation genetic diagnosis (PGD) is a relatively new technology, but one that is becoming more widely recognized as a valid clinical service available in many countries. It is also often a misunderstood concept sometimes charged with creating 'designer babies' and raises wide controversy amongst professionals and the public alike. It is therefore essential that health professionals are aware of the technique and have a basic and accurate knowledge of this new clinical service. Many patients requesting PGD find out about its availability through the Internet or media reports and may in turn request additional information from their general practitioner, midwife or other health professional.

For most couples, the knowledge that they are at risk of having a baby with a genetic condition occurs after they have had an affected child or pregnancy. This discovery is understandably a difficult and traumatic event for a family and is likely to prompt many questions. Once the couple have had the initial information about the diagnosis and what this means for them and their child, one of the issues usually raised is the risk to future offspring. Many will want to consider their future reproductive options.

In general terms, depending upon the mode of inheritance of the specific genetic condition, couples may face between a 1 in 2 (autosomal dominant condition) and 1 in 4 (autosomal recessive or X-linked condition) risk in the next pregnancy. It is usually at this point that they may request referral to a clinical genetics department to discuss this risk and their reproductive options. At a genetics consultation the couple will be given the opportunity to find out about what options may be available to them in the future. Every couple will present with their own individual agenda much of which will depend upon their past experience of the condition and how and when the diagnosis was made. It is the responsibility of the clinician to help assess the needs of the couple and discuss with them their future options (Harper, 1996). These may include:

- taking a chance, becoming pregnant spontaneously and opting to have no confirmatory testing during a pregnancy;
- undertaking prenatal diagnosis following a spontaneous conception;
- taking the decision not to have any (or any further) children;
- considering gamete donation;
- considering adoption;
- undertaking preimplantation genetic diagnosis (PGD).

During this consultation the above issues can be broadly discussed with couples, but it must be recognized that more in-depth discussion may be necessary and that a referral to a specialist in these cases will be warranted. This chapter will focus upon the last reproductive option mentioned above, that of PGD.

WHAT IS PREIMPLANTATION GENETIC DIAGNOSIS (PGD)?

Preimplantation genetic diagnosis is a highly specialized and, some would argue, still an experimental technique, which enables a couple to conceive a pregnancy that is biologically their own and is unaffected by the genetic condition in the family. Embryos are created by using *in vitro* fertilization technology (IVF) and are tested for the relevant genetic condition 2–3 days after fertilization prior to implantation. Thus the aim of the treatment is to help a couple have a child that they know will be unaffected by the condition in question from the moment the pregnancy is established.

The history of preimplantation genetic diagnosis

Preimplantation genetic diagnosis was first introduced for sexing embryos in the case of X-linked genetic disorders in 1990 (Handyside *et al.*, 1990). In 1992 the first case of a live born girl after successful PGD for the single gene disorder, cystic fibrosis, was reported (Handyside *et al.*, 1992). Preimplantation diagnosis for single gene disorders moved on a stage further in 1995 when a centre in Belgium reported the successful outcome of a pregnancy following PGD for Duchenne muscular dystrophy by testing for the dystrophin gene deletion (Liu *et al.*, 1995). This resulted in a successful non-carrier female pregnancy. Since then the worldwide development of this service has expanded. Although it has not been possible to combine accurately all data on an international basis, the European Society of Human Reproduction and Embryology (ESHRE) published its third report, presenting data from 25 centres comprising data from Europe, USA and Australia (ESHRE, 2002).

This publication reports on referrals for and outcomes of 1561 cycles of PGD, giving the reasons for referral, reproductive histories and the outcome of treat-ment. It is clear that most of the couples requesting PGD have had at least one previous pregnancy that resulted in a fetus or child with a genetic disorder and that most of these couples do not have any living unaffected children. Data have been collected on 451 pregnancies resulting in 251 deliveries (156 singletons, 54 twins and 5 triplets) giving a total of 279 babies born. Four cycles resulted in an incorrect diagnosis in the fetus and in one cycle a fetus was found to have a chromosomal problem unrelated to the reason for referral for genetic diagnosis.

Outcome of live-born babies

Evidence suggests that human embryo development *in vitro* is not affected by biopsy at the eight-cell stage (Hardy *et al.*, 1990), but the authors acknowledge that on-going pregnancies should be closely monitored by ultrasound scanning for evidence of fetal abnormality. Verlinsky *et al.* (1994) recommended the need for international collaboration for long term follow up of children born as the result of PGD. In the latest report from the ESHRE Consortium it is noted that there is a lack of data on outcome of the pregnancies reported and that this will be addressed in future data collection. However data were available on 180 of the 279 babies born. The perinatal mortality rate was 3/180 (16.7 per thousand births). Prematurity was the most commonly reported neonatal complication (67/180) which in turn was related to the number of multiple pregnancies. Overall the congenital malformation rate was 6.6% (3.9% major; 2.7% minor) (ESHRE, 2002).

Given that the number of centres offering PGD in the United Kingdom and worldwide is small it is essential that data on the outcome of pregnancies continue to be collected collaboratively so that the information provided is statistically significant and meaningful.

FOR WHAT CONDITIONS IS PREIMPLANTATION GENETIC DIAGNOSIS AVAILABLE?

There are two broad groups of genetic disorders for which PGD is available: single gene disorders (X-linked, autosomal dominantly or recessively inherited) and chromosomal abnormalities. It should be noted that whilst some centres offering PGD for X-linked disorders can offer direct mutation testing in the embryos, many centres will currently only be able to offer embryo sexing with selection of female embryos for transfer. Worldwide, PGD is now available for a wide range of genetic disorders, but as a technically demanding procedure, its application is still limited to fewer conditions than conventional prenatal diagnosis. Table 9.1 is not designed to be an exhaustive list of conditions for which PGD is available, but it does indicate the conditions for which PGD is most widely available.

WHO REGULATES PREIMPLANTATION GENETIC DIAGNOSIS?

The regulation of PGD worldwide varies from country to country (Geraedts *et al.*, 2001). In many countries where regulations do apply, the same bodies responsible for Assisted Reproduction Technology (ART) will regulate PGD.

In the United Kingdom, ART and PGD are regulated by the Human Fertilisation and Embryology Authority (HFEA), which was established in 1990 (Human Fertilisation and Embryology Act 1990). Until recently, although PGD was already being practised in a few centres, the HFEA had not produced any specific guidelines relating to it. However a joint committee was set up between the HFEA and Human Genetics Commission (HGC) to look at issues relating to the clinical application of PGD and they recently published the outcome of a public consultation document (Human Fertilisation and Embryology Authority, 2001). Recommendations were made that now determine good practise in centres offering PGD in the UK (www.hfea.org.uk). Assisted Conception units wishing to practise PGD must apply to the HFEA for a licence to practise PGD and submit details of the genetic conditions for which they are planning to offer treatment. A licence is required for each new single gene disorder and each reciprocal translocation as each is usually unique.

Table 9.1 Conditions for which preimplantation genetic diagnosis is most widely available

Single gene disorders	
Autosomal dominant:	Myotonic dystrophy[a]
	Huntington's disease[a]
Autosomal recessive:	Cystic fibrosis[a]
	Spinal muscular atrophy[a]
	Beta thalassaemia
	Sickle cell disease[a]
X-linked, direct mutation testing:	Fragile X syndrome[a]
	Alport syndrome
	Duchenne muscular dystrophy
X-linked, embryo sexing only:	Duchenne muscular dystrophy[a]
	Hunter syndrome[a]
	OTC deficiency[a]
	Incontinentia Pigmenti[a]
	(the majority of serious X-linked conditions will be considered for PGD by embryo sexing in UK centres)
Chromosomal disorders[b]:	Robertsonian translocations[a]
	Reciprocal translocations[a]
	Other chromosomal disorders (inversions, deletions)[a]

[a] Available in the UK.
[b] Dependant upon the availability of FISH probes.

WHY DO PEOPLE WANT PREIMPLANTATION GENETIC DIAGNOSIS?

Couples requesting PGD do so for a variety of reasons. Many couples will have experienced the loss of a child or a pregnancy and possibly had conventional prenatal diagnosis (PND) in subsequent pregnancies. These may have ended in the termination of an affected pregnancy. Past studies have shown that termination of pregnancy for fetal abnormality or 'genetic termination' carries with it potentially serious psychological consequences (Donnai *et al.*, 1991). The authors point out that termination of pregnancy for genetic reasons is different from social termination as it means the loss of a generally wanted and planned pregnancy. Many women requesting termination for abnormality will have reached the second trimester. In one study of 84 women having undergone termination in the second trimester (White-van Mourik *et al.*, 1992), 20% reported psychological difficulties affecting their general wellbeing 2 years after the termination.

Avoidance of further conventional prenatal diagnosis

The couple may have simply reached the point where they feel they cannot contemplate trying conventional PND again. For them the time between a positive pregnancy test and undertaking PND is a huge emotional burden that they know may end unsuccessfully. Such couples see PGD as relieving them, to an extent, of the burden of having PND and termination of pregnancy, and also giving them the chance of knowing from the earliest possible time that a pregnancy is unaffected. A study published in 1997 reported on attitudes of male and female carriers of recessive disorders to the availability of PGD and other reproductive options (Snowden and Green, 1997). The results indicated that the early knowledge of a pregnancy being unaffected, the genetic link with both parents and the avoidance of termination of pregnancy were all deemed important advantages of PGD.

CASE STUDY   J AND T

J and T were referred for PGD following a 5-year history of miscarriage and fetal loss. J had experienced three first trimester miscarriages followed by two late terminations for abnormalities detected on ultrasound scan. Chromosome analysis revealed that T carried a balanced chromosome translocation. This couple requested PGD as they felt that they could no longer attempt a pregnancy spontaneously that could result in another miscarriage or termination of pregnancy. Following their second PGD cycle they became pregnant and now have healthy twins.

Avoidance of termination of pregnancy

Social, moral or religious beliefs play a major part in many couples' reproductive decision-making. In some cases, termination of pregnancy is not considered to be a tolerable option whereas PGD is an acceptable alternative. In one study, 86% of women stated that avoidance of termination of pregnancy was the main advantage of PGD (Pergament, 1991). As Palomba said 'preimplantation diagnosis is the chosen option when there is a strong desire for pregnancy together with an equally strong desire to avoid abortion' (Palomba *et al.*, 1994).

CASE STUDY   M AND D

M and D had one daughter with cystic fibrosis who was diagnosed at 8 months. Her neonatal course had been problematic and required multiple hospital admissions although currently she was stable and thriving. Her parents wanted a second child who was unaffected, but felt morally against the option of prenatal diagnosis and termination of pregnancy. They had considered the possibility of gamete donation in a further pregnancy but had reservations about having a child that was not biologically their own. They requested PGD, which was successful, and they now have a second child who is not affected with cystic fibrosis.

Infertility related to genetic disorder

Some of the couples seen in the clinical genetics clinics will have fertility problems related to the single gene or chromosomal abnormality that they carry. For example some men who have congenital bilateral absence of the vas deferens (CBAVD) will be carriers of cystic fibrosis mutations (Daudin *et al.*, 2000). Alternatively a man with oligozoospermia may carry a chromosomal translocation (Gardner and Sutherland, 1996). These couples may require assisted reproduction to address their primary fertility problems, therefore the additional step of embryo biopsy would seem reasonable to give the couple the best chance of an ongoing unaffected pregnancy.

CASE STUDY   B AND F

B and F had a history of infertility. After trying to conceive for 2 years without success, semen analysis indicated that F was oligozoospermic. Chromosome analysis revealed that he carried a balanced translocation and this may have been associated with his infertility. This couple required IVF treatment to become pregnant and given that they had an increased risk of chromosomal abnormality in a fetus due to an unbalanced translocation they decided to have a cycle of PGD. The couple became pregnant, but sadly lost the pregnancy in the second trimester due to an unrelated chromosomal abnormality.

HLA tissue typing for bone marrow match for sick sibling

One of the most controversial uses of PGD, for which the HFEA (UK) granted one ART centre a licence to practise in 2002, is that of HLA typing to provide a compatible bone marrow matched child for a sibling with a genetic disorder. The aim of this technology is to analyse the embryos for the genetic disorder concerned and detect an embryo, which is both unaffected, and an HLA type match for the affected sibling (Verlinsky *et al.*, 2001). This procedure is very technically demanding and is unlikely to be available widely in the near future, but demand may grow and this in turn will generate requests for licences from other centres.

THE CLINICAL SERVICE – WHAT CAN COUPLES EXPECT OF THE TREATMENT?

Preimplantation diagnosis is a complex process involving several stages that couples must complete prior to treatment. It is highly invasive and demands a great deal of time and consideration by couples undertaking it. Practice will vary widely, although it has been acknowledged that in order to offer a robust clinical service the centres providing PGD should involve the medical expertise of assisted reproduction and clinical genetics departments (Flinter, 2001). The following will provide a general overview of what is involved in the treatment at the London Centre where the author is based. The stages of the PGD process leading up to pregnancy include:

- consultation with geneticist and confirmation of diagnosis;
- first PGD consultation, hormone profiling and general health checks;
- attainment of consent to treatment;
- ovarian stimulation (woman);
- oocyte (egg) retrieval +/- sperm injection;
- embryo biopsy and genetic analysis;
- transfer of embryos.

Genetics consultation

Prior to attempting PGD it is essential that the diagnosis of a single gene or chromosomal abnormality is confirmed in the family. PGD is a collaboration involving geneticists, embryologists, obstetricians, cytogeneticists and molecular biologists. Once a geneticist has seen a couple and the diagnosis of a single gene disorder or chromosomal abnormality is confirmed, a referral for PGD can be initiated.

First PGD consultation

The aim of this consultation is to establish the background to the couple's request for PGD, ensure that they understand the procedure and discuss the advantages and disadvantages of the technique. Although many couples have read widely about the procedure prior to this consultation, a few have not understood the success rate and limitations of the diagnostic procedure and the complexities and difficulties of undertaking an IVF cycle. Issues raised with couples at this stage include, success rate, misdiagnosis risk, the chance of ovarian hyperstimulation syndrome, the possibility that following the IVF procedure and embryo biopsy there may be no suitable embryos for transfer, and the emotional turmoil of this invasive technique.

Detailed medical histories of a couple will be taken to ensure that there are no underlying conditions which may require treatment or affect the success of IVF treatment. Blood samples will be collected from the female partner for rubella status, virology screening and a 2–6 day hormone profile. This determines if the hormone levels are normal during a woman's menstrual cycle. A semen sample is collected from the male partner for morphology and motility together with a blood sample for virology screening.

Consent to treatment in the United Kingdom

In accordance with the requirements of the Human Fertilisation and Embryology Authority (HFEA) consent forms are required to be signed by the couple for *in vitro* fertilization, intracytoplasmic sperm injection (ICSI), storage of eggs, sperm and embryos and embryo transfer. Consent for permission to disclose information regarding treatment to the general practitioner or other referring doctor is also sought.

Ovarian stimulation

The purpose of stimulating the ovaries by chemical means is to encourage the development of a number of mature follicles so that multiple oocytes are available for retrieval. The success of PGD treatment is correlated with the number of oocytes retrieved. Vandervorst *et al.* (1998) demonstrated that the number of embryos suitable for transfer was significantly higher when more that nine oocytes were retrieved in a cycle. On day 21 of a cycle buserelin is taken by nasal spray or subcutaneous injection. This desensitizes the pituitary gland and prevents spontaneous ovulation. In effect this mimics the menopause and women undergoing treatment can experience mood swings and hot flushes. Fourteen days later (if ovaries are found to be inactive on ultrasound scanning) human menopausal gonadotrophin (HMG) is given by daily injection to stimulate the production of oocytes. HMG comprises follicle stimulating hormone and luteinizing hormone, both required for ovarian maturation (British Medical Association and Royal Pharmaceutical Society of Great Britain, 1998).

Regular ultrasound scanning is performed to assess the development of the ovarian follicles and the date for egg retrieval will be arranged following ultrasound assessment. Thirty-six hours prior to oocyte retrieval, human chorionic gonadotrophin (hCG) is given to allow for final oocyte maturation. A low dose of hCG must then continue as the drug regimen will have inactivated the normal action of the luteinizing hormone which supports corpus luteum development and subsequent progesterone production. Progesterone is essential to the development of the endometrium as it prepares for the reception of the embryo.

One of the reasons behind the frequent and regular ultrasound scanning of women undergoing superovulatory treatment is to assess whether ovarian hyperstimulation syndrome (OHSS) is present. The occurrence of OHSS is relatively common, but can vary in its clinical severity from mild to severe and life threatening. In its mildest form (abdominal swelling, nausea) it is likely to occur in 8–23% of cases, and in its severe form (abdominal swelling and pain, vomiting, diarrhoea, dizziness and breathlessness caused by pleural effusion) 0.1–2% of cases (Li, 1993). In severe cases OHSS can incur a hospital admission for a woman undergoing treatment and this is of specific concern for those undertaking PGD who may have a disabled child at home requiring care.

Oocyte retrieval and fertilization procedures

Following successful ovarian stimulation, oocyte retrieval may take place. Oocytes are retrieved under sedation, transcervically, using ultrasound guidance. As soon as the oocytes have been collected they are transferred to culture medium for incubation. The semen sample is obtained by masturbation and the sample is diluted with culture medium. The motile sperm are then separated from the immotile, washed and placed in a further culture medium solution.

For chromosome translocation and fetal sexing cases, sperm are then added to the oocytes in culture as with routine IVF technology. The embryos will be assessed for signs of fertilization the following morning. Successfully fertilized eggs will be separated and returned to an incubator until they reach the eight-cell stage (usually by the third day following fertilization). Analysis will be done by a technique known as Fluorescence *in situ* hybridization (FISH). FISH is a method of using a fluorescently labelled piece of DNA which attaches to DNA fragments on specific chromosomes and can be visualized using a fluorescent microscope (Strachan and Read, 1996).

When the embryos are to be analysed for single-cell disorders involving polymerase chain reaction (PCR) technology, intracytoplasmic sperm injection (ICSI) of a single sperm is used to ensure that no extraneous sperm around the fertilized embryo compromise the results of the analysis. PCR is used as a method of rapidly amplifying (copying) a selected sequence of DNA for mutation analysis.

Embryo biopsy and single gene or chromosomal analysis

Human genome expression begins between the four- to eight-cell stage of embryo development and therefore analysis of the single cell should not be undertaken before this stage (Braude *et al.*, 1988). Li *et al.* (1998) demonstrated that DNA sequences could be studied on single cells and therefore this analysis could be used for PGD. Embryo biopsy occurs at around the eight-cell stage with the removal of one or two embryonic cells.

Transfer of embryos

Once the PCR or FISH analysis has been performed, the unaffected, morphologically sound embryos are transferred into the uterus. Following evidence of the fetal mortality associated with multiple pregnancies (Winston and Handyside, 1993) and in accordance with the HFEA guidelines, a maximum of two embryos are replaced, although in some circumstances a three-embryo transfer may be considered. The first reliable indication of a successful biochemical pregnancy will be at about 12 days post-transfer, when women are asked to perform a pregnancy test.

WHAT HAPPENS IF TREATMENT IS SUCCESSFUL?

Once a positive pregnancy test has been reported, arrangements are made for an early transvaginal ultrasound scan at around 7 weeks' gestation. On demonstration of a positive fetal heartbeat, the couple will have an opportunity to discuss their options for obtaining confirmation of the diagnosis. This is often a very difficult time for couples and poses a dilemma for many who decided against PND on the basis that they would not want a termination of an affected pregnancy. Other couples are reluctant to put their pregnancy at risk of miscarriage associated with invasive testing and opt to wait until delivery for confirmation of normality. ESHRE (2002) reported less than 50% uptake rate for PND following successful PGD.

As PGD is a new technology and the implications for the health of children born following treatment are not fully ascertained, physical and developmental assessments are arranged at birth, 1 year and 2 years. These data are collected and used for a collaborative European study that will help to provide statistically significant data on the outcome of pregnancies.

WHAT HAPPENS IF TREATMENT IS UNSUCCESSFUL?

A follow up appointment is made for all couples following an unsuccessful treatment cycle. A review of the cycle takes place and the options for the future discussed with them. If necessary a counsellor is available to help support couples at this stage, or indeed at any time before or during treatment.

Disadvantages of PGD

Success rate
The pregnancy and live birth success rates of PGD are comparable with those for infertile couples undergoing ART. The cumulative ESHRE data suggested a pregnancy success rate of 22% per embryo transferred (ESHRE, 2002). This relatively low chance of success must be discussed with couples in detail prior to the start of treatment. It is important to remember that, in contrast to couples with subfertility, many of these couples would not have problems conceiving spontaneously.

Some couples undergoing treatment may have no suitable embryos for transfer. This may be the result of poor ovarian response, failed fertilization, unsuccessful biopsy, all embryos being affected or results that are inconclusive. Couples are counselled that starting treatment does not guarantee transfer of embryos.

Misdiagnosis
There have been reports of misdiagnoses in PGD cycles. The technology of single-cell analysis is complex and demanding and all couples are made aware of the chance of this happening. There are several possible reasons for misdiagnosis, including chromosome mosaicism which may occur if the cell analysed is not representative of the embryo biopsied (Harper *et al.*, 1995) and allele dropout (ADO) when there is failure to detect one of the parental alleles being studied. ADO could lead to misdiagnosis in a dominant disorder because an affected fetus would not be detected if the affected allele were lost (Handyside and Delhanty, 1997). Finally, the need to apply large numbers of PCR cycles to obtain an adequate DNA sample from the single biopsied cell creates scope for contamination.

Cost
Whether publicly or privately funded, PGD is a costly procedure. In the UK funding for PGD is not centrally organized within the NHS. Most local health commissioners will apply their policy for funding IVF treatment to PGD, and this may vary from area to area. Couples who are unsuccessful in their applica-

tion for health service funding will face a costly bill of several thousand pounds per cycle, making treatment inaccessible for many. The UK Department of Health Guidelines can be found at www.doh.gov.uk/genetics.

DIFFICULTIES AND DILEMMAS OF PREIMPLANTATION DIAGNOSIS

Debate around the availability and application of PGD continues. In response to general concerns about PGD technology. In the UK the HFEA and HGC issued a consultation document to look at licensing, extent of clinical application and ethical dilemmas posed by the treatment (www.hfea.gov.uk/pgd/pgdpaper/pdf). The outcome of the public consultation document was revealed in 2001 and recommendations for practice and licensing were made on the basis of this. The difficulties and ethical dilemmas of PGD are rarely out of the public domain and as PGD is such a rapidly progressing technology it is understandable that many people are concerned about its use now and in the future. The last section of this chapter will discuss some of these difficulties and dilemmas in general and in relation to experience gained within the PGD centre which is the author's base.

Severity of the disorder and level of risk

The recommendations of the HFEA in this regard require that the genetic disorder for which PGD is available should have serious clinical implications, the people in question should have a significant genetic risk for it, and that the availability of PND for the condition should be used as guidance for the licensing of PGD. Public response to this issue was divided, the majority believing that whilst the above should apply, the judgement for which conditions PGD should be made available should not be made by clinicians in isolation and that the views of a particular family must be considered. Of those who felt that it should be restricted, concern was expressed that PGD devalued the disabled. Vergeer *et al.* (1998) in a study assessing the psychological and ethical aspects of PGD amongst clinicians, social scientists and ethicists in the Netherlands, found that the groups held similar opinions to those responding to the HFEA consultation document, believing that PGD should be used for serious genetic conditions with high risk.

CASE STUDY   AB

AB had a brother with Duchenne muscular dystrophy (DMD) who died at the age of 18 years. DMD is inherited in an X-linked manner and therefore if AB were a carrier she would have a 50:50 chance of having an affected son. The genetic tests in the family were unable to determine whether or not she was definitely a carrier and as a result she was given a 10% chance of having an affected son. A reliable prenatal test was available, which would have told her whether her male pregnancies would be at virtually 0% risk or 10% risk of DMD. AB's experience of DMD was reflected in her perceptions of DMD being a lethal and severely debilitating condition. She wished to avoid having a son of her own with the condition. While a 10% risk was significant, she could not consider a termination of pregnancy when there was a 90% chance that the male pregnancy would be unaffected. PGD was performed for embryo sexing and AB now has a daughter.

This case illustrates that whilst this was a request for PGD for a serious disorder, the actual genetic risk may be considered relatively low. However it was exactly this risk that made the option of PND for this couple so unacceptable. In this case we felt that it was important to consider how the couple perceived the condition and the risk in the context of what other options were open to them.

Preimplantation diagnosis for social sexing

Although prohibited by law in the UK and by countries that have signed the Convention on Human Rights and Biomedicine (Beyleveld, 2000), some centres around the world are now offering PGD for sex selection. Couples have a preference for one sex of child over another and sex selection by PGD will help them in their goal. Concern has been expressed worldwide about the use of PGD in this category. In one highly publicized case, a couple that tragically lost their only daughter (they have four sons) in an accident, requested PGD for sex selection on the basis that they wished to have another daughter to complete their family. This request was not met by a UK PGD centre so the couple sought treatment overseas. There is concern about the application of sex selection in countries that have a preference for male children and mindful of this the Indian government has just outlawed this practice (Mudur, 2002).

HLA tissue typing

The rationale for requests for PGD for this are discussed above. For many people this raises the issue of using a child as a commodity and that such a child is conceived for the benefit of a sibling and not as an individual in their own right. Concerns have been raised about the effect of a failed stem-cell transplant on the sibling born following PGD. Economists describe a *Pareto optimal state of affairs* as one that is at least as good as all alternative states of affairs in all relevant respects, and better in some respects. Boyle and Savulescu (2001) argued that the concerns raised are outweighed by the benefits for the stem-cell recipient and that the creation of an HLA-compatible embryo with PGD would bring about a Pareto state of affairs, which means that it would be at least as good as, if not better than, any alternatives for that child or family.

Preimplantation genetic screening

In July 2001 the HFEA approved in principle the technique of preimplantation genetic screening (PGS) or aneuploidy screening (Ferriman, 2001). This technique differs from PGD in that it is applied to couples who do not carry a chromosome translocation but who have had repeated IVF failures. It is hoped that by screening the embryos for chromosomal abnormalities it will increase the pregnancy rate amongst infertile couples aged 35 years and over who are having IVF anyway. A large randomized controlled study is yet to be undertaken; therefore conclusive evidence that PGS is beneficial is awaited.

Key points

- Preimplantation genetic diagnosis (PGD) is an alternative early form of prenatal diagnosis acceptable to couples who want to avoid having a child with a genetic disorder, but for whom prenatal diagnosis is unacceptable.
- PGD is a complex procedure that requires in-depth discussion with a couple before treatment can commence.
- There are several disadvantages associated with PGD, including the relatively low success rate, cost and the highly invasive nature of the technique.
- The technology is available for use in a limited number of conditions.
- PGD is a new technology and requires careful regulation to ensure that it is not used inappropriately. The ethical implications of treatment are far-reaching and require careful clinical consideration by those involved.

REFERENCES

Beyleveld D (2000) Is embryo research and preimplantation genetic diagnosis ethical? *Forensic Science International*, 11:113(1–3); 461–475.

Boyle RJ, Savulescu J (2001) Ethics of using preimplantation genetic diagnosis to select a stem cell donor for an existing person. *British Medical Journal*, 323; 1240–1243.

Braude P, Bolton V, Moore S (1988) Human gene expression first occurs between the four and eight cell stages of preimplantation development. *Nature*, 332(31); 459–461.

British Medical Association & Royal Pharmaceutical Society of Great Britain (1998) *British National Formulary*, Vol 36, September 1998.

Daudin M, Bieth E, Bujan L *et al.* (2000) Congenital bilateral absence of the vas deferens: clinical characteristics, biological parameters, cystic fibrosis transmembrane conductance regulator gene mutations and implications for genetic counselling. *Fertility and Sterility*, 74(6); 1164–1174.

Donnai P, Charles N, Harris N (1991) Attitudes of patients after 'genetic' terminations of pregnancy. *British Medical Journal*, 282; 621–622.

ESHRE Preimplantation Genetic Diagnosis Consortium (2002) Data collection 3 (May 2001). *Human Reproduction*, 17(1); 233–246.

Ferriman A (2001) U.K. approves preimplantation genetic screening technique. *British Medical Journal*, 323(7305); 125.

Flinter F (2001) Preimplantation genetic diagnosis needs to be tightly regulated. *British Medical Journal*, 322; 1009–1010.

Gardner RJM, Sutherland GR (1996) *Chromosome Abnormalities and Genetic Counseling* (2nd edition). Oxford University Press, New York.

Geraedts JPM, Harper J, Braude P et al. (2001) Preimplantation genetic diagnosis (PGD), a collaborative activity of clinical genetic departments and IVF centres. *Prenatal Diagnosis*, 21; 1086–1092.

Handyside A, Delhanty J (1997) Preimplantation genetic diagnosis: strategies and surprises. *Trends in Genetics*, 13(7); 270–275.

Handyside AH, Kontogianni EH, Hardy K et al. (1990) Pregnancies from biopsied human preimplantation embryos sexed by Y specific DNA amplification. *Nature*, 244; 768–770.

Handyside AH, Lesko JG, Tarin JJ et al. (1992) Birth of a normal girl after in vitro fertilization and preimplantation diagnostic testing for cystic fibrosis. *New England Journal of Medicine*, 327(13); 905–909.

Hardy K, Martin K, Leese H et al. (1990) Human preimplantation development in vitro is not adversely affected by biopsy at the 8-cell stage. *Human Reproduction*, 5(6); 708–714.

Harper JC, Coonen E, Handyside A et al. (1995) Mosaicism of autosomes in morphologically normal, monospermic preimplantation human embryos. *Prenatal Diagnosis*, 15; 41–49.

Harper PS (1996) *Practical Genetic Counselling* (5th edition), Butterworth Heinemann, Oxford.

Human Fertilisation and Embryology Authority (2001) *Outcome of Public Consultation on Preimplantation Genetic Diagnosis: Summary of Discussions and Recommendations of the HFEA/HGC Joint Working Party and the Analysis of Responses.* www.hfea.gov.uk/pgd/pgdpaper.pdf.

Li HP (1993) Recent advances in hyperstimulation syndrome. In: *Annual Progress In Reproductive Medicine* (eds Asch RH, Studd JWW). Parthenon Publishing, Lancaster.

Li HP, Gyllensten U, Cui X, et al. (1998) Amplification and analysis of DNA sequences in single human sperm. *Nature*, 335; 414–417.

Liu J, Lissens W, Van Broeckhoven C et al., (1995) Normal pregnancy after preimplantation DNA diagnosis of a dystrophin gene deletion. *Prenatal Diagnosis*, 15; 351–358.

Mudur G (2002) India plans new legislation to prevent sex selection. *British Medical Journal*, 324; 385.

Palomba ML, Monni G, Lai R et al. (1994) Psychological implications and acceptability of preimplantation diagnosis. *Human Reproduction*, 9(2); 360–362.

Pergament E (1991) Preimplantation diagnosis: a patient perspective. *Prenatal Diagnosis*, 11; 493–500.

Snowden C, Green JM (1997) Preimplantation diagnosis and other reproductive options: attitudes of male and female carriers of recessive disorders. *Human Reproduction*, 12 (2); 341–350.

Strachan T, Read AP (1996) *Human Molecular Genetics*. BIOS Scientific Publishers, Oxford.

Vandervorst M, Liebaers I, Sermon K et al. (1998) Successful preimplantation genetic diagnosis is related to the number of available cumulus-oocyte complexes. *Human Reproduction*, 13(11); 3169–3176.

Vergeer MM, van Balen F, Ketting E (1998) Preimplantation genetic diagnosis as an alternative to chorionic villus sampling and amniocentesis: psychosocial and ethical aspects. *Patient Education and Counselling*, 35(1): 5–13.

Verlinsky Y, Rechitsky S, Schoolcraft W et al. (2001) Preimplantation genetic diagnosis for Fanconi anaemia combined with HLA matching. *Journal of the American Medical Association*, 285(24); 3130–3133.

Verlinsky Y, Handyside A, Grifo J *et al.* (1994) Preimplantation Diagnosis of genetic and chromosomal disorders. *Journal of Assisted Reproduction and Genetics*, 11(5); 236–243.

White-van Mourik M, Connor JM, Ferguson Smith MA (1992) The psychological sequelae of a second trimester termination of pregnancy for fetal abnormality. *Prenatal Diagnosis*, 12; 189–204.

Winston RML, Handyside AH (1993) New challenges in human in vitro fertilization. *Science*, 260; 932–936.

10 PROBLEMS SURROUNDING LATE PRENATAL DIAGNOSIS

Sally Boxall and Lucy Turner

INTRODUCTION

During the last quarter of a century, prenatal diagnostic techniques have developed with a speed and definition previously unimaginable. However, in the race for medical and technological 'perfection', equal consideration has not been given to the profound ethical, legal and particularly emotional dilemmas raised by the diagnosis of fetal abnormality. These dilemmas, which been explored in previous chapters, are even greater when a diagnosis is made late in the pregnancy, and it could be said that they become more demanding in proportion to the gestational age when diagnosis is made.

All those involved in the provision of prenatal diagnosis should have a close understanding of the immense impact it has, especially when the diagnosis is made after the time of fetal viability, which in the United Kingdom is presently defined as 24 weeks (Human Fertilisation and Embryology Act 1990).

Termination of pregnancy is legal in England and Wales at any stage of pregnancy under ground E of the Abortion Act if 'there is a substantial risk that if the child were born it would suffer from such physical or mental abnormalities as to be seriously handicapped' (Abortion Act 1967). Controversy exists, however, as to how we define 'substantial risk' and 'serious handicap', and this creates an ethical and legal minefield for parents and carers alike. In Holland a different approach is used; third trimester abortion may be considered only if a fetal abnormality is diagnosed which either excludes the possibility of survival after birth or is so serious that postnatal, life-prolonging procedures would be considered futile. A report in the UK by the Royal College of Obstetricians and Gynaecologists' Ethics Committee (1998) suggested that it is not possible to make rules regarding late termination by disease category, as the prognosis can be very variable; each case should therefore be judged on its individual merits.

In the year 2000, in England and Wales, 2555 pregnancies were terminated after 20 weeks of pregnancy, with only 126 being carried out after 24 weeks. Of these, five were for Down syndrome, three for anencephaly, eight for spina bifida and 17 for hydrocephalus. These are small numbers of cases, but for the individual families concerned the event may be one of the most traumatic in their lives.

THE DILEMMA FOR PARENTS

There are several scenarios that can be envisaged leading to a late diagnosis of fetal abnormality.

- A woman may, for whatever reason, present late in pregnancy for prenatal investigations; she may have been away at the usual time for 'routine' investigations, have been unaware of her pregnancy, or concealed it.
- A suspected abnormality may be found at an anomaly scan at about 19 or 20 weeks' gestation; the woman may then be referred on to a specialist centre for further investigation and counselling, which may take some time.
- Clinical indications such as polyhydramnios or intrauterine growth retardation late in the second or into the third trimester may lead to the suspicion of an abnormality.
- A woman may present for a routine investigation, such as a scan for growth or placental site, in the third trimester and be found by chance to have a fetal abnormality, which was not detected or not detectable earlier in the pregnancy.

It is vital that women are aware of the risks and benefits of a particular test before consenting to any investigation in pregnancy. The need for informed consent applies to any screening or diagnostic test, including ultrasound, and women should be informed about the possible sequelae of having tests later in pregnancy. Ultrasound scanning, such a routine part of antenatal care in developed societies, can be a diagnostic test with a potential to discover problems which are very difficult for both the woman and her carers to deal with.

WHAT'S THE NEXT STEP?

Whatever the route that led to the recognition of suspicious findings late in pregnancy, perhaps one of the most difficult problems faced by prospective parents in this situation is deciding how far they wish to go down the path of diagnostic testing. At this stage, their circle of family and friends are often well aware of the impending birth, the parents have been congratulated and have been given gifts for the baby; often the nursery has been decorated and clothes or furniture bought. The baby has made its presence felt by kicking and moving about, a dramatic reminder that he or she is alive. Now there is some possibility that the longed-for event may not materialize or, if it does, it will come about in a way vastly different from that which they had expected and planned for. One part of their consciousness tells them to 'hope for the best' and carry on to delivery without anything definite to cause them to loose hope. The other part is desperate to know what is going on, so that they can prepare themselves as best they can for the outcome.

There are many factors that influence the couple's decision about whether or not to have further prenatal tests following a suspicion of fetal abnormality. These include:

- how the couple saw the size of the risk of abnormality before the suspicion arose and how they perceive it now;
- how the options open to them were communicated to them during counselling;

- their understanding of the condition being investigated;
- their individual circumstances, including social and financial issues;
- their spiritual, moral and ethical beliefs.

All couples should be counselled at their first meeting following the detection of suspicious findings, with information given about the significance of all the tests and the implications of the results if abnormal. At this initial point the couple should be given the opportunity to consider their views on termination of pregnancy, and these should be clarified before any test is performed.

DECIDING ABOUT HAVING FURTHER DIAGNOSTIC TESTS

Considerate and supportive advice is needed to point out the advantages and disadvantages of having the relevant procedures at this late stage. While not making assumptions based on cultural stereotypes, those counselling the parents must take into account the cultures, backgrounds and expressed inclinations of the parents as well as their level of intelligence and understanding. Those caring for the parents should present the alternatives in an objective, unbiased fashion, making it clear they will support them whatever decision is reached. The parents should feel that they can make an informed and personally acceptable decision as regards the diagnostic tests and resulting options, without feeling guilty or under pressure to agree to tests or procedures. The parents may feel confused and isolated when staff talk, often unintentionally, in medical jargon. Parents with limited intellectual ability, or those whose understanding of English is not good, may need a careful explanation in everyday language or via an interpreter if necessary. All parents should be given written information to back up these discussions.

Parents will suffer the emotional stress of considering whether they will terminate the pregnancy if their unborn child is diagnosed with an abnormality, and they should be offered at this pre-diagnostic stage the services of other appropriate counsellors. Support groups for the suspected anomaly, geneticists and religious advisors may all be called upon. Although time is of the essence at this late stage, as test results may take several days to become available, provision should be made for this thorough, sensitive, and in-depth pre-diagnostic counselling, as a hurried decision may cause regret or long-term trauma subsequent to the procedure and related decisions.

WHAT ARE THE OPTIONS?

Further testing

We must not forget that in many cases the parents will be reassured by normal results from diagnostic testing, and can continue with the pregnancy with some degree of relief that their fears have not been confirmed.

The options that will be open to parents who choose to proceed with further tests and whose baby is then shown to have a severe or lethal abnormality include continuing with the pregnancy, or considering ending the pregnancy following feticide.

For some parents, the opportunity to prepare themselves and their family for the birth of a child who may have congenital abnormalities, or who may not live long, is an important reason for undergoing diagnostic testing. The most appropriate place for delivery can be planned, and other medical specialists such as neonatalogists and paediatric surgeons can be involved in preparing the parents for what lies ahead.

No further testing

If the option to continue the pregnancy with no further investigation is decided upon following in-depth consultation, the level of support must be maintained by all concerned, with no hint of recrimination in subsequent discussions. Continuity of care, with the same midwife and obstetrician seeing the couple at each visit, avoids repetition of painful histories and gives the couple a feeling of security and support despite their decision not to proceed with any further investigations. If this is not practically possible, then a small team is the next best option. Once this rapport has been established the parents may feel less inhibited in asking for further help from the people they have now come to regard as friends as well as professionals.

Continuing the pregnancy

Parents who continue with such a pregnancy, with or without further testing, may be faced with a stillbirth or an infant who dies shortly after birth. Chitty *et al.* (1996) discussed some of the experiences of couples who chose to let nature take its course, and emphasized the need for consistent planned antenatal care that is specific to the parents' needs. Any parents in this situation should be given the opportunity to discuss with their key workers a very specific birth plan. This plan should incorporate the optimum place for delivery, whether to monitor the baby during labour, analgesia levels, and the support network to be present. If it is suspected that the baby will be stillborn or die shortly after delivery, provision should be made for their minister of religion to be present if desired and an opportunity made for the parents to have as much time as they want with their dead or dying baby. Sensitive discussion of how the baby will look may be important to help parents prepare themselves and their family, and time should be spent helping to clarify the parents' wishes regarding subsequent events such as post mortem examination. This is always a difficult subject to broach with parents, especially now in the UK in the wake of recent controversies surrounding organ retention, but may provide vital information for the future. It may also be appropriate at this stage to give information surrounding funeral options, to enable them to begin the process of grieving for their child.

Termination of pregnancy

If the parents are considering the option of termination of pregnancy, they need to be given information to prepare themselves for what lies ahead. The overwhelming sadness of undergoing a procedure that will deliberately kill their child must be handled with great sensitivity, and the possibility of emotions such as guilt and anger explored. In order to make this final decision, the parents must be helped to look at all possible aspects. They need to be offered the opportunity to discuss the situation with experts who can give consistent, up-to-date advice on the likely prognosis for their child, backed up with pictures and written explanation to refer to whilst they make their decision. When making this decision, they need to consider not only the extent of suffering for the child, but also the severity of handicap, the effect on themselves, and the burden on others.

The parents need to be made aware of the practical aspects of termination of pregnancy, including the fact that they will have to consent to feticide, a procedure that will cause their child to die. The UK Royal College of Obstetricians' Guidelines (1996) state that, for any termination after 21 weeks, the method chosen should ensure that the fetus is born dead. Most commonly, an injection of potassium chloride is given into the fetal heart, under ultrasound guidance. The labour is then induced and the mother goes through a normal birth process with all the physical and emotional pain that is involved. The baby subsequently has to be formally registered as a stillbirth, itself a distressing procedure. It is hard to imagine how parents are able to go through such an experience with the knowledge that they have had to make the final decision about whether their child lives or dies. Despite the tragedy of the situation, the parents should be encouraged to value the time they have with their baby. Parents may even find that there is a sense of relief that the decision has been made and they can move forward into a new stage of grieving.

IS LATE PRENATAL DIAGNOSIS A 'GOOD THING'?

Health professionals may tend to assume that diagnosing fetal abnormality in the later stages of pregnancy provides the best basis for allowing the parents to make a decision regarding the future of the pregnancy. While prenatal diagnosis will provide a much-wanted choice for many, for others it will be a choice that they would rather not have to confront. Information for the parents about the implications of late diagnosis should be the starting point.

Informed uptake, and equally, informed refusal of late prenatal diagnosis will be increased by the supplying of fuller information by staff to a better-informed client. To achieve this, counselling prior to any prenatal diagnosis should include: the purpose of the test and the likelihood that an abnormality will be detected or missed, an explanation of the test procedure including related risks, the significance of test results both positive and negative, and the options following a positive result so late in pregnancy. A clear discussion of the nature of the potential abnormality and the prognosis for the child will help parents to decide if this is the path they wish to follow.

Ultrasound scanning late in the second and into the third trimester of pregnancy is not usually aimed at identifying fetal abnormality; it is often performed for placental localization or for assessing fetal growth or wellbeing. However the possibilities that a scan may raise some suspicions or diagnose fetal abnormality should be considered, especially if there is cause for concern because of poly-hydramnios or a small fetus. In particular, if there have been no previous scans in the pregnancy, any late second trimester or third trimester scan should include a preliminary discussion about the possibility of unexpectedly detecting a fetal abnormality.

It is crucial that women are adequately informed of the possible findings and the options for further investigation. Jorgensen *et al.* (1985) looked at women who had a diagnosis of fetal malformation in the 32nd week of pregnancy and found that every woman in the sample, having been told of their fetal abnorm-ality, endured mental instability and trauma during the remainder of their preg-nancies. In the event, the imagined 'monster' often turned out to be less horrific than had been anticipated. This also applied to those to whom it had been explained that their child's abnormality was small and correctable.

So, should we all think twice before rushing into performing an ultrasound scan if clinical findings lead us to suspect there may be an underlying anomaly? What do we do if we discover an anomaly? Are we, then, committing ourselves and the woman to further, more invasive investigation at this late stage, and subsequently forcing her to make a desperately difficult and often painful decision? These are all questions without a uniformly correct answer but should provoke thought in all of us. People may argue that this hypothesis taken to the extreme would suggest that simply by making a clinical examination of a pregnant woman we are taking the first step towards perhaps unsought decision-making.

On the other hand, our proscription against infanticide reinforces the perceived desirability of prenatal screening and diagnosis: aborting an abnormal fetus is acceptable; causing newborn babies to die is not (Green *et al.*, 1992). Who is to say what degree of disability means that a child should not be allowed to live? Who decides about quality of life issues? Should the parents have the right to decide or is there room for debate? If a child were born alive at 34 weeks and was found to have Down syndrome, staff would not deliberately cause that child to die; yet feticide of an unborn child with Down syndrome at 34 weeks is legal in the UK. There is not room to fully debate the moral and ethical arguments here, but we must act within the letter of the law and with humanity. Society must make sure that doctors act responsibly and do not exceed the boundaries of what is considered acceptable. In some countries, including the US and the UK, hospital Clinical Ethics Committees may play a role in debating the moral and ethical quandaries associated with late prenatal diagnosis, acting as an independent resource for parents and staff alike.

An awesome burden is put on health professionals today. A couple's expecta-tions of a healthy pregnancy and subsequent birth of a normal baby, allows no room for the unforeseen. Our increasingly sophisticated society expects children to be healthy and free from disability despite the fact that 2–3% of babies will have some form of congenital abnormality. The status of people with disabilities in our society is a subject of continual discussion, and all health professionals will have their own views and personal beliefs.

Faced with the unenviable task of conveying bad news, staff are often reticent and feel very inadequate. This is particularly so when fetal abnormality has been diagnosed late in pregnancy, for whatever reason. The staff members then find themselves in a position in which they are going to deliver the blow that will shatter the hopes and aspirations of the parents for their as yet unborn family member; at the same time they have to deal with their own feelings.

Withholding the information is not an option, however. Women who learn of fetal abnormality once the child is born may feel cheated and let down. Studies of women's responses to false negative results from screening tests such as ultrasound scans or serum screening tests suggest that these women may have more difficulty in adjusting to the birth of an affected child. They are also more inclined to blame health professionals for not having prevented the births of their affected children (Hall *et al.*, 2000). Many women also report that they can tell if there are problems revealed on an ultrasound scan by a change in the staff's attitude, or even their facial expressions. Most women find any delay in being told the truth unacceptable, however unpalatable the truth may be.

CASE STUDIES

Some of the issues discussed so far in this chapter can be illustrated best by looking at individual cases.

CASE STUDY I   MS T

Ms T booked in her third pregnancy at 14 weeks' gestation. She had previously delivered a live healthy boy followed by a spontaneous miscarriage 2 years later. Both she and her husband were fit and healthy and neither had a family history of congenital abnormality.

When she attended for her anomaly scan at her local hospital, polyhydramnios was noted and an accurate demonstration of a four-chamber view of the fetal heart could not be made. These findings coupled with her low maternal serum alpha-fetoprotein raised the possibility of a chromosomal abnormality, and the couple was referred to a fetal medicine unit at another hospital. A scan in the unit confirmed polyhydramnios and demonstrated a short femur, possible micrognathia and an abnormal four-chamber view of the fetal heart. Ms T was counselled regarding the high risk of a chromosome abnormality and prenatal diagnosis was offered. Ms T naturally wished to discuss the findings and the options with her husband.

The couple returned to the fetal medicine unit 5 days later for further counselling and another scan. At this time additional abnormalities were noted, all of which are associated with Trisomy 18. The couple accepted the offer of fetal blood sampling, and this was performed on the same day, since the pregnancy was by then in its 25th week. The karyotype confirmed the suspicion of Trisomy 18.

The couple were devastated and found it impossible to make any kind of decision at that time. They were comforted by staff and the options for the pregnancy were sensitively explained. They left the unit to go home and digest their predicament, somewhat comforted by being able to call key workers on the unit for further advice at any time.

Ms T did call her key worker on several occasions over the ensuing couple of days to voice her anxieties. She felt that the only real option for her and her family was to terminate the pregnancy but was finding it impossible to make the appointment to come in to do so. She was advised to talk to her minister of religion for spiritual support, which she did and found to be helpful. Following this, and with the help of her key worker, Ms T set a time limit of a specific day when she would return to the unit with a decision. She had come to realize that if she did not terminate the pregnancy, this was in fact a decision to continue and that she therefore could not avoid making a decision.

On the morning of the chosen day Ms T rang her key worker giving a history of contractions. She was invited to return to the unit where on examination she was found to be in early labour. The decision had been made for her. She delivered a stillborn male infant later on that day.

The following is a verbatim report of how Ms T felt about the way her pregnancy was handled:

Before they took blood for the alpha-fetoprotein test the reason for the test wasn't explained very well. Down syndrome was mentioned. I felt that by having the test I was doing them a favour. When asked, I replied, 'Yes you might as well do it', I didn't for a minute think of the consequences. It never dawned on me that it would be the start of such a nightmare. When the alpha-fetoprotein test was offered I received conflicting advice as to the value of the test from the medical staff, some saying 'have it', others saying that it was a waste of time. This cheesed us off; we didn't know who to believe and this doubt stayed with us throughout the pregnancy; later causing us to doubt the Trisomy 18 result we were given. If there was doubt between members of the same medical team as to the worthiness of a test, could they have got our result wrong? Should we therefore continue with the pregnancy and take our chances? Maybe, just maybe, they were wrong.

I think it is very important that mothers are told that one of the main reasons for performing ultrasound scans is to look for fetal abnormality; they are not just to make sure that the baby is alive and growing as I had previously thought.

When they scanned my baby following the alpha-fetoprotein test results and the heart defect was discovered, I came away from the hospital convinced that my baby had Down syndrome. I felt extremely angry with the hospital. I felt I had been given conflicting advice, not enough information, inadequate explanations, no support, and having been given this shattering news I was left to sit out in the corridor alone with not so much as a cup of tea or offer of a phone call to my husband. In such a sensitive situation no one even bothered to say good-bye to me when I left the clinic.

I was referred to another hospital where they had a fetal medicine unit. There was a period of a few days between appointments. When asked afterwards whether I found those days useful in coming to terms with what I had so far been told, the answer was 'no'. I would far rather have gone on to the second hospital that same day if at all possible. I was now hungry for more information.

When I was seen at the fetal medicine unit I felt as if people understood how I felt. I felt 'safe'. Their whole attitude was different. They took the time to sit and talk to us to explain in terms that we understood what the problem was, what it meant for our baby and what other tests could be done to find out more. I felt that I hated the sister and the doctor when they told me that my baby had Trisomy 18, although the fact that they were adamant that there was no doubt did help. They were very positive in outlining the situation.

We then had to come to a decision as to what to do. At the back of our minds was still the nagging thought that perhaps they were wrong. Looking back, I don't think we would ever have been able to reach the decision to terminate the pregnancy, and as the sister who helped us at the time kept reminding us, by not making a decision we were in fact making the decision to continue the pregnancy. We obviously talked about it a lot and we both felt deep down, that perhaps we had done something to cause this problem, despite being reassured otherwise.

I was so relieved when I went into spontaneous labour; the decision was taken out of my hands. All I wanted now was to get it all over with. I was very scared though; I wondered what I was about to produce, I thought I was about to give birth to a monster.

The staff on the labour ward treated me 'normally', like I was having a live baby, I felt it was all very dignified and I felt in control. They were very encouraging and it helped me a lot. When our baby was born they took him out of the room cleaned him and dressed him before bringing him back for me to hold. This was a tremendous help. I really don't think I would have coped had they handed me Steven unclean and undressed. His colour shocked me, and it would have helped to have been forewarned. The fact that he looked perfect made me angry as again we both thought, could they have made a mistake.

After discharge from the hospital I felt it was a real anti-climax. We had been showered with so much attention, sympathy and concern leading up to, during and after Steven's birth and suddenly it all stopped. I felt as though I had been abandoned. 'When the community midwife called to see me, I felt very much as if I was just another client on her list; I didn't feel special and I wanted to feel special. I wanted everyone to realize what I had been through and what I was still going through. The midwife told me that she had had two miscarriages, the last thing I wanted to hear. I wasn't interested in her; I was too involved in my own grief.

I now wish I had spent more time with Steven, seen him more. I also wish there had been some facility to see one of the midwives who had been through it all with me. Either a visit at home, or a number to ring at an allotted time when I knew a midwife was allocated to answering calls from women like me would have been a huge help.

CASE STUDY 2   MS M

Another woman, Ms M, was referred to a fetal medicine unit when a fetal renal tract abnormality was suspected on ultrasound at 31 weeks. She had delivered a normal girl with no complications 4 years previously.

In this pregnancy, nothing untoward was detected at a 22-week anomaly scan apart from a low-lying placenta. The pregnancy progressed without complication until a repeat scan for placental localization revealed the renal anomaly.

The findings were not straightforward and further investigations including karyotyping and amniotic infusion were performed. Ms M's case was discussed with a paediatric urologist who subsequently also counselled the couple. The karyotype was normal but Mr and Ms M were told that there was no guarantee about the baby's outcome. They were told that the baby might suffer and die from lung hypoplasia secondary to the lack of amniotic fluid before reaching the paediatricians specializing in renal medicine. They were also told that the baby might need immediate renal dialysis and possibly a kidney transplant. On the other hand, it was explained that there was a chance that the baby might be well and require minimal treatment. Naturally, the decision about continuing the pregnancy was particularly difficult given the wide spectrum of possible outcomes for their unborn child.

They decided to continue the pregnancy and their son was born by caesarean section at 34 weeks' gestation; he died nineteen hours later in his parents' arms, from lung hypoplasia.

Here Ms M recalls her feelings and thoughts at and around the time of the prenatal diagnosis being made, the decision-making and the eventual outcome.

I remember wondering why they were sending me to another hospital. Was it because they had a better scanning machine? I was led to believe, or perhaps I wanted to believe, it would be a case of emptying the baby's bladder and deciding on the right time for delivery. I was totally unprepared for what was to come. I never dreamt in a million years that there was something so wrong and that he would die. I thought it was a straightforward, simple problem that would be easily corrected. I hated the doctor that broke the bad news to us. I felt that she had taken everything away from me. The bottom had fallen out of my world; why me, why now, why wasn't it picked up earlier, why, why, why? I was in a state of shock and total disbelief; I wanted to turn around to find she was talking to someone else.

I now wanted to know everything that could be done, the investigations, the care after he was delivered, everything. The fact that the doctor had given him such a little chance of survival made me think, 'I will prove you all wrong; he is going to survive'. When we found out that he didn't have Down syndrome and that some of the other results were not as expected and therefore difficult to interpret, I thought, 'I'm not going to write my baby off just because everyone else has', which was how I felt at the time.

For a very short time after hearing the bad news, I thought that I didn't want to walk around with what I saw then as a dead baby inside me. When I got home and thought about it, I soon changed my way of thinking and although the sheer horror that something was wrong with *my* baby had hit me, I thought, 'He's still a feeling little person in there'. I then knew that I would carry on and do everything for him and give him every chance.

I'm glad I knew about his problems before he was born; it didn't cushion the blow, but it would have been worse had I not known. It was very difficult to accept his death when looking at him. He looked so beautiful and perfect.

After his death I only wanted to be with my husband and daughter. I didn't even want my mother. I was finding it difficult enough to cope with my own grief without hers as well. I was so distraught; I felt that I had let both my husband and daughter down.

It is now 3 months ago, and I still have this huge hole that I cannot fill, and finding someone who is willing just to sit and listen to me is so helpful.

CASE STUDY 3   MS W

Ms W (a 30-year-old with one normal son) had an anomaly scan that showed an umbilical cord with two blood vessels and mild polyhydramnios. As a result of these findings she was referred to a fetal medicine unit for a further detailed scan and counselling. This next scan confirmed the presence of a two-vessel cord, but there was now also a suspicion of a claw hand.

She returned again to the fetal medicine unit. The previously diagnosed abnormalities were confirmed and both fetal hands were found to abnormal. Ms W had attended this appointment alone and was counselled as to the risks of chromosomal abnormality. At this stage the pregnancy had already advanced into the 28th week of gestation. Fetal blood sampling to determine fetal karyotype as quickly as possible was offered, but Ms W declined, not wishing to put the pregnancy at risk, and stating she would not terminate even if the results were abnormal. The option of amniocentesis was also offered, carrying less of a risk, but taking longer for the results to become available. This was accepted as she felt it might help her to come to terms with the prospect of giving birth to an abnormal child without the higher risk of the fetal blood sample.

Ms W then left to go on holiday with her family. While she was away the karyotype results showed Trisomy 18. On return from their holiday Mr and Ms W were invited to return to the fetal medicine unit to hear the results of the karyotype and to discuss the options for the pregnancy. This they did, and, naturally devastated, they asked for time to think over the options that had been given to them including that of termination of pregnancy following a lethal injection of potassium chloride into the fetal heart. They returned two days later for further discussion and decided, despite their previous beliefs, to opt for termination of pregnancy preceded by feticide by potassium chloride. This was arranged and carried out 5 days later at the parents' request, when the pregnancy was at 33 weeks' gestation.

Ms W recalls her feelings:

I just couldn't believe what I was hearing; my baby that had now been kicking inside me for the best part of 3 months was abnormal. When I agreed to the amniocentesis test I had not really thought that I would find myself in this hellish position; that is why I went for it thinking 'well what will be will be'; we'll cope with a handicapped child. How wrong I was! Now faced with the grim reality of it all, I soon started to realize that I had started something by having that test that would be extremely difficult to finish. We had to think of our little boy. Was it fair on him? Could he cope; could I cope; could we cope?

We went home to mull over our thoughts numbed by the news. We knew we had to make a decision and in the not too distant future. The options were all ghastly – to continue on for possibly another 7 or 8 weeks carrying a baby that probably would not survive, but if it did would be handicapped. The alternative, terminating our baby after the injection that would kill it, was abhorrent. There was no easy way out – that soon became clear – and after 2 days of agonizing we decided to end it then and not prolong the torture any longer.

The day that we went to the hospital for the procedure to be carried out haunts me now – the overwhelming guilt I felt for what I was about to do. The room where it all began with the scan and amniocentesis was now witness to the murder (or that is how I perceived it at the time), of my baby. It was so hard to lie there while they did it. I had to hold on to the bed to stop myself jumping off it or shouting at them to stop. Not that that was what I wanted, it was just the guilt I was feeling and whether I would be able to live with it for the rest of my life. They turned the ultrasound screen away from my view, and although I didn't witness my baby's heart stopping, the staffs' faces said it all – I felt so sorry for them too, what an frightful thing to ask anyone to do.

I don't regret my decision now; a year has past, but the feelings of guilt are no less than they were that dreadful day.

CASE STUDY 4 MS B

Ms B, a 40-year-old woman in her first ongoing pregnancy after several years' infertility and assisted conception, was referred to a tertiary level fetal medicine unit. She had requested prenatal diagnosis for chromosome abnormalities in view of her age, but because of work commitments was unable to attend for amniocentesis until 20 weeks. This was performed without event, and both the routine ultrasound scan and fetal karyotype were normal.

In view of the history of infertility, her obstetrician arranged for her to have a scan for growth at 28 weeks. Tragically this showed that the baby had bilateral cerebral ventriculomegaly and it was at this stage that she attended the fetal medicine unit.

Scanning in the fetal medicine unit confirmed the abnormality and gave rise to suspicions that the baby may have had some bleeding into its brain. The parents had a wide-ranging in-depth discussion with the fetal medicine consultant and specialist midwives. It was explained that the presence of the ventriculomegaly gave cause to be concerned about the potential neurological development of the unborn child, but that the spectrum of disability was uncertain. A paediatric neurologist and a neonatologist were consulted to give further valuable advice for the parents, but no one could accurately predict the prognosis for this baby. The parents' blood was examined for evidence of anti-platelet antibodies, a potential cause for fetal thrombocytapenia, which could precipitate bleeding, and maternal blood was taken to look for evidence of exposure to viruses. All these results were reported as normal within a few days.

The parents were advised that there was a high risk that their child could have a significant degree of handicap in terms of intellectual development. There were no other tests that would add to the multidisciplinary team's ability to give a more accurate prognosis.

What a dilemma for the parents. They had grave concerns about knowingly giving birth to a child with a potentially very severe handicap but were aware that the child may have less severe problems. They left the unit to consider their options, with a further appointment made for a few days time. During this waiting time the parents consulted widely with support groups, their own minister of religion, family and friends. They also searched for information on the Internet. The specialist midwife liased with the parents' own primary care team to enable support to continue away from the tertiary unit, and also kept in close contact with the parents. Ms B expressed some of their agonizing thoughts.

> People think we should just accept that this child will have problems, because of our infertility. They think we should be grateful. They seem to think that a disabled child is better than no child at all. We're not sure that we agree – how can we knowingly sentence a child to a poor quality of life, not to mention the effects on our families and ourselves? We know we may not be able to have another child, but we would rather put ourselves through the worst pain now rather than live with a disabled child and always be thinking.... we could have been spared this.

After several days the parents returned to the fetal medicine unit, having decided to terminate the pregnancy. The pregnancy was by this stage advanced to just over 30 weeks. After further counselling, including discussion about post mortem examination, the fetus was given an intracardiac injection of potassium chloride, and the parents returned to their referring unit for delivery.

WHAT ABOUT THE STAFF?

We have seen how parents feel, but what about the staff? They are, after all, only human.

Staff are not exempt from feelings and may also share in the parents' grief. Repeated exposure in no way lessens the intense feelings. When fetal abnormality is discovered 'late' in pregnancy, the obstetrician and midwife have also felt the baby kicking when palpating the mother's abdomen, auscultated the fetal heart beat, and watched him or her on the ultrasound scan. This makes the task of assisting the couple in making decisions for the future of their pregnancy more demanding.

Although most couples find comfort in knowing that staff are also sorrowful, others prefer more dispassionate medical explanations as this helps them to maintain some self-control and composure.

Staff may need help to gain insight into their non-verbal communication skills. Parents often report that they could tell there was a problem, even before any words were said, by the facial expressions or posture of the staff involved. Counselling skills training may prove beneficial in helping staff to consider how best to communicate bad news to parents.

For staff as well as parents, there is a crucial difference between terminating a pregnancy at 12 weeks' gestation and terminating at 32 weeks. At 32 weeks a birth has the potential of producing a live baby, thus creating a worse scenario for the parents. This then puts the parents and those caring for them in the unenviable position of having to actively kill the baby prior to the induction of labour, thus ensuring no possibility of a severely handicapped live baby being born. It would be distressing for the parents and labour ward staff for such a baby to show signs of life, and it would also put the paediatricians in a very difficult situation. Would they resuscitate a baby who supposedly was 'terminated' and who might survive with little or no quality of life if they did so? This would be quite the opposite of what was intended.

Feticide, however, is also a very emotionally painful procedure for both parents and staff. The fact that the process is carried out using ultrasound means the staff involved witness the life and subsequent death of the baby, as a result of their actions, on the screen. The guilt involved can be overwhelming, despite the decision having not been made lightly, and knowing that the decision and its consequences will produce the most acceptable outcome for the parents. It is at times like these that staff need extra support from each other and often from outside agencies or counsellors.

Before setting up a birth plan with the parents, whether they are delivering a live baby at term with suspected or known abnormalities or giving birth following feticide, the midwives and obstetricians who will be caring for the family should be supported and helped to understand the situation. In the United Kingdom, midwives and doctors have the right to conscientiously object to taking part in terminations of pregnancy but in an emergency would be expected to provide care (Nursing and Midwifery Council, 2002). Staff who have moral objections and who are working in settings where terminations of pregnancy may take place, should voice their concerns with the team caring for the family so that alternative care can be provided without causing distress to the staff or parents.

It is vital that the staff who are helping the couple through the decision process are clear about their own feelings surrounding late termination of pregnancy and feel comfortable with these issues. Staff should feel able to turn to each other for support and may benefit from independent supervision and counselling.

CONCLUSION

Late prenatal diagnosis is here to stay because it can be done. It undoubtedly benefits some people, but the emotional cost to both staff and parents should not be underestimated.

Key points

- The ethical and moral dilemmas associated with late prenatal diagnosis are considerable, especially after the stage of fetal viability.
- A multidisciplinary approach is needed to help parents who are faced with difficult choices in the event of a late diagnosis of fetal abnormality.
- Termination of pregnancy is permissible in English and Welsh law at any gestation if there is a significant risk of serious handicap. Feticide is recommended for any termination of pregnancy after 21 weeks. Most commonly this is performed by intracardiac injection of potassium chloride.
- Whether the parents' decision is to carry on with the pregnancy or to terminate, the emotional burden is huge, and they should be fully supported at all stages.
- Those caring for women undergoing such procedures are also in need of support and emotional care.

REFERENCES

Abortion Act (1967). HMSO, London.

Chitty L, Barnes C, Berry C (1996) For debate; continuing with pregnancy after a diagnosis of lethal abnormality: experience of five couples and recommendations for management. *British Medical Journal*, 313; 478–480.

Green J, Statham H, Snowdon C (1992) Screening for fetal abnormalities: attitudes and experiences. In *Obstetrics in the 1990's: Current Controversies* (eds Chard T, Richards MPM). MacKeith Press, London.

Hall S, Bobrow M, Marteau T (2000) Psychological consequences for parents of false negative results on prenatal screening for Down's syndrome: retrospective interview study. *British Medical Journal*, 320; 407–412.

Jorgensen C, Uddenberg N, Ursing Z. (1985) Ultrasound diagnosis of fetal malformation in the second trimester: the psychological reactions of the women. *Journal of Psychosomatic Obstetrics and Gynecology*, 4; 31–40.

Nursing and Midwifery Council (2002) *Code of Professional Conduct*. NMC, London.

Royal College of Obstetricians and Gynaecologists (1996) *Termination of Pregnancy for Fetal Abnormality in England, Wales and Scotland*. RCOG, London.

Royal College of Obstetricians and Gynaecologists (1998) *A consideration of the law and ethics in relation to late termination of pregnancy for fetal abnormality.* RCOG, London. (http://www.rcog.org.uk/guidelines).

FURTHER READING

Borg S, Lasker J (1982) *When Pregnancy Fails.* Routledge & Keegan Paul, London.

Brock DJH, Rodeck CH, Ferguson MA (1992) *Prenatal Diagnosis and Screening.* Churchill Livingstone, Edinburgh.

Harper PS (1998) *Practical Genetic Counselling* (5th edn) John Wright & Sons, Bristol.

Jolly J (1987) *Missed Beginnings – Death Before Life has Been Established.* Lisa Sainsbury Foundation, London.

Royal College of Obstetricians and Gynaecologists (1993, updated 1997) *Effective Procedures in Maternity Care Suitable for Audit: Antenatal Screening and Diagnosis.* (http://www.rcog.org.uk/mainpages)

Royal College of Obstetricians and Gynaecologists (1991) *Antenatal Diagnosis of Fetal Abnormalities. Report of a Study Group Called by the Royal College of Obstetricians and Gynaecologists* (eds Drife JO and Donnai D). Springer Verlag, London.

Royal College of Obstetricians and Gynaecologists, and the Royal College of Paediatrics and Child Health (1997) *Fetal Abnormalities – Guidelines for Screening, Diagnosis and Management.* RCOG, London.

11 DILEMMAS IN SELECTIVE FETOCIDE AND MULTIFETAL PREGNANCY REDUCTION

Elizabeth M. Bryan

INTRODUCTION

For the 9000 or so couples in the United Kingdom expecting twins each year, the risk of giving birth to a baby with a congenital anomaly is not only doubled because of the two babies but increased further by the average age of mothers of twins being higher than that of singletons. Furthermore twins as such, particularly monozygotic pairs, are at a greater risk of being affected (Doyle *et al.*, 1990).

MULTIPLE PREGNANCIES

The relative risk of some abnormalities in a multiple pregnancy differs from that in a single pregnancy. For instance Trisomy 21 is less common in twins, whereas some neural-tube defects are more common. On the other hand concordancy for neural-tube defects, even in monozygotic twins, is unusual and Down syndrome, although usually concordant in monozygotic twins, rarely affects both of a dizygotic pair (Doyle *et al.*, 1990).

With two fetuses the combined risk of at least one being affected is inevitably higher than in a single pregnancy. Some would therefore argue that amniocentesis should be offered to women with multiple pregnancies at a younger age (Rodis *et al.*, 1990). However, the results of amniocentesis may present a far greater dilemma for parents of twins than of singletons.

If neither baby has a serious abnormality, the parents can feel reassured. If both have serious abnormalities, it is a tragedy but a decision to terminate the pregnancy is probably no more complicated than with a single child. Indeed, many would feel the decision to be easier in that the burden of two children with very special needs would be even greater. In these circumstances most couples who had actually chosen to have the test done will probably proceed to have the whole pregnancy terminated.

If one baby is apparently normal and the other abnormal the dilemma can plainly be agonizing. In the past the choice lay between terminating the whole pregnancy or persisting with it knowing that one baby would suffer from a disability and require special care while the parents were also responding to the healthy child's needs. Many couples who would not hesitate to have a pregnancy terminated for a single abnormal fetus feel unable to do this when the sacrifice of a normal baby is also involved.

There is now another choice, however: selective fetocide. Since the first report in 1978 (Alberg *et al.*, 1978), the intrauterine killing of an abnormal fetus in a multiple pregnancy has been performed for a large number of different conditions where only one twin is affected (Evans *et al.*, 1999). These include chromosomal anomalies (e.g. Trisomy 21 and Turner syndrome), genetic disorders (e.g. cystic fibrosis, haemophilia, beta thalassaemia and Duchenne muscular dystrophy) neural-tube defects (spina bifida and anencephaly) and the twin-to-twin transfusion syndrome. The method most commonly used now (except in monochorionic pregnancies – see below) is the injection of potassium chloride into the heart of the affected fetus. In a few cases the fetus has been removed by hysterotomy, thus sparing the mother the psychologically distressing experience of carrying a dead baby. The risk, however, of precipitating premature labour with this method is considered to be too high by most obstetricians. Various other methods have been used in the past such as cardiac puncture, air embolization and fetal exsanguination.

Chorionicity is one other important consideration. All dizygotic twins and a third of monozygotic twins have dichorionic placentae. For all of these, selective fetocide is technically straightforward. In the two thirds of monozygotic twins who have a monochorionic placenta and therefore a shared circulation, selective fetocide can only be performed by total occlusion of both umbilical arteries and the umbilical vein of the targeted fetus. This is the only way to prevent the unaffected fetus receiving a toxic injection or suffering exsanguination following the fall in blood pressure in the dead co-twin (Deprest *et al.*, 2000).

The decision to proceed with selective fetocide will partly depend on the severity of the abnormality, and this can be difficult to estimate in some conditions associated with variable degrees of intellectual impairment. But it will depend also on whether the child is likely to die at, or soon after, birth or survive, perhaps for many years, with a serious disability. A further consideration must of course be the continuing safety of the unaffected twin fetus. An abnormal fetus may actually jeopardize the life of the healthy child, as in cases where the presence of an anencephalic fetus causes polyhydramnios, and thus induces premature labour.

In cases of anencephaly or other lethal conditions, some would recommend first trimester selective fetocide as being safer than fetocide later in pregnancy. Others would suggest waiting to see if polyhydramnios develops. A further consideration is the parents' wishes about possible organ donation.

The choice of timing of a selective fetocide has become wider in recent years (Evans *et al.*, 1999). On the one hand, with the development of first trimester prenatal diagnosis, a greater percentage of couples can choose to terminate early in the pregnancy. On the other hand, with the introduction of new legislation in the UK and several other countries, parents now have the option to delay selective fetocide until the third trimester with the advantage of avoiding the risk of a death of the co-twin should the procedure precipitate premature labour. It is yet to be established which timing parents find more acceptable. Evans *et al.* (1996) found that gestational age at diagnosis was not a particularly important factor in the decision to abort or not; the main predictor of the decision to abort in singleton pregnancies was the severity of the fetal prognosis. However a third trimester fetocide can lead to conflict between parents and staff, as not all obstetricians personally support pregnancy termination beyond fetal viability.

Selective fetocide is a superficially easy solution but may seem bizarre and horrifying to many doctors as well as to parents. Some parents will not have even heard of selective fetocide before being faced with the option and few, if any, will know another mother who has undergone the procedure. Many will be horrified at the concept and the difficulty of coming to terms with these feelings may be harder when relatives, friends and even doctors show their shock, incredulity or revulsion.

Not surprisingly, there is sometimes disagreement between partners. One or both may have deep religious objections. One may be distressed at the thought of disposing of a potential baby of theirs whereas the other may be equally distressed by the idea of having a disabled child. Partners are very likely to disagree to some extent and there will often be a need to compromise as to what is best for them as individuals, as a couple and as a family. Both partners will need to weigh carefully and sensitively the arguments on both sides. It is sometimes only with the help of a counsellor that they come to understand the views and feelings of their partner.

Professionals need to be aware of their own complex feelings, before offering guidance or support to others. Many parents have been disconcerted by their doctor's ignorance. Parents may seek the advice and help of their general practitioner, who is very unlikely to have come across such a case before in the practice. Communication between primary and secondary care is vital if the general practitioner who knows the family is to be able to offer long-term support.

A careful explanation to the couple of exactly what is involved in the procedure is all the more important because they are unlikely to find much written information about it. Some mothers have, for instance, been disconcerted by the sudden cessation of movements in one part of their abdomen. The side-effects of the sympathomimetic drugs given to prevent the onset of premature labour may be found distressing. It can be very helpful for a couple to meet another couple who have been through the experience.

When parents are offered the option of selective fetocide they must also be told about the potential risks attached to the procedure. These include precipitating an abortion or preterm labour, the introduction of infection and the possibility, however remote, of incorrect selection of the target fetus (Evans *et al.*, 1999). Failure to kill the fetus on the first attempt can be very distressing to parents especially if they are watching the procedure on the ultrasound scan.

It seems that some people who would agree to the termination of a single pregnancy cannot accept selective fetocide either for a congenital anomaly or in order to reduce the number of fetuses (Evans *et al.*, 1991). In addition to the loss of a wanted baby, selective fetocide raises uncomfortable ethical issues and uneasy associations with eugenics (Bryan and Higgins, 1995; Schlotzhauer and Liang, 1999). It is therefore all the more necessary to identify and clarify the emotional issues that are stirred up. For both parents and staff, the termination of a pregnancy, where the fetus dies because it was delivered too soon, may feel easier to accept than selective fetocide. With selective fetocide, it is harder to deceive yourself – the baby is killed in its mother's womb.

BEREAVEMENT

Parents should always be offered counselling for their bereavement and the assurance that this is available not only during the period immediately after their loss but in the longer term.

For many parents the full impact of the bereavement is not felt until the delivery many weeks later of a solitary live baby. This is also when undeniable proof arrives that the couple will not after all enjoy being the parents of twins. Moreover, different to a simple termination, there is much greater awareness of the baby that might have been because of the presence of the survivor. The bereaved parents have the peculiar and painful difficulty of grieving for a lost baby both during the continuing pregnancy and after the live birth.

By the time of the delivery, especially if it is in a different hospital to that in which the selective fetocide had been performed, the mother's carers may have forgotten that it was a twin pregnancy and their consequent failure to respect the dead baby may add to the mother's distress. A follow-up study of the first 12 mothers in the United Kingdom to have a selective fetocide for discordant anomalies in their twins, found that all felt they had made the correct decision but that many thought their loss had been underestimated or even forgotten, and that bereavement support had been inadequate (Bryan, 1989).

When one twin dies and the other survives, not only the bereaved couple but those who care for them are faced with contradictory emotional processes. The mother's celebration of the birth of the live baby, and her increasing emotional commitment to it, contrast with the parallel process of a sorrowful coming to terms with the death of the other baby.

The dead baby may at first seem like a fantasy, particularly if the mother did not see it and has no mementoes of its brief existence, such as an ultrasound picture. Some mothers deeply regretted that they were not allowed to see the baby after it was delivered, even when the fetus had been dead for some weeks. As one mother said, 'I wanted to know – I kept asking – they wouldn't show it – they just took it away'.

The lack of respect for the fetus has upset many mothers. One was outraged that a post mortem should have been performed without even a request for her permission 'How dare he do it without me knowing? As if the baby was nothing to do with me; this was the baby I had been relating to'. Others said that their questions about the fetus seemed to be ignored or avoided.

The bereavement was generally felt more deeply by those who had not expected a problem for one of their much-wanted twins and then discovered an anomaly, such as Down syndrome or anencephaly, than by those who had known all along that they might have to lose the entire pregnancy because of a genetic disorder such as cystic fibrosis or haemophilia.

A mother's full commitment is necessary for the effective physical and emotional nurturing of her newborn live baby. The grief work concerning the lost baby may therefore be postponed and if this process of conscious relinquishment is not resumed later it can give rise to the various syndromes of failed mourning (Lewis and Bryan, 1988). In some cases, however, the mother may grieve compulsively for the dead baby and hence reject the live one. Because there is still a live baby, it is all too common for the relatives, friends and even medical staff to ignore the bereavement. The parents' loss, if acknowledged at all, is usually greatly under-estimated. Ill-considered and insensitive remarks such as 'at least you have got one baby' cause much pain and resentment. Parents of twins are often made to feel guilty about their grief, as if they were being ungrateful for the surviving baby. (Yet which mother of singletons would ever be rebuked for mourning the loss of one of her children?) For those with monozygotic twins in particular, they have the constant reminder of their dead baby in the surviving child.

Parents are too often discouraged, even overtly, from talking about the dead baby. If mothers are not allowed to do this they may silently idealize the dead baby and be positively alienated from the survivor.

In coming to terms with her loss, the mother needs to be able clearly to distinguish the two babies in her mind; otherwise she may think of the survivor, as one mother put it, as 'only half a baby'. Naming the babies can be particularly helpful. It makes it easier for the parents to distinguish the babies in their minds and when they talk about them. For the survivor, later, it is obviously easier if he can refer to his sibling by name. Many parents like to have a funeral service and some form of memorial. One couple whose twins were miscarried at 22 weeks had a memorial service at which the priest baptised the babies 'by intent'.

Even though the babies can hardly look attractive so long after their death, some parents will still wish to have a photograph of them. Clearly the wish should be respected. Sketches and paintings drawn from photographs or from the parents' descriptions assist in providing a visual representation which parents may be more comfortable showing to their friends. A photograph of the ultrasound scan showing both babies may also be – or become – a precious tangible reminder and a unique proof to parents that they ever had a multiple pregnancy.

The pride of being an expectant mother, or father, of twins is enormous and the failure to become one therefore all the greater. Some parents have found it as hard to come to terms with the loss of twin parenthood as they do with the loss of their baby.

MULTIFETAL PREGNANCY REDUCTION

New techniques in the treatment of infertility have resulted in a worrying increase in the number of higher order pregnancies, despite the limitation in the number of embryos that may be implanted (to a maximum of three in the UK). Some parents will choose to have a reduction of a pregnancy of three or more embryos to two by undergoing a multifetal pregnancy reduction at the end of the first trimester. (The term selective fetocide should be limited to a pregnancy where one [or more] of the fetuses has an anomaly.)

In the case of such a higher order pregnancy, each baby has the same potential for a normal healthy life and an apparently arbitrary decision on the fate of a precious baby can be very disturbing. Even though the fetus selection is usually made on the grounds of technical accessibility, parents may feel that they are playing God in sacrificing one baby in preference to another. As one mother said, 'How could you say I'll kill him but not her?' It is therefore all the more necessary to identify and clarify beforehand the emotional issues that are stirred up.

Although the surviving fetus should suffer no physical ill effects, the thought of a live baby lying for many weeks by the side of his dead twin can be very distressing. Moreover, when no fetus has actually been expelled, the natural tendency to deny and forget the sad reality becomes much easier and feelings of loss are postponed.

With multifetal pregnancy reduction, some parents will feel a lasting grief and guilt over the death of one or more potentially healthy children. Nevertheless it appears that the great majority who do proceed with a reduction feel afterwards that they had made the right decision (Garel *et al.*, 1997).

Many will still, however, feel a profound bereavement and will rightly expect this to be respected. Others, of course, will prefer that people 'forget' what has happened and will not wish any reference to be made to it. Particular sensitivity is needed by the carers in helping such couples, especially if they have chosen not to disclose anything to their relatives and friends.

THE SURVIVING TWIN

A surviving twin will usually feel the loss of their twin brother or sister far more deeply than the loss of an ordinary sibling. Strangely enough, this may still be so even when one twin has died before or at birth (Woodward, 1998). This may be due to the intrauterine relationship of twins but little is known about this. Nor is there yet any information on the reactions of the surviving twin following selective fetocide.

It is almost certainly better that the survivor be told about their twin from the start. There have been many accounts of painful and unexplained feelings of loss experienced by surviving twins who had not been told about their stillborn twin. Many felt a sense of relief when these feelings were finally explained, sometimes very many years later.

If the child knows he (or she) is a twin, he can be helped to identify and express his feelings. He may be angry with his parents for 'allowing' the baby to die. He may feel anger towards his twin for causing so much unhappiness. Later he may have to come to terms with a form of survivor-guilt. The surviving child or children may understandably be emotionally bewildered by the apparent arbitrariness of their own survival.

It is vital that we should learn about the feelings of a survivor of selective fetocide as soon as possible so that more appropriate counselling can be given to both parents and children. Follow-up studies need to be carried out on the physical and emotional well-being of both the parents and the surviving children. The results will not only suggest what support should be provided but may well influence policy on selective fetocide and multifetal pregnancy reduction in general.

CONCLUSION

Both selective fetocide and multifetal pregnancy reduction are now becoming more generally available and need the same deep thought and public discussion as the implications and ethics of terminating a single pregnancy. For many couples selective fetocide may be the least painful of the options facing them, but they will still need much understanding and support.

Key points

- The nature and implications of the selective fetocide or multifetal pregnancy reduction procedure should be explained clearly and sensitively.
- Parents should be helped to consider in advance whether they wish to see the fetus and what form of funeral arrangements or memorial, if any, they wish to have.
- Everyone involved with the care of the mother (both during the pregnancy and in the future) should be aware of the parents' loss.
- At delivery, the dead fetus should be treated with respect.
- Parents should be aware that counselling support will continue to be available for themselves and for the surviving baby or babies.

REFERENCES

Alberg A, Mitelman F, Cantz M (1978) Cardiac puncture of fetus with Hurler's disease avoiding abortion of unaffected co-twin. *Lancet*, ii; 990–991.

Bryan EM (1989) The response of mothers to selective fetocide. *Ethical Problems in Reproductive Medicine*, 1; 28–30.

Bryan E, Higgins R (1995) Embryo reduction of a multiple pregnancy: an insoluble dilemma? In *Infertility. New Choices, New Dilemmas* (eds Bryan E, Higgins R). Penguin, London, pp. 130–140.

Deprest JA, Audibert F, Van Schoubroeck D *et al.* (2000) Bipolar coagulation of the umbilical cord in complicated monochorionic twin pregnancy. *American Journal of Obstetrics and Gynecology*, 182; 340–345.

Doyle PE, Beral V, Botting B *et al.* (1990) Congenital malformations in twins in England and Wales. *Journal of Epidemiology and Community Health*, 45; 43–48.

Evans MI, Drugan A, Bottoms SF *et al.* (1991) Attitudes on the ethics of abortion, sex selection, and selective pregnancy termination among health care professionals, ethicists, and clergy likely to encounter such situations. *American Journal of Obstetrics and Gynecology*, 164; 1092–1099.

Evans MI, Sobiecki MA, Krivchenia EL *et al*. (1996) Parental decisions to terminate/ continue following abnormal cytogenetic prenatal diagnosis: 'what' is still more important than 'when'. *American Journal of Medical Genetics*, 61; 353–355.

Evans MI, Goldberg JD, Horenstein J *et al*. (1999) Selective termination for structural, chromosomal, and mendelian anomalies: international experience. *American Journal of Obstetrics and Gynecology*, 181; 893–897.

Garel M, Stark C, Blondel B *et al*. (1997) Psychological reactions after multifetal pregnancy reduction: a 2-year follow-up study. *Human Reproduction*, 12; 617–622.

Lewis E, Bryan EM (1988) Management of perinatal loss of a twin. *British Medical Journal,* 297; 1321–1323.

Rodis JF, Egan JF, Craffey A *et al*. (1990) Calculated risk of chromosomal abnormalities in twin gestations. *Obstetrics and Gynecology*, 76; 1037–1041.

Schlotzhauer A, Liang BA (1999). The ethics of selective termination cases. *The Journal of Legal Medicine*, 20; 441–456.

Woodward J (1998) *The Lone Twin*. London, Free Association Books.

FURTHER READING

Bryan E, Hallett F (1997) *Bereavement Guidelines for Professionals*. Multiple Births Foundation, London.

MBF (1997) *Multiple Pregnancy: Selective Fetocide*. Multiple Births Foundation. London [leaflet].

MBF (2000) *Higher Multiple Pregnancies – Fetal Reduction*. Multiple Births Foundation, London [leaflet].

12 DIFFICULT DECISIONS IN PRENATAL DIAGNOSIS

Christine Garrett and Lyn Margerison

INTRODUCTION

Decisions in prenatal diagnosis are difficult when the diagnosis is clear. How much more difficult it is when there is only a risk of abnormality, or where the effects of the abnormality cannot be predicted. This chapter will explore some of these situations, the ways in which couples come to a decision, and the role of the counsellor in helping them to decide.

UNSUSPECTED CHROMOSOME ABNORMALITIES

Prenatal diagnosis is usually performed because of concern about a particular chromosomal abnormality, most commonly Down syndrome (Trisomy 21). Prenatal diagnosis counselling should include explanation of the possibility that other chromosome abnormalities may also be detected. Trisomy 18 or Trisomy 13, both lethal abnormalities, are conditions where the outcome can be predicted and the choice facing the couple is usually clear. This is not so when a sex chromosome Trisomy, or an apparently balanced structural rearrangement, or mosaicism is detected. In such cases the outcome may be difficult to predict, and while many such babies may be entirely normal some may suffer from significant disability. The counsellor needs to be aware of the effects of these chromosome abnormalities in order to give the couple the most reliable information on which to base their decision as to whether to continue the pregnancy. These problems are considered in more detail below.

Sex chromosome abnormalities

Klinefelter syndrome (XXY)
The XXY chromosome pattern is present in approximately 1 in 1000 male births (Editorial, 1988). Not long ago the traditional textbook description of Kline-felter syndrome was of a mentally retarded male, lacking in male secondary sexual characteristics and with breast enlargement – an alarming prospect for future parents. This picture resulted from a bias in selection, since originally only those with the most severe manifestations were karyotyped, and the true extent of the effects of Klinefelter syndrome have only recently emerged from prospective studies involving long-term follow-up of babies identified by newborn surveys (Leonard, 1990; Linden *et al.*, 1996; Ratcliffe, 1999; Bender *et al.*, 2001).

Performance intelligence quotient scores are normal but there is a 10–20 point reduction in verbal skills, with significant problems in expressive language. While most boys attend normal schools, the speech and language disorder may require speech therapy. Men with Klinefelter syndrome are invariably infertile, although patients with Klinefelter have fathered offspring with the aid of ICSI (intracytoplasmic sperm injection) (Poulakis *et al.*, 2001). Tall stature is a feature but there is no increase in congenital malformations. Gynaecomastia may occur, but rarely requires surgery. The chance of homosexuality or transsexualism is not increased, but diminished potency or libido may require treatment with testosterone replacement. There is a tendency towards passive behaviour characterized by lack of self-esteem, shyness and emotional immaturity. However, preliminary data suggest that most affected males manage well with respect to social adjustment and socio-economic status.

Triple X syndrome (XXX)
In the Triple X syndrome the baby is female and has an extra X chromosome, an abnormality present in approximately 1 in 1000 female births. As with Klinefelter syndrome, early reports tended to exaggerate the effects of the extra X chromosome, because ascertainment was biased in favour of individuals who were karyotyped because of significant problems. Prospective studies on girls diagnosed by screening at birth give a more accurate picture (Leonard, 1990; Linden *et al.*, 1996; Ratcliffe, 1999; Bender *et al.*, 2001). There are no distinguishing features at birth but as they grow older they become relatively tall with long legs, with a slightly reduced head circumference. Sexual development is usually normal and many women with Triple X are fertile. However there may be an increased incidence of infertility and premature menopause, and women with Triple X are probably more likely to have chromosomally abnormal offspring particularly with an extra X chromosome.

The main cause for concern is the possible effects on the child's future intellectual development and personality. Delay in speech and language development is common, and speech therapy is often necessary. Lack of coordination, poor academic performance, and immature behaviour may persist throughout childhood and overall intelligence quotient is reduced by around ten points. Behavioural problems are common, and few achieve academic success (Bender *et al.*, 2001). The risk of psychotic disorders may be increased.

Extra Y chromosome (XYY)
An extra Y chromosome, XYY, is present in approximately 1 in 1000 male births, and is not associated with raised maternal or paternal age. This finding on amniocentesis may present the parents with a dilemma, not least because of the association (in the older medical literature) of this condition with criminality. Again, the true picture is beginning to emerge from data built up from long-term follow up of boys with XYY ascertained by newborn surveys (Leonard, 1990; Linden *et al.*, 1996; Ratcliffe, 1999). Affected boys are physically indistinguishable from the general population, but tend to be taller than average. Behaviour

problems are frequent in childhood, with temper tantrums and hyperactivity, and speech development may be delayed. Intelligence is 10–15 points less than that of their normal siblings and verbal intelligence quotient is affected more than performance. Many XYY men have fathered children who are chromosomally normal but there is probably an increased risk of a chromosomal abnormality, including XYY, in their offspring.

Turner syndrome (45,X)

Absence of a sex chromosome, 45,X, causes Turner syndrome. The main features are short stature, infertility, and mild specific learning difficulties. The incidence is 1 in 2000 in newborn girls, but much higher at conception, representing nearly 2% of conceptions. Over 99% abort spontaneously, most in the first trimester. It should be explained to the parents when a diagnosis of Turner syndrome is made at amniocentesis that less than one fifth will survive to term. For those diagnosed by chorionic villus sampling this figure is probably less than 1% (Connor, 1986). Congenital malformations are found more frequently in Turner syndrome, especially coarctation of the aorta and renal malformations. Mean adult height is 143 centimetres and treatment with growth hormone may be beneficial in increasing final height, but remains controversial (Ranke and Saenger, 2001). The ovaries are present in fetal life, but then degenerate to streaks of tissue, resulting in amenorrhoea and lack of secondary sex characteristics. Occasionally a woman with Turner syndrome may menstruate, and rarely pregnancy may occur, although the offspring may be abnormal. Usually hormone replacement therapy is required in order to produce secondary sexual characteristics. Since the uterus is present, pregnancy is possible using ovum donation (Hovatta, 1999).

As in the other sex chromosome abnormalities, ascertainment bias originally led to an overestimate of the incidence of intellectual problems. The intelligence quotient is normal except that verbal ability tends to exceed performance, and visuo-spatial perceptual difficulties are common (Linden et al., 1996; Bender et al., 2001).

Outcome of pregnancies with a sex chromosome abnormality

When a sex chromosome abnormality is discovered prenatally, the parents should be offered expert counselling. This should include an explanation of the chromosome abnormality, and information about the anticipated effects, based on the prospective studies following newborn surveys.

There is great variation in what different healthcare professionals know, think and say about the same sex chromosome abnormality. It is essential that obstetric units should have an established protocol for giving results and for all staff who communicate results to have accurate, up-to-date information about the condition identified (Abramsky et al., 2001). Healthcare providers have an obligation to explore the meaning the information has for women and their partners to help decision-making, and if this is not within their expertise to refer to a genetic counsellor (Biesecker, 2001). Many parents ask to see relevant literature and photographs, but there is little suitable literature available at present, and textbooks tend to show extreme examples that may give a biased view. Showing photographs of patients whose parents have given their permission presents a more realistic picture (Clayton-Smith et al., 1989).

For parents facing a decision as to whether to continue the pregnancy, the main issues are the possibility of congenital abnormalities, the risk of mental retardation, the concern about behavioural problems, and the prospects for establishing sexual identity, future sexual relationships and a successful family life. In discussions with parents, the future happiness of the child is a major consideration, as are the effects on the wellbeing of the parents and other siblings.

There is wide variation in reports of the outcome of pregnancies with prenatally diagnosed sex chromosome abnormalities. Previous studies have shown rates of termination between 56% and 88% (Nielsen et al., 1986; Holmes-Seidle et al., 1987; Clayton-Smith et al., 1989). There is a tendency for more parents to opt to continue the pregnancy as more information from prospective studies becomes available (Holmes-Seidle et al., 1987; Christian et al., 2000). Currently the termination rate varies between 32% and 66%, but in one study in Germany the termination rate was as low as 13%, and was even lower where the couple were counselled according to information from unbiased studies (Meschede et al., 1998). A recent series from Israel, however, reported a termination rate of 80% (Sagi et al., 2001).

When confronted with a diagnosis of Turner syndrome prenatally, the parents may opt to continue the pregnancy, especially when they have been given the full information (Connor, 1986). In one series, however, all pregnancies with an abnormal ultrasound were terminated. One third of the remainder continued and all of these were mosaics with a normal cell line, who would be expected to show milder effect (Holmes-Seidle et al., 1987). The observation that termination is more commonly chosen for Turner syndrome and for Klinefelter syndrome than for other sex chromosome anomalies, could indicate that the prospect of infertility in an offspring is of major concern (Evans et al., 1990). Where the fetus has an XYY karyotype, decisions as to whether to continue the pregnancy are determined largely by the parents' expectations for their child and their concern that he might be disadvantaged in life and that psychological difficulties may cause him unhappiness. In one series (Holmes-Seidle et al., 1987) a decision to terminate was made more often by younger mothers and younger fathers, by couples with few previous children, in all cases with abnormal ultrasound findings, and when post-amniocentesis counselling was given by an obstetrician.

Parents are concerned as to when the child should be told about the abnormality, and who else might be told. This may lead to discussion as to whether problems are more likely to occur if they are expected – the self-fulfilling prophesy (Puck, 1981). To balance this, there is the view that early intervention to provide help for speech or behavioural problems, while requiring the support of teachers and others outside the family, may nevertheless be beneficial. There is some evidence that the outcome is better where the abnormality is diagnosed prenatally (Robinson *et al.*, 1992). This may be due in part to the supportive family environment and 'positive parenting' of these children, where the parents have made a conscious decision to continue.

It is estimated that less than 10% of males with an extra X or Y chromosome are detected prenatally. Postnatally the commonest indicator for karyotyping in a male with XYY will be developmental delay or behaviour problems and with XXY will be hypogonadism and/or infertility, but the majority will go through life without being karyotyped (Abramsky and Chapple, 1997).

Structural rearrangements

Chromosomes are prone to breakage and rejoining, which may give rise to a structural rearrangement, usually a translocation or inversion. Such rearrangements are found in about 1 in 1600 amniocenteses, and are the cause of considerable anxiety. If the rearrangement appears to be balanced, meaning that no active genetic material has been lost or added, and is found in one of the parents, there should be no harmful effects.

However, if it has occurred *de novo* (out of the blue) and is not found in either parent it could cause congenital abnormalities or mental retardation (Jacobs, 1974). This is because the rearrangement may not really be balanced, a small segment of chromosome having been gained or lost, or the break may have occurred within or close to a gene, causing disruption of its function. The phenotypic effects are unpredictable, and this leads to great difficulty for the parents in assessing whether or not to terminate the pregnancy.

The risk of abnormality is difficult to estimate because of ascertainment bias and can only be assessed reliably by follow-up of *de novo* translocations detected by chance prenatally (Donnai, 1989). The incidence of congenital abnormalities and mental retardation in one follow-up series was found to be increased 2–3 times over the general population risk (Warburton, 1991). This is lower than previous studies which have suggested a risk of up to 10% (Hsu, 1986). Problems common to all these studies have been the small numbers of cases, the short length of follow-up, and the difficulty in assessing the presence of an abnormality if the pregnancy was terminated. In one survey, about 25% of couples elected to terminate the pregnancy following counselling (Warburton, 1991). In another small series from a centre giving an optimistic prognosis only one in eight pregnancies was terminated, and this was for an abnormality detected on ultrasound (MacGregor *et al.*, 1989). Some reassurance can be offered if high resolution ultrasound examination is normal as this would be expected to detect one third of abnormalities (Warburton, 1991).

Supernumary marker chromosomes

A supernumary marker chromosome (an extra chromosome fragment) discovered prenatally causes similar difficulties to a structural rearrangement. Urgent karyotyping of the parents is needed and if one of the parents has the same supernumary marker it is presumed to be genetically inactive, with no increased risk of fetal abnormality. *De novo* markers are found in around one in 2500 amniocenteses and are associated with an increased risk of congenital malformations and mental handicap, but the size of this risk is difficult to assess because of ascertainment bias. Prospective studies of *de novo* markers found at amniocentesis showed an overall risk of abnormality of 13% (Warburton, 1991). Almost half of the pregnancies where a *de novo* marker was identified prenatally were terminated, reflecting the perception of the counsellors that the risk of abnormality is high (Warburton, 1991). Special cytogenetic techniques to identify the origin of the chromosome are now available which allow for more accurate risk estimation to be given (Crolla *et al.*, 1998).

Mosaicism

Chromosomal mosaicism is the mixture of two or more cell lines with different chromosome constitutions. Mosaicism found prenatally can cause difficulties in interpretation in the laboratory and causes anxiety in parents and counsellors. The problem is whether the abnormal cells are present in the fetus, and if so how this might affect the baby. The possibility of finding mosaicism should be explained during prenatal diagnosis counselling. True mosaicism occurs in about 1 in 500 amniocenteses (Hsu *et al.*, 1992), and even more frequently in chorionic villus sampling material since mosaicism is more common in the placenta than in the fetus. This confined placental mosaicism may arise early in embryonic development, or could arise from a vanishing twin (Gardner and Sutherland, 1996).

Specific details about the degree and type of mosaicism will influence the counselling given to the patient, and the extent to which further investigation is performed (Hsu *et al.*, 1997; Wallerstein *et al.*, 2000). The presence of an abnormality on high resolution ultrasound is likely to influence any decision regarding termination. Amniocentesis to confirm mosaicism found at chorionic villus sampling may be useful, but repeat amniocentesis is usually not helpful since a normal result does not invalidate the findings of the previous test. Fetal blood sampling may yield further information but is associated with a small risk of miscarriage and does not exclude mosaicism completely, even if all the cells sampled are normal (Gosden *et al.*, 1988). With certain types of mosaicism involving imprinted chromosomes, molecular studies to identify uniparental disomy may be indicated (Hsu *et al.*, 1997). In one series, termination was performed in 40% of cases of true mosaicism, and was more likely in autosomal than sex chromosome mosaicism (Hsu *et al.*, 1992).

THE FETUS AT RISK OF BEING AFFECTED

There are several circumstances in which the fetus is at risk of having a disability, but it is not known definitely to be affected. Parents may find it very difficult to decide whether the risk is sufficiently serious to warrant termination of the pregnancy, and may find counselling helpful.

This situation may arise if abnormalities are seen on ultrasound which could indicate that the baby has an underlying condition or syndrome associated with serious disability but there is no way of confirming this antenatally.

Similar difficulties occur when the mother is exposed to a possible teratogen early in the pregnancy. Parents need to know what defects might occur and the likelihood of the baby being affected. Some couples feel that any increased risk of abnormality is unacceptable and will opt for termination, whereas others wish to continue unless they are told that the baby is definitely abnormal.

Most couples who are at risk of having a son with Duchenne muscular dystrophy can now be offered accurate prenatal diagnosis, either by direct detection of the mutation or by linkage analysis. There are still couples for whom this is not possible and the only form of prenatal diagnosis is fetal sexing, with the option of termination if the fetus is male. A mother who has grown up with affected brothers may feel very strongly that she does not wish to take any risk, and may be prepared to go through more than one termination rather than have to face having an affected son herself. The options are similar if the mother is at risk of being a carrier for an X-linked condition for which there is no accurate prenatal diagnosis as yet, for example some forms of X-linked mental retardation.

Another situation where couples may opt for termination because of a risk (rather than a certainty) that the baby could have inherited a genetic disorder occurs if one of the couple has a parent with Huntington disease and does not wish to risk passing on the condition to the child. Prenatal diagnosis of Huntington disease can now be achieved by direct detection of the mutation in the gene, but if the partner at risk does not wish to know if he or she has inherited the gene, prenatal exclusion testing using linkage analysis can be offered. If the fetus has not inherited a chromosome from the relevant pair from the affected grandparent, it will be at very low risk of having the Huntington gene. If the fetus is shown to have inherited a chromosome from that pair from the affected grandparent, it will have a high risk, approaching 50%, of having the Huntington gene, and the couple may opt for termination (Tyler *et al.*, 1990). This is acceptable to couples who feel that, although they do not wish to know their own status regarding Huntington disease, they could not risk passing on the condition, but nevertheless have a strong desire for a child. They may be prepared to go through more than one termination to achieve this.

FACTORS AFFECTING DECISIONS REGARDING TERMINATION OF PREGNANCY WHERE THE DIAGNOSIS OR PROGNOSIS IS UNCERTAIN

All parents faced with the choice of whether or not to terminate a pregnancy for fetal abnormality have to make a very difficult decision. Not all will choose termination, even where prenatal diagnosis was done in order to detect the abnormality found (Verp *et al.*, 1988). Many factors influence the parents' decision. When the diagnosis or prognosis is unclear, as in the situations described above, the decision may cause even greater anguish. The counsellor has to provide a full and accurate explanation of the problem, as well as helping in the decision-making process and supporting the parents afterwards. A number of studies have tried to identify factors influencing the decision. While these are able to identify trends, it must be remembered that for each pregnancy the circumstances are unique, and the outcome will depend not only on the abnormality in the baby, but also the significance of the pregnancy to that particular couple, who have invested their future aspirations in their coming child.

The severity of the problem

One of the main factors in the parents' decision is the severity of the abnormality. When the prognosis was severe, such as for autosomal Trisomy, 93% of pregnancies were terminated, whereas in questionable abnormalities, such as apparently balanced translocations, 27% of parents opted for termination (Drugan et al., 1990). As discussed previously, the presence of a congenital malformation and the prospect of future infertility may influence the decision as to whether to terminate the pregnancy for a sex chromosome abnormality. The pregnancy is more likely to continue where mosaicism is present, since the effects would be expected to be milder (Holmes-Seidle et al., 1987; Robinson et al., 1992).

Experience of the condition

The couple's previous knowledge or experience of the condition may affect their decision. It is probably easier if they have experience of the problem in their own family or acquaintance as they will be aware of the burdens involved. This is apparent where a woman who has had a brother with Duchenne muscular dystrophy may prefer to terminate all pregnancies with a male fetus, rather than risk having an affected child. In more variable conditions their view will be coloured by the severity of the condition in the affected person they know. This might not be typical. Because of this variation, it might not always be helpful for a couple contemplating termination for an abnormality to make contact with affected families.

Gestational age

A decision to terminate the pregnancy after diagnosis of a chromosomal abnormality by chorionic villus sampling in the first trimester, when there is less emotional involvement with the fetus, would be expected to be less difficult than following amniocentesis. There is some evidence for this from one series, where 98% of affected pregnancies diagnosed by chorionic villus sampling were terminated, whereas 78% diagnosed by amniocentesis were terminated (Verp et al., 1988). Another survey found no difference, although this could be biased, as the two methods were not randomly assigned (Drugan et al., 1990). Termination might be less difficult in the first trimester, when there is more privacy, and less pressure from family and friends. The procedure is safer and less frightening, and might be expected to lead to less emotional sequelae. This is not necessarily the case, and the baby may be imagined as a real person from very early in pregnancy. Early termination may deny the possibility of seeing and holding the baby, and may make the loss harder to bear (Seller *et al.*, 1993; Statham *et al.*, 2001).

The effect of ultrasound

The presence of structural abnormality on ultrasound, having a more direct impact than an abnormal karyotype, is a highly significant factor in the decision to opt for termination (Holmes-Seidle *et al.*, 1987; Drugan *et al.*, 1990). On the other hand, since ultrasound enhances early parental bonding, a normal ultrasound scan reinforces the decision to continue the pregnancy when the risk of abnormality is low. Couples undergoing prenatal diagnosis who know beforehand that they may terminate the pregnancy (for example, for Duchenne muscular dystrophy) may wish to avoid seeing the baby on the scan, so that the decision to terminate the pregnancy is not made even more difficult. The parents' grief reaction may be more severe following termination of a pregnancy where ultrasound reveals an unexpected abnormality, in comparison to termination of a pregnancy known to be at increased risk of a genetic disorder (Dallaire *et al.*, 1995).

Family structure

Holmes-Seidle *et al.* (1987) found that older parents are less likely to terminate the pregnancy for a sex chromosome abnormality, possibly because they have less chance of having another baby, and more chance of having a severe abnormality next time. Parents continuing the pregnancy had more children than those choosing termination. This could be related to their age, or perhaps it reflects a greater desire for children in some parents. Alternatively, they may not have such high expectations of their new offspring if these have already been fulfilled by their existing children.

Socio-economic and cultural factors

Socio-economic and cultural factors inevitably affect the parents' decision. The more affluent parents in one series from the United States were more likely to terminate the pregnancy with a sex chromosome abnormality (Tannenbaum *et al.*, 1986). The financial circumstances of the family may be influential. One mother who felt unable to continue the pregnancy when the baby was found to have Klinefelter syndrome, was concerned that the demands of a child with behavioural problems or special needs would conflict with her job; as a single parent she would risk losing her only means of economic support.

Psychological factors

There are many other factors regarding the couple's feelings about the pregnancy that might be expected to influence their decision. The pregnancy may have been unplanned and unwelcome, and this may add to feelings of guilt if an abnormality is found and lead to paradoxically greater reluctance to terminate the pregnancy. This may also occur if there is revival of guilt feelings regarding a previous termination for social reasons. The pregnancy may be particularly precious, having been achieved after years of infertility, or after the loss of a previous pregnancy or child, or courageously in the face of a high risk of abnormality, or as a last chance in older parents. The baby's sex may be influential if it fulfils the desire for a boy or girl.

The couple may have strong religious or moral objections to termination, or feel revulsion towards it, or believe that it prevents nature taking its course. There is fear of the physical and long-term emotional burdens of termination, and fear of others knowing and being censorious.

These factors have to be weighed against the fear of having a disabled child, and the desire to prevent it from suffering, and concern about the effect on other siblings and the relationships within the family. Couples question their ability to cope, physically, emotionally, and financially with the extra burdens. They may have very high expectations for their child's future, particularly for a first child, which a disabled child could not fulfil. To quote from our own experience, this may have influenced the decision of one older childless couple to terminate the pregnancy when the baby was found to have an XYY karyotype whereas another mother with fewer socio-economic advantages and several children, one of whom had learning difficulties, decided to continue as she knew she would be able to cope.

Some parents tend to polarize their perceptions of the problem with the baby. Those who feel either that any increased risk of abnormality is unacceptable, or that they would not wish to terminate the pregnancy unless they knew that the baby would be severely affected, seem to find it easier to come to a decision.

The attitudes of others

Couples may be influenced by the attitudes of others. A woman's decision to terminate the pregnancy will partially depend on her partner's feelings, which she may feel have equal weight to her own. A partner may have strong views against termination that may sway her decision. Another may feel that it is for the mother to decide as she is more closely involved. Couples want to know how their decision will be viewed objectively by others, and often ask what the counsellor would do, or what most other couples have done in their situation. The counsellor should try to be non-directive, but information about what others have decided may help the couple to test the validity of their decision. There may, however, be a danger here of seeming to exert social pressures on the couple.

The effect of counselling

The decision to terminate is also influenced by the counselling received. Parents are more likely to continue the pregnancy when counselled by a geneticist rather than an obstetrician (Holmes-Seidle *et al.*, 1987). Geneticists would be expected to be better informed as to the prognosis with a sex chromosome abnormality, and can offer more encouraging information from prospective studies. They may be more inclined to offer non-directive counselling, with the aim of preserving the parents' autonomy.

The task of assisting a couple faced with an unexpected abnormality of uncertain significance in pregnancy is one of the most difficult in genetic counselling. The counsellor should try to see the couple together, without delay, and should try to reduce their level of stress. The information to be communicated is often complex and the lack of certainty is frustrating to both the parents and counsellor. There is often little time for reflection, but the counsellor should try to provide the framework for the couple to make their decision and support them afterwards. The role of the counsellor and the decision-making process itself is explored more fully below.

COUNSELLING IN PRENATAL DIAGNOSIS

It is understandable that when couples attend for genetic counselling, particularly prenatally, they are hoping for reassurance. For some, the term counselling implies a solution to be offered, a panacea. Sadly, often this is not the reality. In fact, as one study found, most are confronted with an inconclusive diagnosis, a chance or estimate of the numeric risk involved and ambiguity about the severity of the potential problem (van Zuuren *et al.*, 1997). It is concluded that the degree of uncertainty in the information provided is in direct contrast to the needs of the client. In view of this, it is not difficult to appreciate that the whole experience of genetic counselling is one likely to lead to client dissatisfaction (Shiloh *et al.*, 1990).

Counselling, at its simplest, can be defined as the process by which one person helps another to resolve a difficulty and decide upon an appropriate course of action. The Oxford Dictionary includes the phrases 'give advice' and 'recommend' within its definition. Currently, the emphasis in most counselling situations is towards a non-directive approach which aims to inform, support and encourage clients and allow them space and freedom within which they can make their own decisions. How far this can apply in prenatal diagnosis is debatable (Clarke, 1991; Pembrey 1991).

A number of approaches exist which define stages in counselling (Egan, 1998); some are more complex than others. Whatever method is employed, the aim should be to assist the client to make a valid and autonomous decision. To help determine whether this has been achieved, the Hastings Centre in the USA proposed the following short checklist of considerations that may be helpful (Miller, 1981):

- There is no such thing as 'free action'. There will always be pressures from somewhere and these need to be recognized.
- There must be a period of effective deliberation.
- The authenticity of any decision must be checked by the client so that they are not acting out of character or contrary to their own needs.
- There needs to be moral reflection in which the client decides whether the action proposed is reasonable, informed, right for them, and something they can live with.

Psychological support is essential throughout and after the prenatal counselling process (Skirton, 1995); it is suggested that follow up 3–6 months after the event may identify couples who would benefit from additional supportive counselling (Frets *et al.*, 1991a).

Trouble with figures

As already stated, genetic counselling deals with people who are in search of some certainty, but often there is none. The most that can then be offered is a possible outcome and a probable occurrence. Consequently, many geneticists, rightly or wrongly spend a significant proportion of their time relaying 'risk' figures to their clients. Therefore it is worth considering how these figures can be presented and how this can affect perceived risk (Thornton *et al.*, 1996).

Counsellors need to appreciate that the language of figures is as fraught with ambiguity as any other. To further confuse matters, there is a lack of consensus among practitioners regarding the level of probability conveyed by the descriptive words such as 'high', 'moderate' and 'low' (Parsons, 1993). The strategies used in comprehending risk figures have an impact on what the figures mean. When interviewed, one person looked at a risk of 10% of one million people as a large number of people and therefore a high risk, another as 10% off in a sale – a small saving and therefore a low risk (Kessler and Levine, 1987). Furthermore, there is no guarantee that the client will be able to understand the meaning of the figures at all, believing that a 1 in 20 risk of abnormality is preferable to 1 in 200. The severity of a disorder can affect the perception of the actual risk figure, and a low risk of a severe disorder may actually be seen as high (Frets *et al.*, 1990).

When communicating figures to clients, it can often be helpful to put them into an understandable context and also to frame risks in two ways, i.e. the chance of being affected *and* the chance of being unaffected. This will give the figures some perspective. It is also worth being aware that those who have had problems themselves, or who have been the 'one' in a 1 in 5000 risk situation, may perceive a low risk as being quite high. In fact, the whole validity of risk measurement is questionable when the actual figure may be of less concern to the patient, than the fact that they are in a state of being at risk (Lippman-Hand and Fraser, 1979).

Decision-making

However great the pressure of time may feel in an urgent prenatal situation, it is still important to ensure that there is some time allowed for reflection before couples make a major decision (Thornton *et al.*, 1996). Having to address a complex problem can be psychologically paralysing. It is common for people to postpone the decision for as long as possible. A decision taken at the last moment will often be impulsive, failing to take account of all the relevant factors. Couples need time to make decisions about termination of pregnancy, but they also need an endpoint, so that a decision to continue is not made by default – in effect having made no decision.

The more complex is the problem, the more difficult it is to resolve. First, short-term memory is stretched by having to keep track of several different alternatives, and people will often forget one aspect while dealing with others. Second, direct comparison between alternative options can be problematic when the outcomes are dissimilar in kind. Parents contemplating termination when the diagnosis or prognosis is uncertain may have to weigh the consequences of losing a healthy baby against the long-term stress of having an affected child.

The literature on decision-making contains a number of sophisticated tools intended to aid the decision-making process. Some of these have been applied to genetic counselling. One resembling Egan's three stage counselling process requires strict, sequential working through in order to reach a 'high quality' decision, with recognition of the effect of stress on the client's ability to make a decision (Janis and Mann, 1977). Another requires that recognition of the five sequential stages of the coping response (shock and denial, anxiety, anger and guilt, depression, and psychological homeostasis) is necessary before a valid decision can be made (Falek 1984). 'Decision trees' can be constructed, the intention being to arrive at a decision which is both 'rational' and 'logical' (Zarin and Pauker, 1984).

However, others (Lipmann-Hand and Fraser, 1979) dismiss such methods, favouring the use of a less structured approach emphasizing the tendency for clients to process complex issues into a binary form and adopt a broad view of the consequences of having an affected child. They advocate the use of 'worst case scenarios'' as a test of the client's ability to cope. Vlek (1987) explores an approach whereby desirability is weighed against expected stress. A situation is analysed in terms of desirable and undesirable outcomes, and the practical and emotional demands and coping abilities associated with them. The client determines the acceptability of various possible scenarios, including the best scenario, which helps to put into perspective other alternatives. For instance, parents need to be aware of the expectations they may have for their offspring in order to assess how they would cope should the disorder make these impossible to fulfil.

Psychological and social factors

Increasingly, there is recognition that decision-aiding processes need to take account of the various medical, psychological, social, religious, familial and financial implications of the decision. Human behaviour is not always a 'goal-oriented intellectual process' but sometimes a simpler or more direct procedure of permitting immediate rewards and punishments to dictate direction (Cross and Guyer, 1980). A client at risk of transmitting Huntington disease, who once felt that prenatal exclusion testing was a moral obligation, changed her mind because of the strain it might put on her new relationship. In this case, the immediate rewards of a stress-free relationship overrode previously held views and the threat of future punishment.

Bearing these factors in mind, another approach is that of the 'interpretive perspective' (Parsons, 1993). This starts with the acceptance of the beliefs and 'prior biography' the client brings to the counselling situation. Parsons points out that the client is not an empty container waiting to be filled with information. She respects the ability of the client to 'negotiate and construct' her life around the consequences of genetic disease. She calls on the genetic counsellor to recognize the many factors other than genetic risk that influence the client.

In a follow-up study of couples who had undergone genetic counselling (Frets *et al.*, 1990), it was demonstrated that the desire to have children remains a major motivator, despite genetic risk. This is confirmed by Wexler (1979) in connection with families at risk of Huntington disease. It is recognized by both, that an element in this, is the unconscious denial of the reality of the situation, countering the loss of self-esteem that results from the hereditary nature of the disorder.

There is conflicting evidence with regard to the impact of the availability of prenatal diagnosis on the decision-making process. Frets *et al.* (1990) found that in cases of high genetic risk, a significant number of couples refrained from having children when prenatal diagnosis was not possible. However, Sorenson *et al.* (1987) found that in the absence of prenatal diagnosis, clients with higher recurrence risks were in fact more likely to have children than those in lower risk categories. Other important factors appear to be experience of the disorder and interpretation of recurrence risks.

In practice, most counsellors will be familiar with what can, at first, appear to be irrational considerations by clients. Frets *et al.* (1991b) encourages acceptance of such considerations as important, as they are likely to reflect the influence of unconscious motives. Therefore it is advocated that genetic counsellors focus primarily on understanding clients' feelings. It is also important to be aware of the role played by guilt feelings towards parents or affected siblings.

Although much of the work in this field remains inconclusive and sometimes contradictory, a broad consensus is beginning to emerge. It is evident from research into reproductive decision-making that there is growing acceptance of a more holistic and client-centred view. The prime need is to be flexible, and to borrow any method that seems appropriate in a given situation. The role of the counsellor then becomes that of a reliable informer and facilitator, who works within the agenda that is set by the pre-existing plans and beliefs that the family hold.

Key points

- Prenatal diagnosis for a chromosome abnormality should include an explanation that an unexpected abnormality may be detected where the outcome is difficult to predict.
- After the discovery of an unexpected chromosome abnormality the parents should be offered expert counselling with up to date information.
- The majority of sex chromosome abnormalities involving an additional X or Y chromosome would not be detected postnatally as the individual would not stand out from the general population.
- Decisions regarding termination depend on many factors, including the severity and previous experience of the condition, gestational age, the presence of an ultrasound abnormality, socio-economic and cultural factors, religious beliefs and the way in which information about the condition is communicated.
- Supportive counselling for women or couples facing the option of termination should focus on their needs and aim to facilitate a positively made decision that they can live with.
- Despite the pressure of time in the prenatal situation, a period should always be allowed for reflection before a final decision is made.

REFERENCES

Abramsky L, Chapple J (1997) 47,XXY (Klinefelter syndrome) and 47,XYY: estimated rates of and indication for postnatal diagnosis with implications for prenatal counselling. *Prenatal Diagnosis*, 18; 303–304.

Abramsky L, Hall S, Levitan J et al. (2001) What parents are told after prenatal diagnosis of a sex chromosome abnormality: interview and questionnaire study. *British Medical Journal*, 322; 441–442.

Bender BG, Linden MG, Harmon RJ (2001) Neuropsychological and functional cognitive skills of 35 unselected adults with sex chromosome abnormalities. *American Journal of Medical Genetics*, 102; 309–313.

Biesecker B (2001) Prenatal diagnoses of sex chromosome conditions. *British Medical Journal*, 322; 463–466.

Christian SM, Koehn D, Pillay R et al. (2000) Parental decisions following prenatal diagnosis of sex chromosome aneuploidy: a trend over time. *Prenatal Diagnosis*, 20; 37–40.

Clarke A (1991) Is non-directive genetic counselling possible? *Lancet*, ii; 998–1001.

Clayton-Smith J, Andrews T, Donnai D (1989) Genetic counselling and parental decisions following antenatal diagnosis of sex chromosome aneuploidies. *Journal of Obstetrics and Gynaecology*, 10; 5–7.

Connor JM (1986) Prenatal diagnosis of the Turner syndrome; what to tell the parents. *British Medical Journal*, 293; 711–712.

Crolla JA, Long F, Rivera H et al. (1998) FISH and molecular study of autosomal supernumerary marker chromosomes excluding those derived from chromosomes 15 and 22: 1. Results of 26 new cases. *American Journal of Medical Genetics*, 75; 355–366.

Cross J, Guyer M (1980) *Social Traps*. University of Michigan Press, Ann Arbor, MI.

Dallaire L, Lortie G, Des Rochers M *et al.* (1995) Parental reaction and adaptability to prenatal diagnosis of fetal defect or genetic disease leading to pregnancy interruption. *Prenatal Diagnosis*, 15; 249–259.

Donnai D (1989) The clinical significance of *de novo* structural rearrangements and markers detected prenatally by amniocentesis. *Journal of Medical Genetics*, 26; 545.

Drugan A, Greb A, Johnson MP *et al.* (1990) Determinants of parental decisions to abort for chromosome abnormalities. *Prenatal Diagnosis*, 10; 483–490.

Editorial (1988) Klinefelter's syndrome. *Lancet*, ii; 1316–1317.

Egan G (1998) *The Skilled Helper*. Brooks/Cole; CA.

Evans JA, MacDonald K, Hammerton JL (1990) Sex chromosomes anomalies: prenatal diagnosis and the need for continued prospective studies. In: *Children and Young Adults with Sex Chromosome Aneuploidy* (eds Evans JA, Hammerton JL, Robinson A). Wiley-Liss for the National Foundation – March of Dimes, New York, pp. 273–281.

Falek A (1984) Sequential aspects of coping and other issues in decision making in genetic counselling. In: *Psychological Aspects of Genetic Counselling* (eds Emery AEH Pullen IM). Academic Press, London, pp. 23–36.

Frets PG, Duivenvoorden HJ, Verhage F *et al.* (1990) Factors influencing the reproductive decision after genetic counselling. *American Journal of Medical Genetics*, 34; 496–502.

Frets PG, Duivenvoorden HJ, Verhage F *et al.* (1991a) Analysis of problems in making the reproductive decision after genetic counselling. *Journal of Medical Genetics*, 28(3); 194–200.

Frets PG, Verhage F, Niermeijer MF (1991b) Characteristics of the post–counselling reproductive decision making process: an explorative study. *American Journal of Medical Genetics*, 40(3): 298–303.

Gardner RJM, Sutherland GR (1996) *Chromosome Abnormalities and Genetic Counselling*. Oxford Monographs on Medical Genetics, No 29 (eds Motulsky, AG, Bobrow M, Harper PS, *et al.*). Oxford University Press, Oxford, p. 315.

Gosden CM, Nicolaides KH, Rodeck CH (1988) Fetal blood sampling in investigation of chromosome mosaicism in amniotic fluid cell culture. *Lancet*, i; 613–617.

Holmes-Seidle M, Ryyanen M, Lindenbaum RH (1987) Parental decisions regarding termination of pregnancy following prenatal detection of sex chromosome abnormality. *Prenatal Diagnosis*, 7; 239–44.

Hovatta O (1999) Pregnancies in women with Turner's syndrome. *Annals of Medicine*, 31; 106–110.

Hsu LYF (1986) Prenatal diagnosis of chromosome abnormalities. In: *Genetic Disorders and the Fetus*, (2nd edn) (ed. Milunsky A). Plenum Press, New York.

Hsu LYF, Kaffe S, Jenkins EC *et al.* (1992) Proposed guidelines for diagnosis of chromosome mosaicism in amniocytes based on data derived from chromosome mosaicism and pseudomosaicism studies. *Prenatal Diagnosis*, 12; 555–573.

Hsu LYF, Yu MT, Neu RL *et al.* (1997) Rare Trisomy mosaicism diagnosed in amniocytes, involving an autosome other than chromosomes 13, 18, 20, and 21: karyotype/phenotype correlations. *Prenatal Diagnosis*, 17; 201–242.

Jacobs P (1974) Correlation between euploid structural rearrangements and mental subnormality in humans. *Nature*, 249; 164–165.

Janis J, Mann L (1977) *Decision Making: a Psychological Analysis of Conflict, Choice and Commitment*. Free Press, New York.

Kessler S, Levine EK (1987) Psychological aspects of genetic counselling. 4. The subjective assessment of probability. *American Journal of Medical Genetics*, 28; 361–370.

Leonard MF(1990) A prospective study of development of children with sex chromosome abnormalities. In: *Children and Young Adults with Sex Chromosome Aneuploidy* (eds Evans JA, Hammerton JL, Robinson A). Wiley-Liss for the National Foundation – March of Dimes, New York. BD:OAS 26(4); 117–130.

Linden MG, Bender BG, Robinson A (1996) Intrauterine diagnosis of sex chromosome aneuploidy. *Obstetrics and Gynecology*, 87; 468–475.

Lippman-Hand A, Fraser FC (1979) Genetic counselling – the post counselling period: 1. Parents perceptions of uncertainty. *American Journal of Medical Genetics*, 4; 51–71.

MacGregor DJ, Imrie S, Tolmie JL (1989) Outcome of *de novo* balanced translocations ascertained prenatally. *Journal of Medical Genetics*, 26; 590–591.

Meschede D, Louwen F, Nippert I *et al.* (1998) Low rates of pregnancy termination for prenatally diagnosed Klinefelter syndrome and other sex chromosome polysomies. *American Journal of Medical Genetics*, 80; 330–334.

Miller BL (1981) *Hastings Centre Report*, 11(4); 22–28.

Nielsen J, Wohlert M, Faaborg-Andersen J *et al.* (1986) Chromosome examination of 20,222 newborn children: Results from a 7.5 year study in Arhus, Denmark. In *Prospective Studies in Children with Sex Chromosome Aneuploidy* (eds Ratcliffe SG, Paul N). Wiley-Liss for the National Foundation – March of Dimes, New York. B.D:O.A.S, 22(3); 209–219.

Parsons EP (1993) Genetic risk and reproduction. *Sociological Review*, 41; 4.

Pembrey M (1991) Non-directive genetic counselling. *Lancet*, ii; 1266–1267.

Poulakis V, Witzsch U, Diehl W *et al.* (2001) Birth of two infants with normal karyotype after intracytoplasmic injection of sperm obtained by testicular extraction from two men with non-mosaic Klinefelter's syndrome. *Fertility and Sterility*, 76; 1060–1062.

Puck MH (1981) Some considerations bearing on the doctrine of self-fulfilling prophesy in sex chromosome aneuploidy. *American Journal of Medical Genetics*, 9; 129–137.

Ranke MB, Saenger P (2001) Turner's syndrome. *Lancet*, 358; 309–314.

Ratcliffe S (1999) Long-term outcome in children of sex chromosome abnormalities. *Archives of Disease in Childhood*, 80; 192–195.

Robinson A, Bender BG, Linden MG (1992) Prognosis of prenatally diagnosed children with sex chromosome aneuploidy. *American Journal of Medical Genetics*, 44; 365–368.

Sagi M, Meiner V, Reshef N *et al.* (2001) Prenatal diagnosis of sex chromosome aneuploidy: possible reasons for high rates of pregnancy termination. *Prenatal Diagnosis*, 21; 461–465.

Seller M, Barnes C, Ross S *et al.* (1993) Grief and mid-trimester fetal loss. *Prenatal Diagnosis*, 13; 341–348.

Shiloh S, Avdor O, Goodman RM (1990) Satisfaction with Genetic Counselling: Dimensions and Measurement. *American Journal of Medical Genetics*, 37; 522–529.

Skirton H (1995) Psychological implications of advances in genetics. *Professional Nurse*, 10(9); 597–598.

Statham H, Solomou W, Green JM (2001) *When a Baby has an Abnormality: A Study of Parents' Experiences.* Centre for Family Research, University of Cambridge.

Sorenson JR, Scotch NA, Swazey JP *et al.* (1987) Reproductive plans of genetics counseling clients not eligible for prenatal diagnosis. *American Journal of Medical Genetics*, 28; 345–352.

Tannenbaum HL, Perlis TE, Arbeitel BE *et al.* (1986) Analysis of decision to continue or terminate pregnancies diagnosed with sex chromosome abnormalities by severity of prognosis, socioeconomic level and sex of the fetus. *American Journal of Human Genetics*, 39; 183A.

Thornton JG, van den Borne MP, de Bruijn AJ (1996) Risk Communication; the patient's view. *Early Human Development*, 47 (Suppl); S13–S17.

Tyler A, Quarrell OJW, Lazarou LP *et al.* (1990) Exclusion testing in pregnancy for Huntington's disease. *Journal of Medical Genetics*, 27; 488–495.

van Zuuren, FJ, van Schie EC, van Baaren NK (1997) Uncertainty in the information provided during genetic counselling. *Patient Education Counselling*; 32(1–2); 129–139.

Verp MS, Bombard AT, Simpson JL *et al.* (1988) Parental decision following prenatal diagnosis of fetal chromosome anomalies. *American Journal of Medical Genetics*, 29; 613–622.

Vlek C (1987) Risk assessment, risk perception and decision making about courses of action involving genetic risk: an overview of concepts and methods. In: *Genetic Risk, Risk Perception and Decision Making* (eds Evers Kiebooms G, Cassiman J, Van den Berghe H, *et al.*). Wiley-Liss for the National Foundation – March of Dimes, New York. Birth Defects Original Article Series. 23(2); 171–207.

Wallerstein R, Yu MT, Neu RL *et al.* (2000) Common Trisomy mosaicism diagnosed in amniocytes involving chromosomes 13, 18, 20 and 21: karyotype–phenotype correlations. *Prenatal Diagnosis*, 20; 103–122.

Warburton D (1991) *De novo* balanced chromosome rearrangements and extra marker chromosomes identified at prenatal diagnosis: clinical significance and distribution of breakpoints. *American Journal of Human Genetics*, 49; 995–1013.

Wexler N (1979) Genetic Russian roulette: the experience of being at risk for Huntington's disease. In: *Genetics Counselling: Psychological Dimensions* (ed. Kessler S). Academic Press, London.

Zarin DA, Pauker SG (1984) Decision analysis as a basis for medical decision making: the tree of Hippocrates. *Journal of Medicine and Philosophy*, 9; 181–213.

13

Continuing a pregnancy after the diagnosis of an anomaly: parents' experiences

Helen Statham, Wendy Solomou and Josephine M. Green

Introduction

The first edition of this book contained a number of chapters on parents' experiences of termination of pregnancy after a prenatal diagnosis of fetal abnormality. Throughout the book it was obvious that there was another choice that could be made after a diagnosis: not to terminate the pregnancy. Parents who made that decision were mentioned: one mother's 'terribly stressful pregnancy' after a diagnosis of anencephaly; another's preference to have a Down syndrome baby rather than no baby (Abramsky, 1994). Yet even in a book that addressed many sensitive aspects around prenatal diagnosis, there was little consideration of what it was like for parents continuing a pregnancy. This chapter seeks to remedy the previous omission. First, however, we will raise two important questions: 'what do we mean by an anomaly'? and 'how do parents come to be *continuing* a pregnancy'?

What do we mean by an anomaly?

When people think about prenatal testing, they usually associate this with the diagnosis of serious conditions. This was highlighted recently when one of the authors was talking about parents who had continued pregnancies after confirmed prenatal diagnoses. A midwife present discussed her prior perception of a continuing pregnancy. She would not have seen a mother whose baby had, for example, cleft lip as 'continuing'; that definition was reserved for mothers whose babies had conditions such as Down syndrome or spina bifida.

We use the word 'anomaly' here to include the full range and variety of conditions that might be detected prenatally, some of which would be thought of as less serious and others as more serious abnormalities. Defining anomalies in terms of severity or seriousness has been a source of concern to us. We use the terms 'serious/severe' and 'less serious/severe' cautiously, not implying any judgement of the decisions that different parents make when confronted with conditions of different prognoses. However, it is the case that for some conditions, e.g. Down syndrome or Edwards syndrome, the large majority of parents choose to terminate the pregnancy, whereas relatively few do for conditions such as cleft lip or unilateral renal agenesis. This finding in itself goes some way to showing how parents themselves define conditions as severe and less severe. The ethos underpinning our interpretation of what parents say is that all parents are deeply distressed by news of any abnormality diagnosed and find subsequent decisions very difficult; none take decisions lightly. Different conditions will have different short- and long-term implications for the babies. However, the immediate impact of a diagnosis for the parents is not dependent on objective measures of 'severity' or 'seriousness'.

What do different anomalies mean for babies?

Parents form their opinion as to the severity of a diagnosed abnormality according to the prognosis for their baby, although in some cases prognosis is uncertain. There is a range of possible outcomes. The anomaly diagnosed can be:

- lethal, such as anencephaly, triploidy or absent kidneys;
- non-correctable, with the prognosis of moderate to severe disability, such as Down syndrome, spina bifida and missing limbs;
- non-correctable, with uncertainty as to the long-term effects, such as sex chromosome anomalies;
- of uncertain prognosis such as some renal anomalies that might disappear after birth or only require antibiotic treatment or which might require risky surgery;
- treatable, but with varying degrees of associated risk, such as diaphragmatic hernia, many heart abnormalities, and cleft lip and palate.

The level of risk associated with treatable conditions varies. Risks of surgery for major heart abnormalities are very high and more than one operation is often required, each carrying a risk of death or damage to the baby. Surgery to correct a diaphragmatic hernia is risky, as is any major surgery on a new-born baby, but mostly one operation will be sufficient and the risks are less than for heart surgery. Surgery for other conditions, such as cleft lip and palate, is more predictable and carries less risk.

What do different anomalies mean for the ongoing pregnancy?

Although in this chapter we will discuss very little about antenatal care for a mother of a baby with an anomaly, this is an important issue (Statham *et al.*, 2001, 2002); different types of malformation require different patterns of care and monitoring of the baby. Where the malformation is lethal, whatever the monitoring, the baby will not live. Monitoring will inform parents as to whether or not the baby is alive, but only the timing of the delivery might be influenced if the baby dies *in utero*. Other conditions (e.g. diaphragmatic hernia, heart malformations) require regular observation to ensure the health of the baby is not deteriorating. Monitoring may identify when intervention *in utero* is needed or when, where and how the baby should be born for optimal wellbeing.

In other situations, there is no need to monitor the baby. Antenatal care can be normal for that pregnancy, once the abnormality has been confirmed. Babies with cleft lip and palate, sex chromosome abnormalities (excluding Turner syndrome) and even Down syndrome are no more likely to develop problems *in utero* than other babies (although babies with Down syndrome may develop hydrops). Specific care may be needed after delivery, but it is not specialized care that has to be ready at the moment of birth.

HOW DO PARENTS COME TO BE CONTINUING WITH A PREGNANCY?

Some parents are not given a choice between terminating or continuing with a pregnancy after prenatal diagnosis, either because the abnormality is not deemed severe enough by clinicians or because the diagnosis is made too late in pregnancy. Severity may be less important in the UK as termination of pregnancy is legal before 24 weeks even when no abnormality is present, and UK law permits termination for serious abnormality at any gestation (Fisk, 2001), but this is not the situation in all countries. These points are discussed further in Statham *et al.* (2000) and Statham (2002). A small number of parents make no choice because they are overtaken by events: the baby may die, or labour start unexpectedly while diagnosis is ongoing or during decision-making. The duration of such an ongoing pregnancy is usually short. These parents have not terminated their pregnancy but neither have they chosen to continue.

Many of the parents who continue with a pregnancy after a prenatal diagnosis do so because that is their choice. They are given the option of termination or continuing and for a variety of reasons they make the decision that they wish the pregnancy to continue.

A number of studies have reported the factors that appear to relate to the decision that parents make (reviewed in Green and Statham, 1996; Marteau and Mansfield, 1998; Statham *et al.*, 2000; Marteau and Dormandy, 2001; Statham, 2002). Factors such as gestation, severity, ultrasound visibility of the abnormality, who counsels the parents, and cultural differences have all been implicated, but there is inconsistency in findings across various studies. Our research (Statham and Solomou, unpublished) based on interview-derived data, suggests that one or more of four main factors influence decision-making for most parents:

- severity of the abnormality;
- parents' prior attitudes to, and beliefs about termination;
- perceived impact (on themselves and others) of having the baby;
- gestation at diagnosis.

It should be noted that perceptions of severity are individual. Prior attitudes, which may derive from religious beliefs, personal morality or prior experiences do not always predict decisions; 'others' that are considered are close family rather than wider society; and very few parents actually invoke gestation as being of major influence. Over and above these main factors, decision-making takes place against a background of situational factors including pressures of time, social relationships, various aspects of information (its consistency, source, accessibility and presentation), whether it is a twin pregnancy, and whether the parents have seen the baby on ultrasound.

WHEN A BABY HAS AN ABNORMALITY: A STUDY OF PARENTS' EXPERIENCES

In describing parents' experiences of continuing with a pregnancy after prenatal diagnosis we will use data from our recent longitudinal study (1996–2001) which explored the experiences of 72 women who had received a prenatal diagnosis of fetal abnormality and did not make the decision to terminate the pregnancy. Full details can be found in Statham *et al.* (2001). Diagnoses were made between 17 and 37 weeks' gestation. Twenty women did not discuss the option of termination and four were 'overtaken by events' with the baby being born before any decision was made. Three women were pregnant with twins and only one of the babies had an abnormality. Parents of 45 singleton pregnancies considered both options and decided to continue with the pregnancy.

Forty-one women were pregnant at the time they were first interviewed. Of the 31 babies already born, 13 were alive, 10 had been stillborn and 8 had died after birth. The babies had been diagnosed with a range of abnormalities, including lethal conditions, Down syndrome, spina bifida, gastroschisis, diaphragmatic hernia, renal abnormalities and facial clefting.

The data presented here have mainly been drawn from interviews that took place soon after diagnosis. Additional data were collected by postal questionnaires and interviews over the following year, when some parents reflected on the pregnancy period as well as discussing their current situation with their baby. We can learn from these 'looking-back' accounts; some parents said it was only then, when the baby was born, and usually (but not always) doing well, that they allowed themselves to acknowledge what had happened and how they had felt:

> M: ... *at the time it was all very overwhelming, and I was only keeping things together by the skin of my teeth really* ... . *I felt if I even talked to anyone about it, it would just open the floodgates, and I just didn't think I would be able to carry on.*
>
> (A year after the diagnosis of omphalocoele)

PREVIOUS RESEARCH

Previous research, which we have reviewed elsewhere (Statham *et al.*, 2000) concentrates mainly on very serious or lethal anomalies and tends to focus on the longer term rather than the pregnancy. The experience of having a less serious anomaly diagnosed has been largely ignored. For lethal abnormalities, parents' feelings have been compared with perceptions of what they might have been had the pregnancy been terminated (Watkins, 1989; Lilford *et al.*, 1994; Chitty *et al.*, 1996; Sandelowski and Jones, 1996a, 1996b; Redlinger-Grosse *et al.*, 2002). The message that emerges from some of these reports is that not to terminate may be better for a woman's emotional well being; women who continue a pregnancy may avoid the guilt they might have felt had they terminated. These studies are mostly small: one woman in the study by Watkins and five in that by Chitty. Where feelings have been measured in larger studies, data show that the nature and course of women's distress following spontaneous perinatal loss and following termination are similar (Zeanah *et al.*, 1993; Salveson *et al.*, 1997; Statham *et al.*, 2001).

It is important to take note of issues raised by individuals, and to consider care and practice in the light of what even small numbers of parents say, as for example the recommendations by Chitty *et al.* (1996) concerning communication, continuity of care, personalized care and training for health professionals. It is equally important not to generalize without sufficient evidence. Thus the woman described by Watkins has been exemplified as evidence that continuing a pregnancy with a lethal malformation is a good thing. It may be, for some women, in some situations. In our own study, parents who had terminated pregnancies had welcomed the opportunity to talk about their options: termination or continuing. When the abnormality was lethal, however, a number of study participants expressed similar views to the mother cited below after a diagnosis of anencephaly:

> M: ... *he then said, you know you have two choices – how can I have choices – you've just told me this child's got no top to its head – and he said you can either have a termination or the other choice is that you leave it and you have the baby, and I'm looking at him thinking are you completely mad?*

Where non-lethal malformations are diagnosed, different issues arise depending on the condition, since these anomalies present with a range of severity and possible outcomes. Again, the literature tells us little of how parents feel about being pregnant after the diagnosis, although there is a growing literature concerning the short-term outcome for the infants. Madarikan *et al.* (1990) and Kemp *et al.* (1998) reported an increase in anxiety levels in both women and their partners after the prenatal diagnosis of structural, and potentially treatable malformations. A mother reported by Armstrong (1996) described knowing prenatally about Down syndrome as 'dreadful' and by the end of pregnancy thought it had been a mistake to know. She resented being admired for her decision and the presumption that her child would be happy.

More recently studies have begun to explore the nature and experience of pregnancy after a prenatal diagnosis (Edwins, 2000; Finnemore, 2000; Redlinger-Grosse *et al.*, 2002). They discuss the implications for health professionals caring for parents and reinforce earlier recommendations; they address issues of communication, sensitivity and organization. Finnemore identified uncertainty as the main characteristic of the experience of continuing; the remainder of the pregnancy is the time to try to resolve uncertainties with psychological coping strategies such as grieving, denial and seeking information. Issues of shock at diagnosis, grief for the loss of the expected healthy baby, and isolation from family and health professionals after the decision to continue have been highlighted.

PARENTS' EXPERIENCES OF CONTINUING A PREGNANCY AFTER PRENATAL DIAGNOSIS

Whatever abnormality is diagnosed, once it is certain that the pregnancy will be continuing, parents enter a world of significant uncertainty, described by one father as 'a voyage of discovery'. A number of themes dominated the accounts parents gave of the pregnancy. Those related to care and how it was, or was not, organized and coordinated are discussed in detail elsewhere (Statham *et al.*, 2001). We will focus here on personal, practical and emotional aspects of the pregnancy.

It is important to remember that for some parents the pregnancy is a time of frequent re-adjustment to changing news even after a 'confirmed diagnosis'; for example about survival or about additional abnormalities which are found.

FEELINGS ABOUT A DIFFERENT PREGNANCY AND A DIFFERENT BABY

Parents' own words describe clearly what it feels like to be expecting a baby with an abnormality:

> M: *I was glad they'd found out, but in another way I didn't, because it spoilt the pregnancy for me.*

> (Heart abnormalities)

> M: *I don't actually feel like a pregnant person. I feel like I've got a baby with a problem.*

> (Diaphragmatic hernia)

> M: *I felt really strange about the baby. I felt like somebody had taken away a healthy baby that I had inside me, and put one there with something wrong with it. It's a horrible feeling.*

> (Cleft lip)

Others spoke of feeling 'in limbo' and 'regret that I had made the decision to have another baby'. Many found it hard to express negative feelings, partly because of optimism that family and friends displayed:

> M: *We had people right up to really the end saying, 'oh, they can be wrong, they can be wrong'. You felt like screaming sometimes, you know.*

> (Lethal chromosome anomaly confirmed by amniocentesis)

After a diagnosis, family and friends, who themselves were upset and anxious, tried to be supportive with optimistic talk. This denied parents the sad reality of their situation. One mother commented about the research interview that it had been helpful to talk to someone with no interest in being reassuring or making things better, who 'wasn't trying to mend anything' as had been her experience of well-meaning family and friends. Health professionals' emphasis on the future was, similarly, not necessarily what parents wanted to hear:

> M: *Like they were saying, 'oh, it will be all right, they can do so much this day and age'. And – but at that time that's not what I wanted to hear, and that's not still what I want to hear.*
>
> (Cleft lip)

This mother wanted her midwife to acknowledge the negative feelings about the diagnosis that went alongside her hopes that her baby could undergo successful treatment.

Knowledge of the sex of the baby could have a special significance for some parents told of an abnormality:

> M: *I rang [consultant] again the next day. I said – I would like to know what sex the baby is, because I've got to really I'd bonded with the baby, but I didn't want to think of it as our Downs baby. I wanted to think of it as him or her. And you [partner] said yes, I agree with that.*

Parents talked about the importance of being able to relate to the baby, to give that baby his or her own identity beyond being just an abnormality or syndrome. In talking about the sex of their baby, parents could envisage a future child as opposed to a future problem.

HAVING EMOTIONAL NEEDS

Throughout the pregnancy, parents described concerns and worries about many issues including:

- ambivalence about the decision;
- differing attitudes of partners;
- attitudes and reactions of other family members, including children;
- their ability to cope in the future;
- other stressful events in their lives.

There appeared little provision to meet parents' needs for emotional support around these issues, unless parents sought this for themselves. However, distressed parents often found it difficult to make a move in asking for emotional help. They were particularly distraught if, as sometimes happened, messages left on a counsellor's answerphone were unanswered.

THE USE OF SUPPORT GROUPS

Many parents talked favourably about the valuable service offered by voluntary sector groups providing information, support, and the possibility of making contact with someone who has been in a similar situation. Not all parents wish for the same degree of contact, but groups are accustomed to meeting the varied and specific needs of those who approach them:

> M: *Good to know that people get through this and end up with a happy normal child. Very clear information (photos – not too graphic), and very*

specific. I didn't want to look at the leaflet, but once I had, I was feeling more positive and less emotional than I had expected.

(Gastroschisis, Exomphalos, Extrophies Parents' Support {GEEPS})

F: I'd phoned the Cleft Lip and Palate Association (CLAPA) up the day after we went to see Dr [X], and spoke to the lady there, and she was brilliant ... she was so friendly and so nice. She really did put me at sort of ease.

M: CLAPA sent me out a load of information, which was brilliant. And it was really good for [partner] because he sat down and read it; then a few days later he'd sit back down and read it again.

M: She was saying about all the help you get, you get occupational therapy – because I didn't know none of this, you know. Nobody had told me at that stage. That's what I find more helpful, is talking to people with Down children, and going to see the baby as well.

(re Down's Syndrome Association)

Provision of information about support groups was erratic. Parents were more often told about groups for well-known conditions. Information about unusual abnormalities was less widely available and harder to find (although the Internet may change this). It was often left to parents to seek out relevant groups. Contact a Family (www.cafamily.org.uk) is a useful organization with information for parents and health professionals about rare conditions and existing support groups.

FEARS AND CONCERNS ABOUT PRACTICAL ASPECTS OF CARE

Many parents described practical concerns associated with the demands of their 'different' pregnancy. These included arranging and affording child care; costs of travel and time off work; worries about getting to the 'right' (i.e. specialist) hospital if they went into labour unexpectedly; and whether the special care unit would have a cot for their baby. Table 13.1 shows how many women (out of 51) identified with each of the concerns listed in a questionnaire at the end of our study period.

Table 13.1 Practical concerns during pregnancy expressed by 51 women

Concern	Number of women	% of women
Costs of travel	15	29%
Costs of time off work	10	20%
Car parking	18	35%
Child care for other children	16	31%
Getting to right hospital if labour started	18	35%
Worry that SCBU would be full	8	16%

Some mothers just commented: 'the whole experience was difficult to cope with' (heart abnormality); 'just very worried about everything' (cleft lip)'; 'I didn't worry about practical things – I was too much in a daze to do so' (maternal infection).

Dealing with non-clinical concerns took second place to determining optimal care for the unborn baby, with health professionals not thinking about these issues and parents doing anything for the health of their baby, whatever the personal costs. We would suggest that recognition of such concerns, addressing them and attempting to ameliorate them could become part of the package of care for parents continuing a pregnancy. For example, costs are less if parents who live far away from specialist centres are given appointment times to fit with reduced price train tickets. More research might usefully determine how much care needs to be in specialist, distant, hospitals as opposed to locally.

The issue of getting to the 'right' hospital (i.e. the one that had been arranged) for the baby to be born, was raised by many parents. For some, concerns could be resolved if the birth took place at the local hospital with immediate transfer of the baby. For others, early admission prevented anxiety. Overall, uncertainty about getting to the right place created a sense of vulnerability for some women who spent substantial amounts of time and energy seeking out ambulance stations for information about where they would be taken if labour started unexpectedly:

> M: *Getting to the right hospital worried me more than anything; I lost a lot of sleep over it. I even went to the ambulance station to ask what would happen as my GP, health visitor and consultant didn't know.*
>
> (A year after diagnosis)

THE UNCERTAIN FUTURE

Uncertainty and anticipation of an uncertain future characterizes pregnancy for all parents with a baby with an abnormality. Even with lethal abnormalities, there is uncertainty about when the baby will die; the implications of other malformations can only be known after birth. Some parents experience conflicting emotions as the pregnancy comes to an end:

> F: *... sort of torn between enjoying life now because we know an extra burden is going to come, and actually wanting that time to hurry up.*
>
> (Spina bifida)

Sometimes, partners react differently as the birth approaches. Fathers appear more likely to 'take it as it comes' while mothers need to plan for all eventualities:

> F: *... for you it seems to be actually getting this period over with as quickly as possible.*

M: Yes, I hate to wish my life away. But on the other hand, the uncertainty that happens after that which, for me, I want to get over and done with . . . .
F: It's just time to get things sorted out. And get a nanny sorted out.
I: What words best describe how you feel now?
M: Well in limbo again, but in more controlled limbo, but I think that we're now going towards a date at which the world is going to explode and still we don't know what, and I think we can prepare for that as well as we can, but I still think that we're in for a very big shock, just actually seeing the baby's going to be an enormous shock. And I don't think you [father] think about things like that at all, which is where – that's fine – but sometimes I feel that if I don't point it out to you at given stages, that the shock's going to be worse for you, so occasionally I do prompt you, whether I'm right or wrong . . . .
I: What about you?
F: I have thought about it. I just don't know – I'll take it as it comes. I suppose I think that I don't tend to get – I don't think of possibilities – I try and deal with more – I don't go through all the permutations of what might happen then.

(Omphalocoele)

ADVANTAGES AND DISADVANTAGES OF PRENATAL DIAGNOSIS

During pregnancy, most parents only talked about advantages of knowing prenatally about the baby's abnormality: having choices, being prepared for the birth and/or death of their child, and for the baby to be born in the right place to give the optimum chance of a good outcome. A year later, these benefits were often contrasted with the disadvantages of knowing: preparation versus a spoilt pregnancy, the opportunity to make a choice versus the difficulty of having a choice.

When parents talked about 'being prepared' during the interviews, they gave the impression that they were thinking about emotional preparation, and about preparation for the future as well as making practical preparations for the birth. We have, however, questioned the extent to which parents really do prepare:

> *. . .what actually happened was they actually put [baby] on my stomach and the first time we both realized that we hadn't prepared ourselves for having a baby, was at that point.*

(Oesophageal atresia)

This and similar comments led us to question what parents mean when they say that prenatal diagnosis allows them to prepare (Statham *et al.*, 2001). They are spared the shock of diagnosis at birth and, for those whose baby has a lethal abnormality, given time to prepare themselves emotionally for the birth of a baby who will die rather than one who will live. For those whose baby has a treatable anomaly, they can prepare for the distress around surgery. Many, however, do not focus on the longer-term health implications of the abnormality, the possibility of some permanent impairment, and the impact of the baby on themselves as parents.

PREPARATION FOR BIRTH

For most parents, part of being pregnant is about preparing for the birth of their baby. Parents whose baby has a known malformation endure a stressful pregnancy anticipating an uncertain future, in which a baby might not figure: hardly anticipation of a happy event. These parents talked very little before delivery about plans for the birth or, afterwards, about the experience of birth. Perhaps this reflected their feeling that birth was almost an incidental occurrence to get the baby out so that they knew what they were facing:

> M: Um, yes, there are lots of questions. I mean stupid questions like, I'd like to breastfeed my baby. I mean it's not even necessarily going to be alive, and when its born, what can I possibly expect? What sort of humane – I mean you learn about giving birth and the idea of closeness between mother and baby at the beginning, and this vision of the baby being born, whisked away, and me blinking, and God only knows where I'm going to be or what sort of – I mean it's not even important. I mean it's something that was a major, major part of my life, which was giving birth, is taking a back seat to the fact that this baby actually needs a lot of attention as soon as it's born....
>
> (Diaphragmatic hernia)

Preparations for birth tended to concentrate on aspects specific to the baby's abnormality. Attention was focused around the baby rather than the mother. Meeting the team who will care for their child, knowing what will happen when the baby is born, and visiting SCBU, if this is where care will take place, are of course important for parents. If this aspect of care was unsatisfactory or delayed, then parents reported feelings of upset and anxiety. However, the more usual preparations that pregnant women might make, focusing on themselves as mothers about to give birth, were largely ignored. Women gave a number of reasons for not going to antenatal classes, especially not wishing to attend alongside other women with normal pregnancies and not wishing to confront other pregnant women with their problems. Non-attendance at antenatal classes deprived women of the opportunity to build relationships with community health professionals and other women at similar stages of pregnancy, relationships that could be invaluable after the birth of the baby.

KNOWING THE BABY WILL DIE: A PARTICULAR PERSPECTIVE

Few parents make the decision to continue a pregnancy to term if there is no possibility of the baby living. Management of such pregnancies is inevitably demanding and challenging for health professionals. They get little opportunity to develop skills in understanding the parents' perspectives on their choices, their reasons for making those choices and their needs for support as they await the certain death of their baby. Such choices are often, but not always, underpinned by the moral certainty that termination is wrong. If termination is not an option within parents' moral framework, the certainty of the prognosis and the knowledge that they will not to have to care for a severely handicapped child can engender a sense of peace within the sadness:

> F: *I think throughout we got a bit of a feeling that people were making assumptions that we should be feeling a lot more upset and devastated by it all than in fact we were ... [there was] a sense of awkwardness on our part in not wanting to minimize the sadness of the situation because it was very sad but we also wanted to communicate that actually we were at peace with the decision we'd made and it was in God's hands ....*

> M: *... life has suffering in it ... people do lose babies and in terms of the suffering in the world ... while obviously very very important to us, this was not something to focus in on, and become engulfed by.*

CONCLUSION

We have not discussed in detail here the issues to do with the organization of care for parents whose baby has an abnormality but it was clear within our study that this was important for parents. They appreciated care that was supportive both physically and emotionally, which gave them the information they needed about their baby, and which recognized the woman as a pregnant mother-to-be. Accessing the right care presented many parents with difficulties, especially when they were feeling vulnerable. In particular, care focused on the baby and his or her needs. Parents also focused on the baby, and were anxious, with additional concerns about practical issues. It is important to recognize the impact of continuing the pregnancy for all parents, regardless of the abnormality discovered.

The parents' group Antenatal Results and Choices (ARC) has recently launched a new service and handbook (ARC, 2003) that begins to address the issues around the needs of a parent when a pregnancy is continuing after an abnormality has been diagnosed.

Key points

- Parents will be upset and anxious and may grieve the loss of the healthy baby they were expecting.
- Health professionals, family and friends can underestimate the impact of less-serious abnormalities.
- All parents need care that is well coordinated in an environment that allows them to establish relationships with their carers and where the emotional impact of continuing the pregnancy is recognized.
- It is easy for parents to be forgotten in a pregnancy where the baby has an abnormality.

Acknowledgements

We would like to thank the NHS R and D (Mother and Child Health Initiative) and the Wellcome Trust for generously supporting the studies on which this chapter is based; our fellow grant-holders – Lenore Abramsky, Susan Bewley, Lyn Chitty, Joanie Dimavicius, Nicholas Fisk, Phillipa Kyle – for their encouragement and their practical and intellectual support; and Frances Murton and Sally Roberts from the Centre for Family Research for all their help throughout the study. Most especially, we are grateful to all the parents who took part in the study and who shared with us their experiences of having a baby with an abnormality.

REFERENCES

Abramsky L (1994) Counselling prior to prenatal testing. In: *Prenatal Diagnosis: The Human Side* (eds Abramsky L, Chapple J). Chapman & Hall, London, pp. 70–85.

Armstrong P (1996) *Beating the Biological Clock: The Joys and Challenges of Late Motherhood*. Headline, London.

Chitty LS, Barnes CA, Berry C (1996) Continuing with pregnancy after a diagnosis of lethal abnormality: experience of five couples and recommendations for management. *British Medical Journal*, 313; 478–480.

Edwins J (2000) From a different planet: women who choose to continue their pregnancy after a diagnosis of Down's syndrome. *Practising Midwife*, 3(4); 21–24.

Finnemore P (2000) Future Imperfect: Coping and communication in continuing pregnancy after diagnosis of fetal abnormality. PhD thesis, University of Middlesex.

Fisk NM (2001) Prenatal screening. In: *Risk Management and Litigation in Obstetrics and Gynaecology* (ed. Clements RV). The Royal Society of Medicine Press, London, pp. 103–141.

Green J, Statham H (1996) Psychosocial aspects of prenatal screening and diagnosis. In: *The Troubled Helix* (eds Marteau T, Richards M). Cambridge University Press, Cambridge, pp.140–163.

Kemp J, Davenport M, Pernet A (1998) Antenatally diagnosed surgical anomalies: the psychological effect of parental antenatal counseling. *Journal of Pediatric Surgery*, 33(9); 1376–1379.

Lilford RJ, Stratton P, Godsil S *et al.* (1994) A randomised trial of routine versus selective counselling in perinatal bereavement from congenital disease. *British Journal of Obstetrics and Gynaecology*, 101; 291–296.

Madarikan BA, Tew B, Lari J (1990) Maternal response to anomalies detected by antenatal ultrasonography. *British Journal of Clinical Psychology*, 44(11); 587–589.

Marteau TM, Dormandy E (2001) Facilitating informed choice in prenatal testing: how well are we doing? *American Journal of Medical Genetics*, 106; 185–190.

Marteau TM, Mansfield CD (1998) The psychological impact of prenatal diagnosis and subsequent decisions. In: *Yearbook of Obstetrics and Gynaecology* (ed. O'Brien PMS). Royal College of Obstetrics and Gynaecology, London, pp. 186–193.

Redlinger-Grosse K, Bernhardt BA, Berg K *et al.* (2002) The Decision to Continue: The Experiences and Needs of Parents Who Receive a Prenatal Diagnosis of Holoprosencephaly. *American Journal of Medical Genetics*, 112; 369–378.

Salvesen KA, Oyen L, Schmidt N *et al.* (1997) Comparison of long-term psychological responses of women after pregnancy termination due to fetal anomalies and after perinatal loss. *Ultrasound in Obstetrics & Gynecology*, 9; 80–85.

Sandelowski M, Jones LC (1996a) Couples' evaluations of foreknowledge of fetal impairment. *Clinical Nursing Research*, 5(1); 81–96.

Sandelowski M, Jones LC (1996b) 'Healing fictions': stories of choosing in the aftermath of the detection of fetal anomalies. *Social Science Medicine*, 42(3); 353–361.

Statham H (2002) Prenatal diagnosis of fetal abnormality: the decision to terminate the pregnancy and the psychological consequences. Centre for Family Research, University of Cambridge.

Statham H, Solomou W, Chitty L (2000). Prenatal diagnosis of fetal abnormality: psychological effects on women in low-risk pregnancies. *Bailliere's Clinical Obstetrics and Gynaecology*, 14(4); 731–747.

Statham H, Solomou W, Green JM (2001) *When a Baby Has an Abnormality: A Study of Parents' Experiences.* Centre for Family Research, University of Cambridge, Cambridge.

Statham H, Solomou W, Green JM (2002) *When a Baby Has an Abnormality: A Study of Health Professionals' Experiences.* Centre for Family Research, University of Cambridge, Cambridge.

Watkins D (1989) An alternative to termination of pregnancy. *The Practitioner*, 233; 990–992.

Zeanah CH, Dailey JV, Rosenblatt MJ *et al.* (1993) Do women grieve after terminating pregnancies because of fetal anomalies? A controlled investigation. *Obstetrics and Gynecology*, 82(2); 270–275.

14 INFORMATION AND MISINFORMATION – MAKING OUR DECISION

'Craig and Sally' – One couple's account as told by the father

INTRODUCTION

We ('Sally' and 'Craig') are the parents of a daughter (Jennifer) who was diagnosed before birth as having a sex chromosome abnormality known as Triple X syndrome (47, XXX). This is our account of the information provided to us and of our experiences and feelings from the initial diagnosis in 1996 through to Jennifer's sixth birthday.

BACKGROUND

We are both from a middle-class background, living in the south of England, and have followed professional careers since getting married in the early 1980s. At the time of this pregnancy Sally was 44 and I was 37. We had two daughters aged 9 and 5 and had all enjoyed good health apart from the usual common colds and flu viruses. Both daughters are of average intelligence, outward looking, bright and mix well with other children.

THE THIRD PREGNANCY

Sally was somewhat surprised when she discovered, at the age of 44, that she had fallen pregnant for the third time. While she hoped for a brother for the two girls, my concern was that all should go well for a 44-year-old mother-to-be and that the new addition to the family would be as healthy as the previous babies. Having first overcome the surprise factor of the pregnancy news, we both felt rather proud and excited, and the news was met with equal excitement by the two girls, who both wanted a brother! We decided not to share the exciting news with others until the 16-week mark when we knew all was well.

Because of Sally's age when she conceived each of the children, her obstetrician had on all occasions advised that she underwent an amniocentesis to routinely check for Down syndrome and other common congenital disorders. Having been through this process with the same obstetrician on two previous occasions, Sally had little concern over the process and never really expected anything other than good news. With my experience of two previous pregnancies, I did not have the concerns that a father has during a wife's first pregnancy.

We were devastated by the news that the results of the amniocentesis had shown a condition known as Triple X syndrome. We were due to leave on holiday for a couple of weeks when Sally received a phone call from her obstetrician early one evening, to inform her that we were expecting a daughter who had been diagnosed as being Triple X, and that this was a chromosome disorder/condition. He regretted that he was unable to provide us with any detailed information of the condition but was aware that it was linked to behavioural problems in children and adults with these chromosomes. Arrangements had been made for us to visit a genetic clinic to meet with a consultant who would provide us with further information. It turned out that this meeting would not take place for 10 days.

Thus we were presented with a condition that we did not know existed, given little or no supporting information, and were unable to get further information until we attended the clinic in 10 days time. I can only describe our emotions at this time as being a mixture of confusion, despair, frustration and total devastation.

Having watched Sally go through hell for a couple of days, my immediate mission was to find out as much as possible about the Triple X condition and to this end we spoke to our local general practitioner and midwife, and we visited the hospitals where the girls had been born. We were astounded to find out how little knowledge existed on the condition anywhere. The period that followed, leading up to our appointment at the clinic, was the most frustrating that we had both ever experienced. We didn't know the severity of the condition; Sally understandably imagined the worst scenario, and I felt unable to help her. We did not know where to look, who to contact or how to build our own body of knowledge about the situation we found ourselves in.

THE CONSULTATION

The genetics consultation finally came. Looking back, neither of us had any idea of what to expect from the meeting or what was to follow. We were shown into a room and introduced to a genetic specialist and a counsellor who we were told would be there to help us with counselling if required. I could only surmise from this offer that we were indeed dealing with a very serious issue. The specialist explained that the result of the amniocentesis showed that the baby had a genetic disorder in her chromosome make-up, resulting in Triple X syndrome. The mention of the word syndrome only added to my feeling that we were dealing with a serious condition.

The specialist explained that while some research had been done on the condition, little information existed. She outlined the condition as one in which our daughter would have learning difficulties, may have difficulty in feeding as an infant, would be late in walking and was likely to be reserved and quiet. Thus, for the first time since we had been told of our daughter's condition, we had some real information upon which to understand what we were dealing with. We were given a photocopy of a research paper written by a genetics professor who had done some research in Scotland on the condition. Throughout our meeting, many of our questions could not be answered, so it was still particularly difficult to put a scale to the severity of the condition. If we could have been advised where on a scale factor of 1–10 the condition sat (1 being mild and 10 being severe) it would have helped immensely in understanding how it would affect our lives.

Then the full impact of what we were dealing with (or so we believed) became apparent. In summing up, the specialist told us that we were able to abort the pregnancy because of the chromosome condition and that a couple recently faced with a similar diagnosis had chosen to do so. The offer to abort confirmed our first thoughts that the condition was at the '10' end of the scale rather than the '1' end and that we were now faced with a decision in a very short period of time.

GETTING MORE INFORMATION

Having returned home and gathered our thoughts, we read the research paper that we had been given. We still seemed to have so little information but we were faced with literally a life and death decision. It was at this point we decided to carry out our own research and turned to the research paper that we had been given. The paper concluded that while Triple X babies may have slow physical development (for example, they may sit up and talk a little later than non Triple X girls), they would have no other special physical characteristics apart from a tendency to have long legs and blue eyes! (I would point out at this point that Jennifer sat up at nine months and talked around 11–12 months like both of her sisters.) The paper also stated that Triple X girls' IQs tended to be below that of their parents, brothers and sisters, that they were likely to require remedial help with both reading and maths, that they might have low self-esteem and self-confidence and might have behavioural problems.

I managed to trace the author from an old post held in Scotland to a current post in England, only to be told that she had now retired. I contacted the hospital where she had held her last post and through an amazing stroke of luck found out that she visited once a week to pick up mail. Having found the one person who perhaps could give us some further knowledge we felt that it would be unlikely that we would be able to make contact with her. However we left a message and were extremely surprised to receive a call within a day.

I outlined the whole situation to her culminating in the decision that we were now faced with. She was completely appalled at the fact that we had been offered a termination and could not understand why this should have been offered. After a very detailed discussion of her research on the Triple X condition, we began to understand that in real terms the severity of the condition was indeed at the lower end of the scale of 1–10. To help us understand further we were provided with the contact details of the parents of another Triple X child who since birth had taken part in the research conducted by the professor and who was now 18 years of age. To our amazement we were able to establish that although the child had been slower in a number of learning stages she was now heading for university to undertake a degree course! Once again the parents could not understand why we were ever offered a termination and were deeply disturbed by this fact.

Our contact in Scotland also put us in touch via the genetic clinic with the parents of a young (age 5) Triple X girl who lived within one hour of our house. We made contact immediately with further hope of supporting the fact that the condition was indeed not so severe that a termination would be an option. Both parents listened to our situation and within hours came to see us with their daughter, again greatly disturbed by the option we were faced with. This was the key turning point in our lives and as such will never be forgotten. Here with us was the most wonderful little girl, completely normal, somewhat shy but pretty with blue eyes and our decision was made.

THE FIRST 12 MONTHS

As might be expected, Jennifer's progress during her first 12 months attracted perhaps more attention than that of her sisters, but it soon became evident that there was no difference in abilities at key stages. From the point that she was born her condition became irrelevant, as we both knew that we had made the correct decision. We could have easily made the wrong one without our determination to build a greater body of knowledge from a limited resource. We decided that her chromosomes would remain a private matter between parents, as we did not wish for her to become the focus of attention and for relations and friends to be constantly comparing her childhood progress with that of others.

NURSERY SCHOOL TO TODAY (AGE 6)

Jennifer attended nursery school from the age of 3, has remained at the same school and is currently heading into the second form. Both her reading and speech development have remained behind that of 70% of the children in her class, but she is in the upper end of the lower quartile. She loves sports, and while initially very shy, she has become more outward and has recently been awarded a distinction in her first speech and drama exam. She does ballet, takes part in school plays and events and has an aptitude for art and crafts. She is loved dearly (but no more than her sisters) and is without doubt a special little girl.

CONCLUSION

Research shows that as many as 1 in 1000 females may have a Triple X condition without ever knowing that they have the condition. We, as parents, needed more information from medical professionals so that we could make an informed decision. Our own education led us to insist that we found more information prior to making a life or death decision. Had we not done so and based our decision on the initial understanding ... it's a thought we wish not to think about.

EDITOR'S NOTE:

It was stories such as this which inspired one of the editors (LA) to do a small study investigating how parents are first informed that a sex chromosome anomaly has been prenatally diagnosed (Abramsky *et al.*, 2001). We know that in some places practice has improved; in particular, some cytogenetic laboratories now fax the relevant patient information leaflet to the clinician when reporting a sex chromosome anomaly.

REFERENCE

Abramsky L, Hall S, Levitan, J *et al.* (2001) Telling parents about a prenatally detected chromosome anomaly: a telephone interview study. *British Medical Journal*, 322; 463–466.

15 THE PARENTS' REACTIONS TO TERMINATION OF PREGNANCY FOR FETAL ABNORMALITY: FROM A MOTHER'S POINT OF VIEW

Helen Statham

INTRODUCTION

The aim of prenatal diagnosis is to determine whether or not a fetus has an abnormality. Most parents undergoing testing are told that their baby is not affected by the disorders that have been looked for. Parents told that their unborn baby has an anomaly have a number of options, depending on the nature of the anomaly, the gestation at diagnosis and the legal framework for abortion in the country where the mother lives (Statham *et al.*, 2000; Statham, 2002). The main choices are between terminating or continuing the pregnancy. There are additional choices for those who continue, which may include considering the time, place and method of delivery, treatment (see Chapter 13 in this volume) and then whether or not to keep the child or place him or her for adoption. Although the official language around prenatal testing focuses on giving parents choices (Marteau and Dormandy, 2001) it is unlikely that prenatal diagnosis would have been resourced as it is, just to give parents reassurance, or if most parents with an abnormality chose to continue the pregnancy. The 'enormous potential for the avoidance of serious genetic disease and congenital malformation' (Weatherall, 1992) can only be realized in most cases if women who conceive fetuses with such a genetic disease or malformation terminate the pregnancy.

There are a number of practical issues around prenatal diagnosis and termination that are important to parents who, given a diagnosis of fetal abnormality, choose to terminate the pregnancy. How should a diagnosis be given? How long should there be between diagnosis and termination? Should the termination happen on a labour or a gynaecology ward? Should parents see, hold, photograph and bury their babies? What aftercare do parents need? How do staff cope with this difficult area of their work? These important issues are addressed in detail elsewhere (Statham, 1992; ARC, 1999; Statham *et al.*, 2001). Here, I would like to explore some of the attitudes and emotions of parents and health professionals to the process of diagnosis, the detection of abnormality and to termination.

WHAT IS A TERMINATION FOR ABNORMALITY?

In the early 1980s, I worked in a tissue culture laboratory; sometimes we would receive tissue samples from fetuses aborted because they were at risk of having

Duchenne muscular dystrophy. We were always quite pleased to be getting samples of fetal tissue, although we usually had a few concerns: would it be in good condition; what time would it eventually arrive? We also used to think how lucky the woman was *not* to have to give birth to this (possibly) disabled child.

A few things have changed since that time, especially with the developments around the Human Genome Project. Research into Duchenne is not dependent on fetal tissue; prenatal diagnosis is more accurate, so fetuses are not aborted just because they are male and at risk, and I gained some insight into how these 'lucky' women had probably felt when, following amniocentesis, my second child was diagnosed as having Down syndrome. I realized then just how completely I had absorbed the existing medical perspective on termination for abnormality: a baby with an abnormality is a problem; the problem can be solved by the cause being taken away.

Such a view was understandable (Statham, 1992): perinatal deaths had previously not been recognized as traumatic; attitudes to abortion were increasingly liberal, and early (non-medical) abortion of an unwanted pregnancy was not related to serious morbidity (Adler *et al.*, 1992; Gilchrist *et al.*, 1995; recently confirmed by Major *et al.*, 2000). Attitudes to prenatal diagnosis drew on both of these perspectives. Those developing the prenatal diagnostic techniques also were aware that they were presenting real alternatives for families who knew that a pregnancy had a high risk of resulting in the birth of a disabled child. The other available options were either risking a pregnancy or restraint from all pregnancies, including those that would result in the birth of a healthy baby. For parents who wanted the chance to have a child without a particular abnormality, the advent of prenatal testing and termination of affected pregnancies helped them to do this. They were, therefore, more likely to choose to become pregnant (Laurence and Morris, 1981).

In only a few minutes, my science-based attitudes to detection and termination of disabled fetuses were shaken. Immediately the consultant gave me the news, I lost the healthy baby that I had been expecting; that baby was gone, whatever decision I would subsequently make. Parents who choose to terminate experience a second bereavement, the physical loss of the baby who was not healthy.

> *So I have two griefs really: loss of my Down baby whom I saw on the ultrasound screen and whose heartbeat I heard with sonicaid, and loss of the fantasy 'perfect' baby we all imagine when we're pregnant.*

(ARC mother)

These two losses are united through a third factor, making this bereavement unique; parents choose to cause the loss:

> *The pain of loss, and the pain of having to be the one to make the choice, is the hardest thing I ever have or want to have to go through.*

(ARC mother)

Clearly, a termination for abnormality is not the taking away of a problem. Rather it is the process of adjusting to the knowledge that you have a baby who has a problem, making a difficult and painful decision about what to do, and learning to live with consequences of that decision. One problem for parents has been to ensure that these aspects of their experience are recognized, while not denying that, usually, the choice is one they welcome the opportunity to make: 'Every day I say thank God that they do these tests because I don't know what people did years ago' (Rothman, 1986).

WHY DO WOMEN CHOOSE TO HAVE TESTS?

Some would argue that the question 'why do women choose to have tests?' ignores an important issue; women do not choose tests. Either they are not given the information on which to make a decision or they do not even know they are having a test. Thus women undergo scanning 'aware' that abnormalities can be detected but 'somehow, when you go for a routine scan for size, you can't believe that they'll find something so dreadful' (ARC mother). Twenty-seven percent of women in a study in a London teaching hospital did not know that they had undergone maternal serum screening for neural-tube defects (Marteau *et al.*, 1988). Early work on informed choices focused on women's knowledge of and attitudes to testing, but more recently, Marteau *et al.* (2001) have suggested the need to consider patients' values as well when seeking to measure whether decision making about prenatal screening is 'informed'. Using a scale developed to measure informed choice about serum screening, they classified 18 out of 42 women as having made an informed choice, and 24 as having made an uninformed choice. We do not know if women who have not made an informed choice are particularly vulnerable when given a diagnosis of abnormality. In a report of the South Wales pilot project of neonatal screening for Duchenne muscular dystrophy (Bradley *et al.*, 1993) the family who reacted most adversely to the diagnosis of Duchenne had apparently not been given information about the test and said that they would not have undergone testing if they had been fully informed.

Two weeks after terminating the pregnancy, I wrote:

> *It did not occur to me that the amniocentesis was for any other reason than to remove just one of the worries that as a pessimist had haunted me throughout my first, successful pregnancy. Until the birth, I would still worry about all the other problems that could beset my baby but at least I would know that he or she did not have Down syndrome ... . Once I knew I was not going to miscarry, I stopped worrying.*

(Statham, 1987)

Did it mean that I had not understood the reason for the amniocentesis? Had I been peculiarly naive, even stupid, not to have dwelt more seriously on the possibility of the alternative, and eventual, outcome? Of course I knew my reason for having the test. If I was naive, I was not unusual. Many studies have shown that women undergo tests for reassurance (Farrant, 1985; Marteau *et al.*, 1988;

Green *et al.*, 1993; see also Green, Chapter 5 of this volume). I was embarking upon what Press and Browner (1997) called a 'ritual of reassurance'.

It is usual at this point to contrast women's hopes for reassurance with the alternative view often ascribed to the service provider: looking for abnormalities. This is an important distinction, but is it relevant when an abnormality is discovered? Although there is evidence in the studies listed above that women who undergo diagnostic tests following an adverse screening test result are particularly anxious awaiting results of the test, I know of no evidence that shows that these women react any differently to other women when given the news of a confirmed abnormality. The discovery of an abnormality is always devastating.

DIAGNOSIS OF AN ABNORMALITY

Diagnosis of an abnormality is the immediate loss of a healthy baby. For the parents, being told their baby has an abnormality is just the beginning of a long process. The person breaking that news, feeling that this is probably the most devastating piece of news the parents have ever been given, may wonder if it really matters what is said and how. The answer is, quite definitely, yes, it does matter. At the end of the process, the parents will only have memories. Many relive over and over again the words that were used to them and the way in which they were said; those words are the starting point of the memories (Statham and Dimavicius, 1992; ARC, 1999). Our recent study (Statham *et al.*, 2001) found that a simple measure of satisfaction with how a diagnosis was made and communicated was strongly related to how mothers felt in the year after a termination. For professionals, however, a conflict may be experienced at diagnosis. A radiologist once described her sense of achievement when she spotted something unusual on an ultrasound scan, while knowing that because she had done her job well, the parents were going to be given devastating news.

Rothman (1988) suggested that the availability of prenatal testing has made women see their pregnancies and therefore their fetuses as 'tentative'. She argued that women do not form attachments to fetuses in early pregnancy in case tests show there to be abnormalities; a fetus to which they are not attached will be easier to discard through termination. We have argued previously (Green and Statham, 1996) that there is little empirical evidence for this observation, although some women try to suspend a relationship with their fetus when test results suggest possible problems. In a recent study (Statham *et al.*, 2001), the following comments were made by parents about their feelings while awaiting the results of amniocentesis after a high-risk serum screening result:

F: *I never touched [baby referred to by pet name] after that, really, physically. That all stopped. It wasn't – it wasn't a kind of – it wasn't a coldness. It was just like – it was almost like a – it was put on ice.*

M: *... it didn't feel like I had – was having a baby. It felt like I had a problem. That there was – that it was all going wrong, that it wasn't kind of*

– you know, that it wasn't right, that there was something wrong, you know? And I didn't feel – I kind of felt very unattached to my tummy and to the baby, and to how I was kind of, you know, physically, and emotionally I, you know, felt really dislocated, almost instantaneously – well, not instant, but very – it seemed, in a matter of a couple of days, I began to not – you know, I couldn't enjoy being pregnant, and there didn't seem to be anything positive about that any more.

(After the termination)

Suspended pregnancies are understandable: parents trying to protect themselves from the pain they know will be associated with the news of an abnormal baby. The concept of the tentative pregnancy has been widely accepted as a truth of pregnant women's attitudes and one that has been used to support arguments that prenatal testing promotes the commodification of babies and pregnancies (Lippman, 1991; Davis, 1999). There are, however, no data (including those in Rothman's book) that suggest that women given a diagnosis of abnormality ever commented that the pregnancy had been in any way tentative.

MAKING A DECISION

Bourne and Lewis (1984), describing parents' reactions to the stillbirth of a baby with abnormalities, wrote, 'Congenital abnormalities involve parents in exceptional conflict of revulsion and attachment towards the dead baby, towards themselves and each other'. When the abnormality is diagnosed during pregnancy, parents can experience the same conflicts along with the burden of the decision-making. Such life and death decisions are usually dealt with by fate or by God; it is essential in this situation that parents reach the right decision for them. Can a 'good' decision be made in which the range and consequences of each alternative are explored (Janis and Mann, 1977), when those making the decision are in shock and under pressure to decide quickly?

Marteau and Dormandy (2001) have confirmed recently the 'dearth of research on women's decisions following the diagnosis of a fetal abnormality'. A number of studies have reported the factors that appear, quantitatively, to relate to the decision that parents make: gestation, severity, ultrasound visibility of the abnormality, who counsels the parents and cultural differences. These findings have been reviewed in Green and Statham (1996), Marteau and Mansfield (1998), Statham *et al.* (2000), Statham (2002) and Marteau and Dormandy (2001). The front cover of all SATFA (now ARC) newsletters used to carry the statement: 'The decision to terminate a wanted baby because of fetal abnormality is one made out of care for the unborn child and in consideration of existing family. It is not a decision taken easily or lightly'. Some preliminary findings about how people make these decisions from as yet unpublished qualitative research are described in Chapter 13. Not surprisingly, the major predictor of the decision is severity of the abnormality. Such a bald statement, however, ignores the pain in reaching a 'logical' decision.

Perception of severity is subject to individual interpretation; for some parents, Down syndrome is serious and the only decision they would wish to make, given a diagnosis, is to terminate the pregnancy. Others do not consider Down syndrome as serious enough for them to consider termination.

There are many conflicts that parents must resolve in reaching their decision. The baby was wanted 'Our baby boy, wanted so much, already loved so much and for whom we had such expectations ...' (from Statham, 1992); yet the decision to terminate says that the baby has become unwanted. Judgements are made on the quality of many lives, including that of the unborn baby: '... if he survived the birth, it would mean an operation as soon as he was born and a series of operations which were unlikely to be very successful' (SATFA, 1993). Parents are concerned for the baby when he or she becomes older, and for existing children:

> *We finally decided that at 41 years old the worst thing for us to do would be to die and leave an adult with a mental age of six or less behind to fend for himself ... a Downs child would never be company for our little boy, and it would be an enormous responsibility to put on his shoulders in later life.*
>
> (ARC mother)

In the first edition of this chapter (written nearly 10 years ago) I felt it important to emphasize how women seldom mentioned their own quality of life as a factor in decision-making. We all have hopes for our futures. Those of us who intentionally become pregnant recognize some of the demands that parenting will make on us but see a time when those demands will lessen as the child becomes more independent. Mothers of disabled children will often not experience the independence of their child and the associated independence for themselves. Available evidence in 1994 suggested that it was difficult for many women to admit to the selfishness implicit in not wanting to accept a child who would not allow them to become an independent being again. However our recent, as yet unpublished, data (Statham and Solomou) has clearly identified 'impact of the baby on self' as one of the main factors that influence decisions.

The debate around decision-making has been extensive in recent years. Do parents make their own decisions after a diagnosis or are they pressurized to terminate either directly by doctors or indirectly by a society that does not provide adequate facilities for disabled people? What information guides decisions? Clearly the study of Abramsky et al. (2001), in which health professionals reported what they told parents about little known conditions shows that some are uninformed about some of the disorders they must discuss with parents. Some parents describe their experiences as though they were directed: 'She was very sympathetic but strongly recommended us to consider termination' (SATFA, 1993). Other parents might say they 'had no choice' when their child had a lethal abnormality. Obtaining information about what takes place in consultations is methodologically and ethically difficult and, furthermore, it was clear in our own recent study that parents' own perceptions of their decision sometimes changed over time.

Wertz (1993) examined the arguments (Rothman, 1986; Lippman, 1991) that society creates needs for women to be mothers of perfect children, such that while women think they have choices they are forced into actions which are determined by social class interests and by society's rejections of people with disabilities. Wertz is unsympathetic to these views, believing that parents' preference for a child who is healthy is quite normal, but says:

> *If freedom of choice means absence of legal coercion, a woman carrying a fetus with a severe genetic disorder is free to abort or carry to term. If choice means being able to live with the consequences of this decision, many women may feel that they 'have no choice' because the economic and social costs of raising the child could be unbearable.*

There is a substantial literature by disabled-rights activists arguing that disability is socially constructed (i.e. medical problems are less significant than social attitudes). This debate is omitted here because the purpose of this chapter is to present the perspectives and feelings of parents who have chosen termination. Interested readers might wish to refer to Asch and Geller (1996), Shakespeare (1998), Davis (1999), Buchanan *et al.* (2000), Williams *et al.* (2002), and the reference lists to be found in those papers.

It has been assumed that early terminations of pregnancy are easier for women than later ones, that the distress that women experience is because the baby has been felt moving and has been seen on a scan. Most studies of perinatal loss in general have found relationships between gestation and grief (reviewed in Lasker and Toedter, 2000), but those studies that have investigated the relationship between mothers' feelings after termination for abnormality and gestation at termination are less consistent. Two reports suggest an association (Black, 1989; Iles, 1989) and two find no such relationship (Zeanah *et al.*, 1993; Salveson *et al.*, 1997). Our own study found no effect of gestation. Why do I raise this issue here, in a section on making a decision? If the assertion is true that terminations for abnormality differ from other pregnancy losses because parents make the decision, and that this is the difficult aspect for parents, we must remember that parents have to make a decision, whenever the abnormality is discovered. This might explain why gestation does not matter. A woman whose baby was found to have Down syndrome at 12 weeks pregnant wrote:

> *It may have been early, it certainly is not easy. The decision to terminate may be straightforward, but living with it is possibly the hardest thing a woman and her partner will ever have to do.*

(ARC mother)

THE TERMINATION

After the shock of a diagnosis and the pain of decision-making, going to hospital for the termination can almost be a relief, but only if it happens at the right time, in the right place and if the mother is fully prepared for what will happen to her. There is also the question of how the pregnancy is to be terminated: surgically or through induced labour. For most women this will be gestation-dependent and not something they can decide about. Where women are given the choice they make different choices. Some opt for induced labour with the knowledge that they can see their baby and have a post-mortem. It is widely believed that having a body to grieve is helpful:

> M: *And they advised, which I think in retrospect is the best thing that they can do, they advised me very strongly to have the baby, if you like, naturally, to give birth to the child. They said because – and the midwife said this, and she was a very sort of straight – not a sort of like, you know, counsellor-type person, it was the midwife who said, it will help you grieve.*

In the same way that gestation at termination of pregnancy was unrelated to how women felt in the year after a termination, neither was there an effect of method of termination in our study (Statham *et al.*, 2001). Feeling informed and able to make the right choice is clearly important:

> M: *... and it was incredibly timely and useful to have it [the ARC parents' handbook, ARC, 1999] at that point, because I read about the two methods of termination, and I just straight away thought – well, no, not straight away. I'd been thinking about going through a labour, because it just felt like a gentler, more natural thing to do, and as soon as I read this book, I read that it was – the book was very factual and very straight, and just said, you know, what would happen at each operation, and I just realized from reading that that having a labour would be unnecessarily traumatic and that I just thought, no, I'll go for an operation and have it done under general anaesthetic.*

Where there are choices to be made, making the right choice is more likely if there is someone who has developed a relationship with the woman and her partner since the diagnosis, and informed them of the options available. As for all of the issues discussed here, when the termination should take place is a very individual decision. Some women wish to 'get it over with' as soon as possible, others welcome a delay:

> *It did give us time to establish beyond doubt that we wanted a termination, it allowed us to grieve quietly together and to make arrangements for our other child.*
>
> (ARC mother)

In most aspects of our lives we often make *post hoc* rationalizations that what happened to us was what should have happened. It is likely that most parents look back at the process of the termination in this way, but one woman wrote after an admission within 24 hours:

It seemed humane at the time. Now, looking back, I realize we didn't have time to be fully prepared for what was going to happen, me physically and both of us emotionally and mentally.

(ARC mother)

Her preparation was not helped by the registrar who told her the amniocentesis results. He said that labour was to be induced, it was to be a 'fairly straightforward process' especially as 'the worst part is over now'. She went on to say: 'He must have been told sometime in his career that waiting for the amnio result is agonizing, and if the outcome is a happy one, then it was the worst part'. With the widespread free distribution of the ARC parents' handbook (ARC, 1999) to all hospitals in England and Wales since 1991, there is little reason why parents should be uninformed and unprepared for labour and delivery of the baby. The handbook offers parents and their supporters a common language to discuss how the termination will take place, including how long labour might take and pain relief. The handbook was found to be invaluable to parents in our recent study (Statham *et al.*, 2001) with criticism made if it was given too late.

Hospitals vary in their policies as to where terminations take place. My personal view of this is that the right place is where there is a private room, where the woman and her partner can be given all the practical and emotional support that they need. The carer should be competent in all aspects of delivering tiny babies, some of whom will be obviously malformed; there should be continuity of care with protocols to ensure that someone has discussed seeing the baby, holding the baby, photographs, funerals, post mortems, possible retention of the placenta. Whether such care can best be provided in a maternity unit or on a gynaecology ward will vary with facilities in different hospitals, with staff expertise and attitudes and, if she is given a choice, with the woman herself. In our recent study (Statham *et al.*, 2001), satisfaction with care while undergoing a termination did not relate to the ward that women were on. However, parents do find it particularly difficult if they can hear women in labour and babies:

F: ... *at least two occasions where you could hear a baby crying as if it had just been delivered. And that was hard.*

The events around the point of delivery are worrying for parents and for staff, with unknowns like whether the baby will be born alive, and what it will look like. There is also fear of the baby being born and the abnormalities not appearing as severe as the parents had expected. The delivery of babies who show signs of life should be an infrequent occurrence as terminations that take place after 22 weeks of pregnancy will mostly be preceded by an injection to ensure the baby is not born alive.

This is an area of concern for staff fearful of, or opposed to, post-24 weeks terminations (Devane and Devane, 2000). Parents' responses to feticide vary: for some it is one part of the process of termination, for others a deeply distressing additional procedure (Statham *et al.*, 2001).

A big fear for parents at this time is about what the baby will look like:

At first I was unsure whether to see him because I didn't want to be left with a horrible picture in my mind as facial abnormalities had been mentioned.

(ARC mother)

It is rare for parents to regret seeing their baby but not rare for parents to regret not seeing him or her (Statham, 1992; Statham *et al.*, 2001). In some hospitals fetuses are kept for some time after delivery in case parents who have originally declined to see their baby change their minds, although obviously the situation is different if a post mortem is done. Most parents are offered photographs, hand and footprints, and sensitive and respectful disposal. Parents having earlier terminations under general anaesthetic cannot have some of these mementoes and some parents may find it harder to 'say goodbye':

M: I realized the psychological differences, that in some ways you've got to say goodbye, you know. A natural birth might have been better for me now. But I just couldn't face it. I'd been through so much shock that I just couldn't.

It must be remembered however, that a small group of women will choose to avoid rituals around the death of their baby and there is a growing body of evidence that those who do choose to adopt a more distant attitude to their baby and become less involved with the use of mementoes and rituals around the death may have higher emotional wellbeing (Sitrin, 1994; Rich, 1999; Lasker and Toedter, 2000; Statham *et al.*, 2001; Statham, 2002).

AFTERWARDS

Many women experience a tremendous feeling of relief on going home after the termination, a sense of having survived. There is no statutory requirement to provide aftercare but some doctors, midwives and health visitors do so. For the many women who are left alone, there are questions which must be asked: am I a mother or not? Have I had a baby or not? The answers are confusing: there is no baby; breasts are unexpectedly full of milk. A midwife would come to see a woman with the same bodily symptoms of bleeding, lactation and depression, if there was a baby as well. Why not when there is no such baby? The isolation that women may have felt throughout the whole process of diagnosis and termination is reinforced by their isolation from carers when discharged from hospital.

There are resource implications of visiting the woman, but she would have been visited throughout the pregnancy and afterwards if it had continued. Occasionally, midwives will comment that they asked a woman if she would like a visit and the woman said no; it is likely that if they had just visited, they would have been welcomed. At the time when they feel vulnerable but with no self-esteem, women may not feel worthy of a visit in spite of their desperate need for one. Other women do not want any aftercare; this is clearly an area where sensitivity and understanding on the part of a midwife with a prior relationship with a mother will enable her to provide appropriate care.

Occasionally, contacts are made that are particularly inappropriate, as in the case of a midwife phoning a woman some weeks after the termination to question why she had not been at her antenatal classes which had just started. Examples of similar administrative disasters can be found more often than today's communication channels should allow; it is distressing for parents and staff alike and is an area where simple protocols could be established to ensure that appropriate people are told of events.

Aftercare also means good genetic counselling, post mortem results and a physical check-up for the woman, not in an antenatal clinic. The result of these should be that the parents have all the information they need to make the right decision about another pregnancy. If that pregnancy occurs, it is a very stressful time (Cote-Arsenault et al., 2001); those involved in the care of parents at this time should be aware of the significance of particular rooms, particular dates and even particular personnel.

CONCLUSION

The way in which the feelings experienced by parents undergoing a termination were slowly recognized by those involved in offering prenatal testing has been described previously (Statham, 1992). Even as early as the 1970s, Blumberg *et al.* (1975) reported on post-termination depression, guilt because of decision-making and loss of self-esteem because of the conception of an abnormal child. Over the next 10 years, further studies confirmed these findings, (Donnai *et al.*, 1981; Leschot *et al.*, 1982). Stillbirth, neonatal death and the birth of a disabled child were increasingly recognized as distressing events for parents, and Lloyd and Laurence (1985) and Jorgensen *et al.* (1985) likened the experiences of women undergoing abortion for fetal abnormality to those of women experiencing a perinatal death. Jorgensen added:

> *A decisive difference between stillbirth and abortion of a malformed fetus is that in the case of abortion, the parents have actively decided to terminate the pregnancy, thereby causing the death of a living fetus. The fact that the fetus was malformed might result in even stronger self-accusations and feelings of guilt.*

Professionals were beginning to understand that parents terminating pregnancies because of abnormality were experiencing a bereavement and needed support: Laurence (1989) suggested it was unethical to offer terminations without support. As a number of authors highlighted 'adverse psychiatric sequelae' it became clearer what was 'normal': high psychological distress in the short-term after termination, with some 40% of those taking part in studies showing symptoms of psychiatric morbidity (Black, 1989; White-van Mourik *et al.*, 1992; Iles and Gath, 1993; Zeanah *et al.*, 1993; Hunfeld, 1995; Salvesen *et al.*, 1997; Rona *et al.*, 1998). It would be wrong to assume that support will or should prevent features of grief that are normally found with bereavement and that last for varying amounts of time: anger, sadness, guilt, disbelief, numbness. Mostly, distress falls over time, although some aspects of the loss can cause distress in the longer term and some women remain distressed.

The literature concerning which women might be more likely to remain distressed and possibly in need of clinical input is inconsistent (reviewed in Statham *et al.*, 2000 and Statham, 2002). The factors most consistently associated with post-termin-ation mood disturbance that might be considered 'abnormal' are those related to poor social support from the woman's partner or family and friends and mental health problems: both of these may, however, predate the termination. Research is now needed to identify and evaluate therapeutic interventions for parents whose longer-term reaction after termination is a cause for personal and professional concern (Suslak *et al.*, 1995).

Attitudes to and care for parents terminating pregnancies after the detection of a fetal abnormality has changed, and we believe those changes are for the better. In believing we are doing 'the right things' for parents it is important that the personal nature of parents' experiences, and the impact on individual parents of the death of their baby and their role in deciding its death are not forgotten:

> *Although I have had an abortion and it was ultimately my choice, I feel that the scrambled conception and Trisomy 21 was a cruel blow of fate. After all, when I conceived the child, I was expecting the best Christmas present I have ever had.*

(ARC mother)

Key points

- The discovery of an abnormality is always devastating. Although much is made of the fact that women are not prepared for a positive diagnosis because prenatal testing is seen as there to give reassurance, there is no evidence that prior awareness conveys any benefit.
- When an abnormality is diagnosed, parents immediately lose the healthy baby they had hoped for: numb, in a state of shock and acute grief, they have to make the most difficult decision about whether or not to choose to end the life of their own child.
- Little is known about how parents make their decision after prenatal diagnosis. Available data suggest that they consider the impact that the abnormality will have on the baby, themselves and their existing and future family.
- Attitudes to and care for parents terminating pregnancies after the detection of a fetal abnormality have changed over the years and termination is recognized as a perinatal bereavement. Care should acknowledge the personal nature of parents' experiences, and the impact on individual parents of the death of their baby and their role in deciding its death. Carers should not make assumptions, such as earlier is easier.

AUTHOR'S NOTE

Most quotations in this chapter are from women who wrote directly to me, some via ARC, about their experiences. Others are from parents who took part in a recently-completed study reported in Statham *et al.* (2001). ARC (Antenatal Results and Choices; www.arc-uk.org) is the UK voluntary sector group working with and for parents around prenatal screening, diagnosis and decision-making, and through termination or a continued pregnancy. ARC was previously known as SATFA (Support After/Around Termination for Abnormality) and offers support to parents and training for health professionals.

Acknowledgements

I am grateful to all those parents, health professinals and colleagues who have talked through the issues in this chapter with me over so many years. Many of the contacts with parents have been made through ARC, other through a recent study funded by the NHS R and D Mother and Child Health Initiative. I am particulary grateful to my co-workers on that study, Wendy Solomou and Jo Green, for many very helpful discussions. Responsibility for the views expressed here are, however, mine: they may not always reflect those of ARC or my colleagues on the study.

REFERENCES

Abramsky L, Hall S, Levitan J *et al.* (2001) What parents are told after prenatal diagnosis of a sex chromosome abnormality: interview and questionnaire study. *British Medical Journal*, 322; 463–466.

Adler NE, David HP, Major BN *et al.* (1992) Psychological factors in abortion. A review. *American Psychologist*, 47(10); 1194–1204.

ARC (1999) *Antenatal Results and Choices.* Antenatal Results and Choices, London, pp. 1–32.

Asch A, Geller G. (1996) Feminism, bioethics, and genetics. In *Feminism and Bioethics: Beyond Reproduction* (ed. Wolf SM). Oxford University Press, New York, pp. 318–350.

Black RB (1989) A 1 and 6 month follow-up of prenatal diagnosis patients who lost pregnancies. *Prenatal Diagnosis*, 9; 795–804.

Blumberg BD, Golbus MS, Hanson KH (1975) The psychological sequelae of abortion performed for a genetic indication. *American Journal of Obstetrics and Gynecology*, 122; 799–808.

Bourne S, Lewis E (1984) Pregnancy after stillbirth or neonatal death. *Lancet*, ii; 31–33.

Bradley DM, Parsons EP, Clarke AJ (1993) Experience with screening newborns for Duchenne muscular dystrophy in Wales. *British Medical Journal*, 306; 357–360.

Buchanan A, Brock DW, Daniels N *et al.* (2000) *From Chance to Choice: Genetics and Justice.* Cambridge University Press, Cambridge.

Cote-Arsenault D, Bidlack D, Humm A (2001) Women's emotions and concerns during pregnancy following perinatal loss. *American Journal of Maternal Child Nursing*, 26(3); 128–134.

Davis A (1999) A disabled person's perspective on prenatal screening. *MIDIRS Midwifery Digest*, 9; 8–10.

Devane D, Devane M (2000) Termination for fetal defects? The debate must go on. *British Journal of Midwifery*, 8(8); 475–479.

Donnai P, Charles N, Harris R (1981) Attitude of patients after 'genetic' termination of pregnancy. *British Medical Journal*, 282; 621–622.

Farrant W (ed.) (1985) *Who's for Amniocentesis? The Politics of Prenatal Screening*. Gower, London.

Gilchrist AC, Hannaford PC, Frank P *et al.* (1995) Termination of pregnancy and psychiatric morbidity. *British Journal of Psychiatry*, 167(2); 243–248.

Green JM, Statham H (1996) Psychosocial aspects of prenatal screening and diagnosis. In: *The Troubled Helix* (eds Marteau T, Richards M). Cambridge University Press, Cambridge, pp.140–163.

Green JM, Snowdon C, Statham H (1993) Pregnant women's attitudes to abortion and prenatal screening. *Journal of Reproductive and Infant Psychology*, 11; 31–39.

Hunfeld J (1995) The grief of late pregnancy loss: a four year follow-up. PhD thesis, Erasmus University, Rotterdam.

Iles S (1989) The loss of early pregnancy. *Bailliere's Clinical Obstetrics and Gynaecology*, 3(4); 769–790.

Iles S, Gath D (1993) Psychiatric outcome of termination of pregnancy for foetal abnormality. *Psychological Medicine*, 23; 407–413.

Janis IL, Mann L (1977) *Decision Making: A Psychological Analysis of Conflict, Choice and Commitment*. Free Press, New York.

Jorgensen C, Uddenberg N, Ursing Z (1985) Ultrasound diagnosis of fetal malformation in the second trimester: the psychological reactions of the women. *Journal of Psychosomatic Obstetrics and Gynaecology*, 4; 31–40.

Lasker JN, Toedter LJ (2000) Predicting outcomes after pregnancy loss; results from studies using the Perinatal Grief Scale. *Illness, Crisis and Loss*, 8(4); 350–372.

Laurence KM (1989) *Sequelae and Support for Termination Carried Out for Fetal Malformation*. The Free Woman, Amsterdam.

Laurence KM, Morris J (1981) The effect of the introduction of prenatal diagnosis on the reproductive history of women at increased risk from neural-tube defects. *Prenatal Diagnosis*, 1; 51–60.

Leschot NJ, Verjaal M, Treffers PE (1982) Therapeutic abortion on genetic grounds. *Journal of Psychosomatic Obstetrics and Gynecology*, 1–2; 47–56.

Lippman A (1991) Prenatal genetic testing and screening: constructing needs and reinforcing inequities. *American Journal of Law & Medicine*, 17; 15–50.

Lloyd J, Laurence KM (1985) Sequelae and support after termination of pregnancy for fetal malformation. *British Medical Journal*, 290; 907–909.

Major B, Cozzarelli C, Cooper ML *et al.* (2000) Psychological responses of women after first-trimester abortion. *Archives of General Psychiatry*, 57(8); 785–786.

Marteau TM, Dormandy E (2001) Facilitating informed choice in prenatal testing: How well are we doing? *American Journal of Medical Genetics*, 106; 185–190.

Marteau TM, Mansfield CD (1998) The psychological impact of prenatal diagnosis and subsequent decisions. In *Yearbook of Obstetrics and Gynaecology* (ed. O'Brien PMS). Royal College of Obstetrics and Gynaecology, London.

Marteau TM, Johnson M, Plenicar M *et al.* (1988) Development of a self-administered questionnaire to measure women's knowledge of prenatal screening and diagnostic tests. *Journal of Psychosomatic Research*, 32; 403–408.

Marteau TM, Dormandy E, Michie S (2001) A measure of informed choice. *Health Expectations*, 4(2); 99–108.

Press N, Browner C (1997) Why women say yes to prenatal diagnosis. *Social Science and Medicine*, 45; 979–989.

Rich D (1999) The relationship between type and timing of post pregnancy loss services and grief outcome. PhD thesis, University of Minnesota, MI.

Rona RJ, Smeeton NC, Beech R *et al.* (1998) Anxiety and depression in mothers related to severe malformation of the heart of the child and foetus. *Acta Paediatrica*, 87; 201–205.

Rothman BK (1986) *The Tentative Pregnancy: Prenatal Diagnosis and the Future of Motherhood*. Viking Penguin, New York.

Rothman BK (1988) *The Tentative Pregnancy: Amniocentesis and the Sexual Politics of Motherhood*. Pandora, London.

SATFA (1993) *SATFA News*, February. Support After Termination For Abnormality. SATFA News (February).

Salvesen KA, Oyen L, Schmidt N *et al.* (1997) Comparison of long-term psychological responses of women after pregnancy termination due to fetal anomalies and after perinatal loss. *Ultrasound in Obstetrics & Gynecology*, 9; 80–85.

Shakespeare T (1998) Choices and rights: eugenics, genetics and disability equality. *Disability & Society*, 13(5); 665–681.

Sitrin (1994) Parental copying after miscarriage, still birth, neonatal and infant death (unpublished thesis).

Statham H (1987) Cold comfort. *The Guardian*. 24 March.

Statham H (1992) Professional understanding and parents' experience of termination. In *Prenatal Diagnosis and Screening* (eds Brock DJH, Rodeck CH, Ferguson-Smith MA). Churchill Livingstone, London, pp. 697–702.

Statham H (2002) Prenatal diagnosis of fetal abnormality: the decision to terminate the pregnancy and the psychological consequences. *Fetal and Maternal Medicine Review*, 13; 213–247.

Statham H, Dimavicius J (1992) How do you give the bad news to parents? *Birth*, 19; 103–104.

Statham H, Solomou W, Chitty L (2000) Prenatal diagnosis of fetal abnormality: psychological effects on women in low-risk pregnancies. *Bailliere's Clinical Obstetrics and Gynaecology*, 14(4); 731–747.

Statham H, Solomou W, Green J (2001) *When a Baby Has an Abnormality: A Study of Parents' Experiences*. Centre for Family Research, University of Cambridge, Cambridge.

Suslak L, Scherer A, Rodriquez G (1995) A support group for couples who have terminated a pregnancy after prenatal diagnosis: recurrent themes and observations. *Journal of Genetic Counselling*, 4; 169–178.

Weatherall DJ (1992) Foreword. In: *Prenatal Diagnosis and Screening* (eds Brock DJ, Rodeck CH, Ferguson-Smith MA). Churchill Livingstone, Edinburgh.

Wertz DC (1993) Providers' gender and moral reasoning: a proposed agenda for research on providers and patients. *Fetal Diagnosis & Therapeutics*, 8; 81–89.

White-van Mourik MCA, Connor JM, Ferguson-Smith MA (1992) The psychosocial sequelae of a second-trimester termination of pregnancy for fetal abnormality. *Prenatal Diagnosis*, 12; 189–204.

Williams C, Alderson P, Farsides B (2002). Is nondirectiveness possible within the context of antenatal screening and testing? *Social Science and Medicine*, 54; 339–347.

Zeanah CH, Dailey JV, Rosenblatt MJ *et al.* (1993) Do women grieve after terminating pregnancies because of fetal anomalies? A controlled investigation. *Obstetrics and Gynecology* , 82(2); 270–275.

16 THE PARENTS' REACTIONS TO TERMINATION OF PREGNANCY FOR FETAL ABNORMALITY: FROM A FATHER'S POINT OF VIEW

Ray Hall

A PERSONAL PERSPECTIVE

As the author of this piece I do not bring any professional expertise to the subject. Nor am I drawing on any research that has been undertaken on the experience of fathers who find themselves in this situation; indeed I am not aware that there is very much relevant research. I was the father of a malformed baby that was terminated, and what I have written largely reflects my own experience. Following the termination, my wife Celia and I became involved with a group which was then called Support After Termination For Abnormality (SATFA), and is now called Antenatal Results and Choices (ARC), a charity which provides support for parents who have had a termination because of an abnormality. This has brought me into contact with a number of men who have talked about their experiences. I have, to a certain extent, been able to draw on what I have heard from others to try to say something of more general interest.

I am sure that there is much that can be said about how men fare when there is a termination for abnormality. I have not attempted to try to cover all the ground, but there were two problems that I experienced that I know have also troubled other fathers. The first arose from trying to cope with the termination, while at the same time giving support to my wife. The second is the reluctance that I, and I suspect many other men, feel to talk about the termination or our feelings about what happened.

PROVIDING SUPPORT

The first that I knew of a problem was when Celia called me at work. This was our third child and, like our others it was a planned pregnancy, and we were looking forward to the new baby. Although the pregnancy was not yet halfway through I had already fitted the baby into my picture of the world. Celia had been more uncomfortable this time around, with much stronger bouts of morning sickness, but we had no thought that anything might be wrong with the baby. She had gone to the local hospital for a routine ultrasound scan to check her dates and the baby's development. We were not anxious, and I did not give the possibility of any problem even a passing thought.

As soon as Celia spoke I knew that there was something wrong. It took me a few moments to understand what she was saying. There was something wrong with the shape of our baby's head and Celia would have to have further tests at a hospital with a more sophisticated ultrasound device. We had an appointment in a few days. Nothing was certain, but from what she had seen and the reaction of the hospital staff, Celia was sure that there was a serious problem.

That phone call marked the start of a rush of events and, looking back, set the pattern for the coming weeks. This whole period, from the time of the diagnosis, until shortly after the termination, was very intense and difficult for both of us. Finding out that the baby had spina bifida came as a profound shock to both of us. We talked over what we had been told again and again, trying to come to terms with what was happening. Celia was distraught and later, with the physical trauma of the termination to recover from, she was in a particularly distressed state. I could barely believe what was happening; it all seemed out of focus. But although I was in a bad way, I felt that Celia's pain and distress was more acute than mine. She had carried the baby and had undergone the termination. It therefore seemed perfectly natural that I should adopt a supportive role and try to help her through what was happening to us. My reaction was reinforced by the idea that as a man I should be strong and provide a shoulder to cry on, and that I should keep a grip on my own emotions.

This is by no means bad. Someone has to take on that role, if for no other reason than to deal with the practical side of life. Celia was in no condition to continue with her teaching job, and could not cope with running the home or with our other two children. I had to 'keep the family going' as well as support her emotionally. Taking on those responsibilities while at the same time balancing the demands of a job was very stressful.

It also meant that I made sure I was always at subsequent hospital visits. My initial feeling, on hearing about the results of the ultrasound scan, had been one of guilt. I felt that I should have been there at the hospital. Being present at later visits not only assuaged those feelings but it also helped in understanding the abnormality and what it would mean for our baby if it were born. Seeing ones child and the deformity (which in this case was a severe form of spina bifida), confirmed at first hand that there was a problem and gave us the opportunity to talk through its implications with the doctor. In that way we were both in a position to take responsibility for what was happening to us. The burden was shared.

For me, the down-side of taking on a strong supportive role was that I felt inhibited about expressing, and perhaps even experiencing, my own feelings of grief. I submerged my feelings, and that was harmful to my emotional wellbeing and also to our relationship. There were days when I was trying to support Celia without 'being there' myself. This, I am afraid, meant that at times I appeared unaffected by what had happened and perhaps uncaring.

I know from hearing others talk, that I am not the only father that has found himself in this position. Finding a way of handling these situations without falling into this trap is difficult. The force of circumstance and perceptions about how men are supposed to behave are not easy to overcome. I doubt that there is any general answer to this 'problem', but many things can be done to help. Doctors, hospital staff and other professionals can help by their handling of the father. It is natural that the woman is the focus for treatment, attention and sympathy when there is a termination for abnormality; but it is important not to underestimate the impact of these events on men. Discovering that you have fathered a deformed baby, deciding what you should do about it, being present at the termination, and seeing the baby born, are as emotionally painful for men as for women.

Couples in our position have a variety of experiences with professionals: some good and some not so good. In our case the sympathy and compassion with which we were treated made a tremendous difference to the way in which we coped at the time, and to how I recovered. The termination itself can be a long and solitary ordeal for the father. I could not share Celia's pain; I tried to give her what support I could but, as she was being treated with pain killing drugs, for much of the time I could do no more than sit there holding her hand. This was a draining experience. The care and support of the nursing staff who, despite being busy delivering healthy babies, still found time to come and talk to me, kept me going. Later on we had the help of a midwife who talked to us about the baby after she was born, and about how the deformity would have affected her development. She helped by taking a photograph and giving us the opportunity to touch and hold our daughter. For me those moments are some of my clearest recollections, and because of the compassion we were shown, have been the most helpful in enabling me to come to terms with what happened. It is of course important for a hospital to provide the right treatment, but looking after both the mother's and the father's needs in a sympathetic way, is too important to exaggerate. This kind of event is rare for most people, and it is important to have someone to lead you through it.

Being caught between coping with tragedy and at the same time supporting others is not of course a problem unique to a termination for abnormality; it arises wherever there is grieving within a family or community. Nor is it a problem that faces the man alone. Women will also have to balance their own grief against the need to provide support. Such mutual support is a natural part of any close relationship, but I think that circumstances and the traditional 'strong' role that most men still see themselves as having, gives a different twist to the problem for men.

The dilemma that I found myself in was not of course hard and fast, but it was a tendency that I slowly became aware of and tried to overcome. While my wife needed support and I tried to give it, there were also times when it was important for us to share our grief and those were opportunities for me to bring out those feelings I had submerged. For us, one such moment came when we sat in the car outside the hospital and, having had confirmation of the diagnosis, we both broke down and cried. This brought us closer together. Other times arose when we talked.

TALKING

When we first learnt about the abnormality, talking was not a problem. I may have been in shock, but there was a clear, factual agenda. Relatives, friends, colleagues and others needed to be told what had happened. This can be a strain if the burden is not shared, but the talk is straightforward, if painful. For ourselves, we had to talk about the baby, about what might have caused the abnormality, about what we should do and what was right.... But afterwards, most people, particularly men, seem to find more difficulty, or are more reluctant to talk about what happened and about how they feel about it. You do not want to burden others with this kind of problem, or you do not know how to bring the subject into a conversation, or how others will react if you do. I think everyone who has been through this kind of experience has had those sticky moments when they have talked about what happened and found it a complete conversation stopper.

There is a danger that, for a while at least, you may convince yourself that you have coped and that you can get on with your life, but I suspect this is rarely right. Fathering a malformed baby and then deciding, out of love, to end that life is a decision that has a deep emotional cost. Looking back I can see that it had effects that lasted for a long time, long after I believed I had got over it. As the months and then years went by, I may not have thought about the baby everyday, but the termination put me under stress which not only affected my performance at work, but my relationship with my wife and my health. This is, I suspect, a common experience.

Coming to terms with this loss is a matter of grieving and finding a place for these events in your life, and there is no universal answer about how to do this. People are different and have different personal histories. I have, however, been struck by the fact that few men get involved with self-help groups or seem very willing to talk about their experiences. This may have something to do with the male role of being a source of strength or maybe there is some deeper reason to do with the psychology of men that makes them more reluctant to talk. This is not to say that they will not talk in the right circumstances, but they are reluctant. This seems to be a difference in the way that men and women react. From my experience, there seems to be something in the generalization that while women want to talk about what happened, men want to put it behind them and to get on with their lives. If men experience problems in coming to terms with the termination, there is also the belief that they can solve it themselves and do not need to turn to others for help.

I saw something of this in myself. Celia wanted to get in touch with SATFA (now ARC). I had no objection to that, but I was reluctant to get involved myself; I didn't think I needed to. I knew I had problems with coming to terms with the abnormality and our decision to have a termination, but I thought I could sort those out myself without anyone else's help, and perhaps like many men in this situation I wanted to put the experience behind me and get on with my life.

Why was I, and why are other men reluctant to talk in these situations? I have no evidence to support my view but I believe it can arise from a number of things. The whole episode might be seen as the woman's problem; it was she who bore the child and had the termination. Soon afterward men return to work, and although this will bring stress, the air of normality can crowd out the worries and emotions about the termination. Men may, therefore, appear unaffected and may not recognize their own needs.

My own experience was that whatever reluctance I felt about re-living the experience, once I started to talk it became easier. Although I did not realize it at the start, I found that I did need to talk about how I felt. Talking was painful; at times I just wanted to shut the memories away, but then I discovered that it could be a release. I became more honest with myself and articulated emotions that I had not always been fully aware of. Talking helped me to grieve, to understand my own actions and to find a place in my life for all that had happened.

The reluctance that many men feel about talking is also not helped by circumstances, because they do not often find themselves in situations with appropriate opportunities to talk about what has happened. Certainly one can talk about these things with your partner, but as I have already said, in circumstances where a father may find that he has to adopt a supportive role, this may not be easy. Anyway, what may be needed, for both, is to talk to someone else. However, unless he is fortunate, a man is much less likely to find opportunities to talk than is a woman. The kind of subject that might naturally lead to talk about a termination is much more likely to arise in discussion between women than between men.

Men will also usually return to work shortly after the termination. That is not a place where the topic of a termination for abnormality will be likely to arise, or one that is likely to encourage talk of that kind. Even where there is goodwill, if you have to be tough and hard-nosed in your job it is difficult to unburden your inner feelings at the same time. That is not to say that employers are always lacking in compassion, but while at work demands are made of you, and after the initial expressions of sympathy, a prolonged problem or absence may itself become an issue. No matter how good your relationship with your colleagues, it is a different one to personal relationships you might have outside work. I talked to my colleagues and explained what had happened and what we had decided. It helped to talk, but at the same time I was not entirely sure that I wanted to go into all this with those I worked with. In an environment in which you are expected to perform, and are judged on that performance, people will be wary about disclosing matters of this personal kind.

If I am right about male psychology and the lack of opportunities men have to talk, can anything be done to help? I believe that counselling would be of value but comments from fathers suggests that few are offered any professional counselling. I did not receive any counselling, but through SATFA I became involved with a self-help group which my wife was helping to organize. I had doubts about joining in, but despite those doubts, and inhibitions, I found that it was a beneficial experience. We had all been through the experience, and were there just to talk and listen. In that supportive atmosphere I found that I articulated emotions and feelings that I had not fully recognized before. Even listening to other people was helpful because it not only enabled me to recognize my own feelings, but meeting other people who had come to terms with their grief helped one to see that it was possible to work through this tragedy.

Although I found enormous benefit from that self-help group it is not the answer for everyone, and they have their limitations. Women are in the majority in most meetings and this itself will deter some men from talking or even attending. The composition of a group will also affect the atmosphere. On the few occasions I have been in an all-male group there has been a difference in tone and topic. If nothing else, being away from your partner can give some extra freedom to talk.

A REFLECTION 6 YEARS ON

Some 6 years have now passed since our termination and although the pain has largely gone, one does not forget. As a parent I value the medical advances which enable the detection of fetal abnormality, but such developments have a cost. Ordinary and usually unsuspecting people are put in a position where they have to take a most difficult decision. I believe that parents should have that right, but it is important to remember that while ending the life of an unborn baby may avoid one tragedy, it may, unless both parents are cared for, create another.

A FINAL REFLECTION

A further 8 years have now passed since the termination of our baby, Alison. With the passage of time and another baby the painful memories are not as sharp. There have of course been times when I have wondered what life would have been like if we had made a different decision when we heard about Alison's condition. From time to time I still think about the awfulness of the termination and that she had no life at all. We have not forgotten Alison and always make a point of remembering her every year at the time of her death and encourage our other children to do so as well if they are at home with us. But I believe we made the right decision and we have come to terms with that and all it means. We helped each other and I am sure that talking to other parents at the time and afterwards also helped me. I do not think I would have coped without that help. It was not a happy time but we have been able to move our lives on.

FURTHER READING
O'Dowd T (1993) The needs of fathers. *British Medical Journal*, 306; 1484–1485.

LOOKING IN FROM THE OUTSIDE – REACTIONS TO TERMINATION OF PREGNANCY FOR FETAL ABNORMALITY FROM THE VIEWPOINT OF THOSE WHO CARE

Margaretha van Mourik

INTRODUCTION

Judge no man before you have walked a mile in his moccasins.

(Indian proverb, Arizona)

Couples who embark on a pregnancy expect to have a 'normal' child, yet 2% will, often unexpectedly, have an abnormal outcome. Until a few decades ago there was no choice but to accept the risks distributed by nature. If fate gave you a child with severe problems you accepted it as well as you could and then learned to live with the consequent, often perpetual, grief. Parents who were aware of a genetic problem within their family may have avoided having any children because frequently their fear of having a child with severe problems outweighed their desire for offspring. They subsequently suffered the sadness of not realizing their desired family.

Developments in obstetric ultrasound, biochemistry, cytogenetics and molecular genetics, concurrent with the introduction of laws that allow abortion for fetal abnormality, opened the road to antenatal screening and prenatal diagnosis. These combined advances now provide couples with choice. In some cases, and at a few centres, preimplantation diagnosis may now be offered, but procedures and outcomes are still complex. Testing a baby during pregnancy for genetic or other major abnormalities therefore remains a growing and constantly changing field of medicine. At the same time, however, these tests continue to raise agonizing ethical dilemmas; despite the scientific advances, intervention still usually provides merely one choice; to terminate a pregnancy or to continue.

In this chapter we will examine what happens to couples when fate transforms into an act of their own choosing, and what practical, ethical, spiritual, emotional and social issues are involved in trying to live with the decision to terminate a pregnancy for fetal abnormality. We will explore how as carers and as society as a whole we can try to support couples in coping with the emotional burden of this choice.

AN OUTSIDER'S CONFRONTATION WITH THE PSYCHO-SOCIAL CONSEQUENCES OF A TERMINATION OF PREGNANCY FOR FETAL ABNORMALITY

In the 1980s I was asked to take part in a large medical study which brought me in touch with about 1200 couples who had a termination of pregnancy for fetal abnormality. Over the next decade I visited many of these couples at home and had the opportunity to stay in touch with a number of them over the subsequent 10 years. I learned about the intensity of grief felt by many, a grief that for some was as painful and vivid 5 years after the event as it had been at the time. I noticed that there were great variations in coping with the intervention and its aftermath, but that there were certain emotions and difficulties that many had in common. I wondered at the time about the medical care, follow-up and support given to these couples and will refer to studies reporting on these issues. I observed the difficulties for carers too.

Some couples chose to decline support, and for many this was the right decision. Others, however, found it extremely difficult to ask for help or accept support after the intervention in spite of experiencing problems. They found it easier to accept this support when it was offered in the framework of a research programme and reflected years later on how helpful it had been and how much they had needed it. In this chapter we will explore the reasons for these reactions and try to discover ways to overcome difficulties in providing care.

IDENTIFICATION WITH THE FETUS

Some sections of our society are astonished by the grief reactions of couples after fetal loss. One of the reasons for this may be that Western cultures have still not decided officially on the status of the human embryo (Dunstan, 1988). Some other cultures have traditionally had personification of the fetus before birth. The relationship with the fetus starts after the awareness of pregnancy; thus the Siriona of East Bolivia perform the same bereavement ritual for a miscarried fetus as for a deceased adult. In Cambodia the dead fetus is believed to have magical protective powers and is honoured after birth (Walter, 1980).

Cranley (1981), reporting on the relationship of parents with their 'unborn', noted that there was a wealth of interaction between the mother and her fetus. She observed that both father and mother developed bonding behaviour towards the fetus. She perceived that this phenomenon reflected the fact that the fetus is experienced as a future child.

Although the infant–mother relationship develops gradually, quickening (first maternal awareness of the fetal movements between 14 and 20 weeks of pregnancy) has often been seen as a milestone (Hollerbach, 1979). New developments in diagnostic techniques have been shown to induce an earlier and more intense involvement with the fetus (Reading et al., 1981; Fletcher and Evans, 1983; Blumberg, 1984). Fetal life is now audible (fetal heart sounds) and visible (ultrasonography) from 8–10 weeks, and these techniques present the parents with undeniable evidence of fetal life (Lumley, 1980). It is not unusual for the home pregnancy test to be seen as confirmation of the start of a new phase of life and the first ultrasound picture to be saved as the first photograph of the child.

FETAL LOSS, GRIEF AND MOURNING

With parental awareness of the fetus as an independent identity it is not surprising that the loss of a wanted and planned pregnancy is experienced as the loss of a child. Many women who abort spontaneously experience anguish, loneliness and depression following the realization of pregnancy loss (Borg and Lasker, 1988). Where there was ambivalence toward the pregnancy, there could be guilt feelings. A sense of physical inadequacy and responsibility for the loss is shared by many.

The response to fetal loss is appropriately viewed as a form of bereavement (Lloyd and Laurence, 1985). Grieving is not a pathological symptom but a normal, and even necessary, reaction after fetal loss (Pedder, 1982). The duration of the reaction depends on the success with which the individual does 'grief work', which chiefly entails the acceptance of the feelings of intense distress. Avoiding these feelings and denying what has happened may lead to 'morbid grief', which is either a delayed reaction precipitated by specific circumstances or events sometimes years later, or a distorted reaction which may be difficult to recognize as the original grief. This unresolved grief may in turn have an adverse effect on health (Stroebe and Stroebe, 1987).

It is often assumed that the longer the period of gestation, the closer the bonding to the fetus and therefore the greater the feelings of bereavement after pregnancy loss. However, just as not all births of live healthy babies result in immediate and ideal attachment, so women with first or second trimester pregnancy loss must not be assumed to have a less severe reaction to bereavement. More important criteria are:

- the significance of the pregnancy to the parents;
- their previous experience of loss and adaptation to it;
- their personalities;
- their perception of social support from their partner and others.

TERMINATION OF PREGNANCY FOR FETAL ABNORMALITY

Prenatal diagnosis is now available for many couples with a family history of genetic disease, thus enabling them to dare consider further pregnancies. Antenatal maternal serum screening for detection of neural-tube defects and Down syndrome is offered to an increasing number of pregnant women and cystic fibrosis screening to some. Furthermore, detailed ultrasound scans are increasingly becoming part of routine pregnancy care. In all these programmes there is the option of terminating the pregnancy if an affected fetus is diagnosed. The emotional implications of screening and prenatal diagnosis are many and complex and are discussed in other chapters. I will therefore concentrate on professional observations of the couples who were subjected to the acute trauma imparted by the discovery of fetal defect and who chose the option of termination of pregnancy.

The realization of an unfavourable result triggers an immediate grief response that may be characterized by disbelief, shock and anger (Donnai *et al.*, 1981; Adler and Kusnick, 1982; Dallaire *et al.*, 1995; Marteau and Mansfield, 1998). Hopes and expectations may be dashed by the revelation of the fetal abnormality. A medico-legal necessity of a quick decision either to continue or terminate the pregnancy can add to the burden of the already distressed couple. Previous abstract attitudes towards abortion appear to provide little guidance for couples trapped in this moral dilemma. The parents' understanding of the specific defect affecting the fetus is a significant determinant of their decision and course of action (Blumberg, 1984; Korenromp *et al.*, 1992).

PSYCHO-SOCIAL CONSEQUENCES OF A TERMINATION OF PREGNANCY FOR FETAL ABNORMALITY

In contrast to the mostly positive reactions of women after an abortion for psycho-social indications (Doane and Quigley, 1981; Adler *et al.*, 1990), many authors (Lloyd and Laurence, 1985; Thomassen-Brepols, 1985; Black, 1989; Frets *et al.*, 1990; Korenromp *et al.*, 1992; White-van Mourik *et al.*, 1992; Dallaire *et al.*, 1995) have observed the opposite following a termination of pregnancy for fetal abnormality. When the findings in the literature are collated, the reasons for the increased distress emerge. The majority of women who agreed to antenatal screening or prenatal diagnosis had planned and/or welcomed the pregnancy. Many were in the second trimester of their pregnancy and those who agreed to screening had often not seriously considered an abnormal result. The intervention thus had the psychological meaning of the loss of a wanted child. Loss implies mourning, yet coping and grieving were complicated by other problems which needed attention, such as the perceived loss of biological, moral and social competence and the associated loss of self-esteem. Conflicting emotions were complicated by contradictory images: that of the wished for, fantasized baby and that of the damaged or disabled child (Thomassen-Brepols, 1985).

ASPECTS OF COPING IN THE SHORT TERM AFTER A TERMINATION OF PREGNANCY FOR FETAL ABNORMALITY

The first reaction reported by most couples immediately after the termination of pregnancy was a feeling of relief that it was over. Many felt numbed by the diagnosis and the agonizing decisions that had been made in the previous few days. For some this numbness continued during their stay as an in-patient; others became painfully aware of their loss during their time in hospital. Because many women are cared for in postnatal wards, this awareness was reinforced by hearing other women's babies cry while seeing their own empty cot. Especially painful were questions regarding the baby's wellbeing from fellow patients and well-meaning auxiliary staff. Low self-esteem was sometimes reinforced by ward policies and the attitude of staff. One woman told me that she had spoken to a fellow patient who had had a stillbirth.

Although we both left hospital with empty arms, she had had the opportunity to hold her baby, which had been presented to her dressed and washed in a little Moses basket. She had keepsakes and her baby would be buried. The name of the baby was put in a hospital memorial book. I was offered none of these memories and I would have liked them. Although I could see the baby after asking for it, the midwife held my baby as if it was something distasteful. A request to have my baby's name put in the memorial book was refused because I had had a termination of pregnancy and it was against hospital policy.

Thankfully this kind of story is heard less often now, as maternity units and staff have gained awareness of the grief experienced by couples after this specific kind of loss. The improvement was observed by Statham *et al.* (2001) in a study about parents' experiences when a baby has an abnormality.

Low self-esteem was further reinforced for some on return home. Studies reported that half of the couples were not contacted by any member of the primary care team (general practitioner, midwife, health visitor), nor were they invited to the surgery or visited at home; yet 60% of the women in studies experienced breast engorgement and lactation lasting over 5 days (Lloyd and Laurence, 1985; White-van Mourik *et al.*, 1990; Statham *et al.*, 2001). One woman mentioned; 'I felt that the medical profession had lost interest in me. The faulty fetus was terminated, so that was the end of the problem. But for me my problems were just starting'.

The realization of an unfavourable result triggered an immediate grief response and this was frequently characterized by disbelief, shock and anger. It was in this frame of mind that couples had to make decisions about their fetus. It is therefore not unusual for some newly bereaved parents to start to experience feelings of doubt shortly after the termination of pregnancy. In one study (White-van Mourik *et al.*, 1992), half of the women admitted that they felt ambivalent about their decision. This was often linked to a lack of understanding of the fetal defect. There were fears that the medical professionals might have made a mistake, and that they were disapproved of for the act of terminating the pregnancy.

Mothers whose fetus' abnormality had been identified through investigations done following maternal serum screening, frequently had only a vague comprehension of the fetal condition for which they had been offered the intervention. Dallaire *et al.* (1995) also noted a different response in women who had been taken by surprise after a screening programme from that of those with a known family history of a genetic condition. The latter seemed more able to put a distance between themselves and the pregnancy. The authors mentioned, however, that almost all couples sometimes forgot the seriousness of the disease or malformation and convinced themselves that the infant could, with care and treatment, have recovered after birth. Doubts appeared particularly common in very young women (16–20 years), those who left school at a very young age, and those in whom the severity of the defect was uncertain.

When fetal abnormality was identified by routine ultrasound, most women did not perceive the burden of choice as a consequence of having the investigation. This was in contrast to the women who were identified as being at high risk through a maternal serum screening programme and who felt that they had not fully considered the implications of accepting the test. Doubts in these groups were significantly decreased if, at a post-termination consultation, time was taken to explain the condition of the fetus, the nature of the anomaly or illness, and the likely prognosis. Two years after the intervention, even where there had been initial doubts, the great majority of couples felt at peace with their decision (Thomassen-Brepols, 1985; White-van Mourik *et al.*, 1992; Dallaire *et al.*, 1995).

EMOTIONAL AND SOMATIC REACTIONS IN THE FIRST 6 MONTHS AFTER TERMINATION OF PREGNANCY

It is common for a feeling of deep sadness to be shared by both partners after the termination of pregnancy for fetal abnormality. Depression, anger, fear, guilt and failure were the other most frequently mentioned strong emotions. The anger was often a reaction to the feeling of helplessness for not having been able to protect their child from harm. The feeling of responsibility for this new life was mentioned by some men (see Chapter 16), but was expressed principally by women. Feelings of guilt could be focused on various objects: towards the child, because a decision was made that it should not live, towards a previous child with a similar defect and towards one's partner. When expressing their feelings about fear, couples stressed the possibility of recurrence of the abnormality and the idea of having to repeat the whole decision-making process. Having to face the consequences of that choice was, and for some remained, terrifying.

Some women complained of prolonged numbness, panic spells and palpitations, but in the studies only men admitted to feeling withdrawn and being excluded (Korenromp *et al.*, 1992; White-van Mourik *et al.*, 1992). One male partner typically explained; 'Of course it hurts and making such a decision was emotionally draining, but I can't see how talking about it helps. I want to be left alone'.

In many societies, reproduction and reproductive failure are still frequently perceived as the woman's purview. One husband explained:

Everyone asked how my wife felt but nobody seemed to consider that I had feelings too. Even when things went wrong, the obstetrician explained all about it to my wife and her mother and by the time I came home from work (they did not want to worry me) they had more or less decided to terminate my baby. I felt so angry and redundant, but could not show it as my wife was upset and needed me.

As well as coping with strong feelings, many couples report somatic symptoms. Listlessness, loss of concentration, irritability and crying are mentioned frequently. Lack of concentration in the first few months can lead to mistakes at work and to unexpected failures in exams.

Reported nightmares commonly have one or more of the following elements:

- Replay – in which the termination procedure is repeated night after night, and sometimes continues intermittently for up to a year after the termination of pregnancy.
- Persecution – in which the parent runs away to prevent pursuers from taking the baby.
- Blame – in which the baby, or family members appear and accuse the parent of murder.

Despite these dissonant feelings and complaints many couples feel reluctant to bring them up in discussion with health professionals, family or friends for fear of being judged mentally unstable or weak. This reticence may be overcome by carefully formulated questions asked as part of the routine post-termination protocol.

LONG-TERM PSYCHO-SOCIAL AND COPING ASPECTS

In one study (White-van Mourik et al., 1992), 2 years after the termination of pregnancy, most couples reported that they had regained equilibrium. For some this happened less than 6 months after the intervention. However, most continued to experience sadness about the loss of the baby and to fear recurrence of the condition in a subsequent pregnancy. The feeling of continuing relief was especially mentioned by those families familiar with a distressing disability or genetic disease.

In two studies (Thomassen-Brepols, 1985; White-van Mourik et al., 1992), about 20% of women continued to feel angry, guilty, a failure, irritable and tearful. They felt that these strong emotions had a disruptive impact on their lives and relationships. Men appeared to come to terms with their loss more quickly than did their spouses. The same observation was made by Statham et al. (2001) and Martinson et al. (1980) who reported that, after the loss of a child, fathers were twice as likely as mothers to say that the most intensive part of grieving was over in a few weeks. However, their response may have reflected the social expectations of the father 'to take it like a man'. Men appear to have a greater need to keep their grief private (De Frain et al., 1982) and this may even give their partners the impression that they are not affected by the loss; yet it was often the male partners who were more apprehensive about the idea of a further pregnancy.

THE MARITAL OR PARTNER RELATIONSHIP

Many partners reported an initial closeness after the termination of pregnancy. They found that the procedure and the deep emotions after the intervention had brought a new dimension to the relationship. Where there had been a close relationship before the intervention, partners generally were able to be understanding and supportive. Where difficulties were experienced, these were reported to be most pronounced after 3–6 months. They appeared to be due to lack of communication, irritation and an intolerance of the different coping mechanisms used in coming to terms with the bereavement. Severe difficulties appeared where there were unspoken attributions of guilt and blame between the partners.

Sexual problems arose where the partners experienced different needs and were unable to communicate them. The woman might have difficulties separating the sexual act from pregnancy and conception, while the man might want to reinforce emotional closeness, or vice versa. In a few cases, sexual difficulties had continued over many years post-termination without help being sought (White-van Mourik *et al.*, 1992). Chitty *et al.* (1999) observed that the severity of grief in a woman was closely linked to whether or not a she felt she was getting the support she would like from her partner.

THE OTHER CHILDREN IN THE FAMILY

About half the couples noticed a change in their behaviour towards their other children. The majority treasured them more but felt overprotective and allowed them less freedom. The realization that it was possible for bad luck to strike twice was strong. For some the feeling of over protectiveness became a worry and they had difficulties coping with their anxiety. About 20% of the women interviewed were so preoccupied with their grief that their children were a source of irritation for them. In rare cases there was a feeling of total indifference towards the other children in the family and some children were cared for by other relatives for weeks or months. When the women felt negative about their children, they felt extremely guilty and never brought up the subject without being asked about it, yet discussing this guilt was reported to be a great relief.

FRIENDS AND FAMILY

In times of stress and uncertainty, many people turn to their close friends and relatives for support. The majority of couples in our study looked for different aspects of support in different relationships. Understanding, consideration and warm contact were hoped for in the relationship with their close family. Good listening, understanding and thoughtfulness were felt to be the most valued aspects of support from friends and to a lesser degree from colleagues and neighbours.

Couples expressed the need to feel that others were sensitive to their anguish and shared their feeling of loss. It was the relationships that meant the most to the couple that produced most friction. Friends and relatives were often unsure how to help. In other situations a grieving couple might indicate what help is needed, but in the case of a termination for fetal abnormality they too are bewildered. Couples reported conflicting feelings, of feeling grateful and angry, supported and isolated, of rationally recognizing the prevention of the birth of a disabled child and emotionally mourning the wanted baby. These conflicts were instrumental in the reluctance to instigate discussion, which was evident in many couples.

People often prefer to avoid the subjects of genetic inheritance, disability and abortion, especially when they come 'too close to home'. This means that couples who already found it difficult to talk about their intervention were actively discouraged from doing so. When expressing grief and loss they were sometimes reminded by supporters that they had been lucky to have had the choice. This further created feelings of guilt and failure. Other supporters kept a well-intentioned silence that was readily misinterpreted as disapproval. It was frequently assumed by outsiders that a strong grief reaction was linked to regretting the termination, and silence was employed to prevent guilt in the couple. However, follow-up after 2 years showed that most grieved but, on reflection, few regretted the termination (White-van Mourik *et al.*, 1992; Dallaire *et al.*, 1995). As time passed, women found it painful when those around them seemed totally unaware of the expected date of delivery and the anniversary of the termination.

MORAL DILEMMAS

Grieving after a termination for fetal abnormality is complicated by a loss of moral self-esteem, because there is an awareness of personal contribution to the pregnancy loss. In particular, those with strong religious convictions were troubled by the fact that unlike miscarriage or stillbirth, the loss was not unavoidable but had been chosen. There is a confrontation with one's own morality in making decisions about life and death. Even the knowledge that the fetus would have died anyway does not take away the overwhelming sense of responsibility for this new life and the feeling of having abandoned the fetus.

The decision to terminate the pregnancy frequently conflicted with previously held beliefs about right and wrong. I interviewed women who had been staunch 'Pro-Lifers' who, before the intervention, could not have imagined being able to make a decision to terminate a pregnancy. This ethical conflict and the moral pain of having to choose against life or for possible suffering was strongly illustrated by the fact that many couples were searching for purpose or reason. Even parents who normally did not have strong religious convictions reported preoccupation with a higher being; either to be angry with or to plead care for the child that they had not been able to protect. As a carer I found this deep anguish and continuing care for the lost child extremely moving, but I felt it difficult to give the right expression of support for this spiritual disturbance. Very few women got in touch with a religious leader (Thomassen-Brepols, 1985; White-van Mourik *et al.*, 1992).

SUPPORT FROM THE MEDICAL COMMUNITY

Although hospital staff were generally reported to be kind and caring (White-van Mourik *et al.*, 1990; Stratham *et al.*, 2001), few hospitals appeared to have an accessible protocol concerning the discharge and follow-up procedures after the termination of pregnancy. This meant that it was not uncommon for the woman to turn up in the surgery of her family doctor, only to be asked how the pregnancy was progressing. This was extremely painful for the bereaved women and embarrassing for their general practitioners who had not been informed.

There is reluctance in both men and women to report emotional disturbances or somatic complaints to the family doctor for fear of being put on tranquillizers or antidepressants or even being admitted to a psychiatric hospital. Couples greatly appreciated it when members of the primary and obstetric care team provided empathy, good listening and an understanding of the subjective qualities of the experience, as well as clear, factual information about the fetal condition and disorder, preconception care and the recurrence risk for future pregnancies. Equally important was consideration and understanding of different cultural backgrounds and religious belief systems (Alkuraya and Kilani, 2001).

CONSIDERING FURTHER PREGNANCIES AFTER A TERMINATION FOR FETAL ABNORMALITY

Loss of biological self-esteem is one of the factors that affects couples after a termination for fetal abnormality. As with fetal loss, the birth of a disabled child is still, if at times subconsciously, perceived to be reproductive failure. Feelings of shame and failure were frequently reinforced by the family and in-laws, who would fervently declare that this abnormality could not come from their side of the family. This only exaggerated the bereaved parents' loss of self-value at a time when, as observed in the literature about grief response (Thomassen-Brepols, 1985), self-esteem is an important ingredient in the coping strategy. A further complication is an increased incidence of fetal abnormality in subsequent pregnancies for many parents.

Most couples have a planned family size but the wish for more children may be amended by circumstances. In the past, couples at risk of genetic disease were often deterred from planning further pregnancies (Emery *et al.*, 1972; Emery *et al.*, 1973; Reynolds *et al.*, 1974; Klein and Wyss, 1977). Many authors reported changed reproductive behaviour after the introduction of prenatal diagnosis, in that couples dared to try to achieve their planned family (Kaback *et al.*, 1984; Modell *et al.*, 1984; Scriver *et al.*, 1984; Evers-Kiebooms *et al.*, 1988; Modell and Bulyzhenkov 1988). The decision-making process was perceived to be more burdensome by the couples who decided to have children using the option of prenatal diagnosis than it was by those for whom prenatal diagnosis was not available (Frets *et al.*, 1990).

The literature about the sequelae of a termination for fetal abnormality provides anecdotal information about couples refraining from further pregnancy. Only a few studies examined the reproductive behaviour of couples after a termination for fetal abnormality (De Frain et al., 1982; Thomassen-Brepols, 1985). In the Thomassen-Brepols study, where 40% of the women were 38 years and over, half the women experienced a reproductive conflict. In another study (White-van Mourik, 1989) the mean maternal age was 27 years and only 6% of the women were over 38 years of age. Perhaps for this reason only 14% experienced a reproductive conflict. The women in conflict were torn between their desire for another child and their fear of recurrence of the abnormality and the subsequent decision process.

These studies confirmed Lippmann-Hands and Fraser's view (1979) that neither the objective interpretation of the recurrence risk, nor single factors such as religious conviction, negative feeling about the termination procedure or lack of support post-termination, necessarily deterred couples from further reproduction. She concluded that the deciding factors in the reproductive conflict after a termination for fetal abnormality are:

- maternal age;
- an unexpected diagnosis;
- the presence of children in the family;
- a subtle combination of factors.

Frets et al. (1990) made similar observation in genetic counsellees.

The reason that the risk of procreational conflict was largest amongst women with advanced maternal age was that for them time was running out with the approaching end of fertility. Not only did this group have to contend with the losses described in the sequelae of termination for abnormality, they frequently experienced disapproval for their desire for further pregnancies from their spouse, relatives and friends, especially if they had other older children. Another group who wanted more children but often decided against further pregnancies were women who had received an unexpected diagnosis; i.e. one different from the one for which they may have requested prenatal diagnosis (Leschot et al., 1982; Thomassen-Brepols, 1985). Previous knowledge of fetal abnormality was not only helpful during the decision-making process, but also in attempts to come to terms with the termination of pregnancy; thus a surprise diagnosis reinforced the perceived loss of biological competence and decreased the feeling of self-value.

Help can be offered to couples with such a conflict by providing focused counselling. In this, the counsellor focuses on the counsellee's feelings concerning the reproductive decision, accepts apparently irrational considerations (because these feelings indicate the influence of unconscious motives) and understands the role which guilt plays in the decision (Frets et al., 1990).

All women who subsequently became pregnant in the Thomassen-Brepols (1985) and White-van Mourik (1989) studies chose prenatal diagnosis.

LIVING WITH THE CHOICE

The issue brought up most frequently after the termination was that of confusion concerning the ethical status of their decision. Directions may have been given regarding tests, the condition of the fetus, the admission to hospital and the termination procedure. This may not have been done very well but at least there was a system. However, when the termination was completed, all became vague. Medical and social responsibility frequently seemed to have come to an end. The choices had been offered and the couples themselves had made the decisions. As has been discussed, for many couples and especially for those unfamiliar with the diagnosed fetal abnormality, the long process of realization, grieving and resolution was just starting. Unfortunately, few hospitals had a protocol for psycho-medical after-care or, where desirable, long-term follow-up. Few couples were given the information about the psycho-social sequelae of the intervention or helped to explore the coping strategies for coming to terms with the decision. Barbara Katz Rothman (1986) observed:

> *These women are victims of a social system that fails to take collective responsibility for the needs of its members, and leaves individual women to make impossible choices. We are spared collective responsibility, because we individualize the problem. We make it the woman's own. She chooses, and so we owe her nothing. Whatever the cost, she has chosen. It is her problem not ours.*

Often, new directions in screening and prenatal diagnosis have been funded for their scientific development whilst research into the psycho-social consequences frequently has been under-funded. Surely it should be an integral part of all pregnancy screening programmes and diagnostic services, not only to provide choice but to support couples learning to live with this choice.

CARE PROGRAMMES

No care, however thoughtful and thorough, can take away the pain of loss; neither can reassuring remarks take away moral anguish. Resolution of grief does not mean forgetting the event, as many women who lost babies decades ago could testify. Support can be provided by recognizing that the turmoil of feelings after a termination of pregnancy may be disabling, but is not usually pathological, and by helping those couples who are having difficulties in unravelling their ambivalence.

This was confirmed in the perinatal mortality programmes that started to gain popularity in the mid-1980s (Bourne and Lewis, 1984; Kellner *et al.*, 1984; Kirk, 1984). These programmes were instigated to gain greater awareness of psychological problems of families after a stillbirth or neonatal death. They allowed, and then encouraged, bereavement processes to run their course until a resolution of grief. An immediate pregnancy to counteract the grieving process was discouraged. Forrest *et al.* (1982) mentioned that the duration of bereavement reactions was appreciably shortened by support and counselling.

An important strategy was to encourage parents to hold and see their dead baby so that farewells could be said and thus provide an end to a process that started with the discovery and confirmation of the abnormal pregnancy. The reality of the farewell facilitated the grieving process, which made resolution possible. In another study (White-van Mourik, 1989), the women who most deeply regretted not seeing their fetus were those too frightened or too tired to request a viewing after the termination of pregnancy procedure. They would have welcomed a picture of the fetus on file. It is indeed not uncommon for women to ring the hospital a decade after the intervention to request a picture of the fetus. Others, however, who had not wanted confirmation of their loss by mementoes had not regretted this decision after 2 years. Statham *et al.* (2001) noted that women who specifically did not want care and had a less ritualized approach to grieving, had the higher emotional wellbeing scores.

Parents should be allowed and encouraged to do what they wish and state what care they would like. No rigid regime about the 'right way' to grieve, should be imposed (Zinner, 2000). Although coping strategies could be suggested, parents' preferred coping style should be recognized and respected.

Self help groups (such as ARC in the UK) have been seen as invaluable in supporting women by reducing isolation (Vachon *et al.*, 1980). Their additional role in public relations and their help in the education of professionals has done much to raise public awareness of the problems and achieve change in the way care is provided.

COUPLES' PERCEPTIONS OF GOOD MANAGEMENT

When couples were asked for their recommendations on good management, three themes clearly emerged: recognition, information, and hope (White-van Mourik *et al.*, 1992).

Recognition was described in several ways:

- as the confirmation of the couple's status as parents by medical staff, relatives and friends;
- as perception and comprehension of their grief and the impact the diagnosis and intervention had on them;
- as an insight into the fact that apparent choice is often perceived by the couple as no choice at all, but as the only possible action under the specific circumstances;
- as an understanding of the fear of social disapproval and the subsequent reticence to ask for help when required;
- as perception of the turmoil of ambivalent feelings and the time it may take to come to terms with the event.

Recognition helps to boost the couple's self-esteem by making them feel normal under the circumstances. It prevents trivialization and the use of platitudes.

Information and communication were found to be of enormous value in coming to terms with the termination of pregnancy for fetal abnormality, but it was important that the information provided by professionals was accurate and not guessed at. Explanations, using appropriate language, about the fetal abnormality, the termination of pregnancy procedure and preparation for the physical, psycho-social, short- and long-term sequelae were considered essential. An exploration on how to cope with feelings of anger, depression and irritability was appreciated. Better and continuing communication minimized the feeling of being out of control and reduced misunderstanding.

Understanding of parents' religious and cultural background and the influences of this on their coping strategies were essential in communication and providing information. Equally important was facilitating an understanding of the various issues involved for translators and ethnic minority patient-advocates.

Good communication between the caring professionals in the hospital and community services promotes appropriately timed care and prevents the embarrassment of having to explain the sequence of events and the pregnancy loss, time and again. Statham *et al.* (2001) observed that many needs would be met more easily if a single individual were to coordinate a woman's care.

Hope for another pregnancy was felt to be of great importance to those wishing to achieve their planned family. A successful subsequent pregnancy counterbalanced the loss of biological self-esteem and to some extent restored a sense of social competence. Couples attached great importance to discussions about the implications of the fetal abnormality for further pregnancies, prenatal diagnosis, and preconception health care.

THE NEW BABY

The birth of a new baby was frequently the climax to a worrying time, as anguish experienced after the diagnosis of an affected baby re-emerged (Rillstone and Hutchison, 2001). Most parents were totally delighted with their healthy child. Unfortunately, frequently this delight was coloured with sadness by the memory of the delivery of the affected fetus. A few women admitted to having a pregnancy too soon after their loss in order to try to alleviate the pain of their grief. The birth of a healthy child may in these cases start a renewed grieving pattern. One woman said:

> When my healthy baby was put in my arms I suddenly realized what I had missed last time, and the only thing I could do was cry. I must have cried for weeks and felt so ungrateful for feeling so intensely sad. My husband and parents were totally bewildered, because I had been so good after the termination of pregnancy.

Understanding of these feelings by those carers attending the parents postnatally was found extremely helpful. Rillstone and Hutchison (2001) in their study of women with a pregnancy subsequent to one complicated by fetal abnormality, found that health professionals could assist parents at this time. They found that facilitating parents' efforts to develop emotional armour, limit disclosure, delay attachment to the baby and enlist support from health care professionals and support groups can mitigate social and psychological discomfort for these parents.

PRACTICAL CONSIDERATIONS FOR THOSE WHO CARE

All couples should be given information about possible sequelae. They need an assessment of their coping strategies and encouragement to take steps to counteract their lack of self-esteem, but not all couples need long-term counselling. Within the context of continuing medical care, professionals have a responsibility to understand this new kind of grief and to recognize the signs that may indicate a need for further counselling or professional mental health intervention. Some groups may have particular problems in expressing their anxieties. Men, especially from some 'introvert" northern European cultures, are inclined to find it hard to open up for fear of showing emotions and tears. It is therefore important to see the couple together. Those without a support network and those with a vulnerable personality need extra care. Those who have not coped with a previous bereavement experience appear to have an increased risk of a poor outcome. For young immature couples (between 16 and 20 years), it is often particularly hard to come to terms with the termination. Their moral convictions are frequently more inflexible, their self-esteem is often lower and their peers have less experience or interest in bereavement processes. In addition, they are frequently patronized by parents and medical professionals and are more timid about expressing themselves. Others who may need more time are couples who have communication difficulties and those with a reproductive conflict after the termination for fetal abnormality.

It should not be presumed that those with a termination of pregnancy in the first trimester gestation need less support than those with a second or third trimester intervention. It is important to address individual needs and wishes (Chitty *et al.*, 1999).

Use of perinatal grief scales adapted to the special issues surrounding the sequelae of a termination for fetal abnormality, may aid professionals in identifying those men and women who may need follow-up and support over a longer period. Such a scale should however be robust and undergo vigorous prospective testing.

CONCLUSION

In our multicultural society, carers must be particularly aware that psycho-social sequelae of fetal loss, grief and pre- and postnatal decisions may be influenced by the country or culture from which the parents come (Toedter *et al.*, 2001). Further in-depth studies are needed to provide carers with information so that they can respond appropriately to these differences.

Carers must ensure that they have channels to unload themselves as the intense pain and distress experienced by many couples can, at times, have a cumulative effect on one's own outlook on life.

Finally, regional audit of communication, provision of information and criteria of service will ensure that standards are being upheld.

Key points

- Following a termination of pregnancy for fetal abnormality, parents grieve for the loss of the hoped-for baby.
- This loss is complicated by the loss of biological, moral and social competence and the associated loss of self-esteem.
- Conflicting emotions oscillate between the image of the wished-for, fantasized baby and the image of the damaged or disabled child.
- Most parents do not need long-term counselling but those without a support network, with communication difficulties and reproductive conflict may need extra care and support.
- Understanding and empathy, knowledge about the sequelae, clear and accurate information and the hope for another pregnancy were reported as helpful by parents.
- Although coping strategies could be suggested, parents' preferred coping style should be recognized and respected at all times.
- In a multicultural society carers must be particularly aware of assumptions, as different countries and cultures may have a different psychosocial sequelae after a termination for fetal abnormality.

REFERENCES

Adler B, Kusnick T (1982) Genetic counselling in prenatally diagnosed Trisomy 18 and 21. *Paediatrics*, 69; 94–99.

Adler NE, Henry PD, Major BN *et al.* (1990) Psychological responses after abortion. *Science*, 248; 41–44.

Alkuraya FS, Kilani RA (2001) Attitude of Saudi families affected with haemoglobinopathies towards prenatal screening and abortion and the influence of religious ruling (Fatwa). *Prenatal Diagnosis*, 21(6); 448–451.

Black RB (1989). A 1 and 6 month follow-up of prenatal diagnosis patients who lost pregnancies, *Prenatal Diagnosis*, 9; 795–804.

Blumberg BD (1984) The emotional implications of prenatal diagnosis. In: *Psychological Aspects of Genetic Counselling* (eds Emery AEH, Pullen IM). Academic Press, London, pp. 202–217.

Borg S, Lasker J (1988) *When Pregnancy Fails: Families Coping with Miscarriage, Ectopic Pregnancy, Stillbirth and Infant Death* (rev. edn). Bantam Books, New York.

Bourne S, Lewis E (1984) Delayed psychological effects of perinatal deaths: the next pregnancy and the next generation. *British Medical Journal*, 289; 147–188.

Chitty LS, Statham H, Solomou W *et al.* (1999) Termination of pregnancy at different gestational ages: the grief response of mothers. *Ultrasound in Obstetrics and Gynaecology*, 14(suppl. 1); 24.

Cranley MS (1981) Roots of attachment: the relationship of parents with their unborn. In: *Perinatal Parental Behaviour: Nursing Research and Implications for the Newborn Health* (eds Lederman RP, Raff BS, Caroll P). Alan Liss, New York, pp. 59–83.

Dallaire L, Lortie G, Des Rochers M *et al.* (1995) Parental reactions and adaptability to prenatal diagnosis of fetal or genetic disease leading to pregnancy interruption. *Prenatal Diagnosis*, 15; 249–259.

De Frain J, Taylor J, Ernst L (1982) *Coping with Sudden Infant Death*. Lexington Books, D.C. Heath; Lexington, MA.

Doane BK, Quigley BG (1981) Psychiatric aspects of therapeutic abortion. Review article, *Canadian Medical Association Journal*, 125; 427–432.

Donnai P, Charles N, Harris R (1981) Attitudes of patients after genetic termination of pregnancy. *British Medical Journal*, 282; 621–622.

Dunstan G (1988) Screening for fetal and genetic abnormality: social and ethical issues. *Journal of Medical Genetics*, 25; 290–293.

Emery AEH, Watt M, Clark ER (1972) The effects of genetic counselling in Duchenne muscular dystrophy. *Clinical Genetics*, 3; 147–150.

Emery AEH, Watt M, Clark ER (1973) Social effects of genetic counselling. *British Medical Journal*. 1; 724–726.

Evers-Kiebooms G, Denayer L, Cassima JJ *et al.* (1988). Family Planning decisions after the birth of a cystic fibrosis child: impact of prenatal diagnosis. *Scandanavian Journal of Gastroenterology*, 143(suppl.); 38–46.

Fletcher JC, Evans MI (1983) Maternal bonding in early fetal ultrasound examinations. *New England Journal of Medicine*, 308; 392–393.

Forrest GC, Standish E, Baum JD (1982) Support after perinatal death: a study of support and counselling perinatal bereavement. *British Medical Journal*, 285; 1475–1479.

Frets PG, Los FJ, Sachs ES *et al.* (1990) Psychological counseling of couples experiencing a pregnancy termination after amniocentesis. *Journal of Psychosomatic Obstetrics and Gynecology*, 11(Special Issue 1); 53–59.

Hollerbach PA (1979) Reproductive attitudes and the genetic counsellee. In: *Counselling in Genetics* (eds Hsia YE, Hirschorn K, Siverbrg RL, *et al.*). Allan Liss, New York, pp. 155–222.

Kaback M, Zippin D, Boyd P *et al.* (1984) Attitudes towards prenatal diagnosis of cystic fibrosis amongst parents of affected children. In: *Cystic Fibrosis; horizons* (ed. Lawson D). John Wiley and Sons, New York, pp. 6–28.

Kellner KR, Donnelly WH, Gould SD (1984) Parental behaviour after perinatal death: Lack of predictive demography and obstetric variables. *Obstetrics and Gynecology*, 63; 809–814.

Kirk EP (1984) Psychological effects and management of perinatal loss. *American Journal of Obstetrics and Gynecology*,149; 46–51.

Klein D, Wyss D (1977) Retrospective and follow up study of approximately 1000 genetic consultations. *Journal of Human Genetics*, 25; 47–57.

Korenromp MJ, Iedema–Kuiper HR, van Spijker HG *et al.* (1992) Termination of pregnancy on genetic grounds; coping with grieving. *Journal of Psychosomatic Obstetrics and Gynaecology*, 13; 93–105.

Leschot NJ, Verjaal M, Treffers PE (1982) Therapeutic abortion on genetic indication; a detailed follow-up study of 20 patients. *Journal of Psychosomatic Obstetrics and Gynaecology*, 1; 47–56.

Lippman-Hands A, Fraser FC (1979) Genetic counselling: the provision and perception of information. *American Journal of Medical Genetics*. 3; 113–127.

Lloyd J, Laurence KM (1985) Sequelae and support after termination of pregnancy for fetal malformation. *British Medical Journal*, 290; 907–909.

Lumley J (1980) The image of the fetus in the first trimester. *Birth and the family* 7; 5–14.

Martinson I, Modow D, Henry W (1980) *Home Care for the Child with Cancer. Final report* (Grant no. Ca 19490). US Department of Health and Human Services, National Cancer Institute, Washington DC.

Marteau T, Mansfield CD (1998) The psychological impact of prenatal diagnosis and subsequent decisions. In: *Yearbook of Obstetrics and Gynecology* (ed. O'Briens PMS). Royal College of Obstetrics and Gynaecology, London.

Modell B, Bulyzhenkov V (1988) Distribution and control of some genetic disorders. *World Health Statutes Quarterly*, 41; 209–218.

Modell B, Petrou M, Ward RH *et al.* (1984) Effect of fetal diagnostic testing on birthrate of thalassaemia major in Britain. *Lancet*, ii; 1383–1386.

Pedder JR (1982) Failure to mourn, and melancholia. *British Journal of Psychiatry*, 141; 329–337.

Reading A, Sledgemere CM, Campbell S *et al.* (1981) Psychological effects on the mother, of real-time ultrasound in antenatal clinics. *British Journal of Radiology*, 54; 546.

Rillstone P, Hutchison SA (2001) Managing the reemergence of anguish: pregnancy after a loss due to anomalies. *Journal of Obstetric, Gynaecologic and Neonatal Nursing*, 3; 291–298.

Reynolds BD, Puck MH, Robinson A (1974) Genetic counselling: an appraisal. *Clinical Genetics*, 5; 177–178.

Rothman BK (1986) *The Tentative Pregnancy*. Viking Penguin, New York.

Scriver CR, Bardanis M, Cartier L *et al.* (1984) Beta–thalassemia disease prevention; genetic medicine applied. *American Journal of Human Genetics*, 36; 1024–1038.

Statham H, Solomou W, Green JM (2001) *When a Baby Has an Abnormality: A Study of Parents' Experiences*. Centre for Family Research, University of Cambridge, Cambridge.

Stroebe W, Stroebe M (1987) Bereavement and health, the risk of psychological and physical consequences of partner loss. In: *Risk Factors in Bereavement Outcome*. Cambridge University Press, Cambridge, pp.168–223.

Thomassen-Brepols LJ (1985) Psychosociale aspecten van prenatale diagnostiek (Psycho–social aspects of prenatal diagnosis). PhD thesis, Erasmus University, Rotterdam.

Toedter LJ, Lasker JN, Jansen HJEM (2001) International comparison of studies using the Perinatal Grief Scale: a decade of research on pregnancy loss. *Death Studies*, 25; 205–228.

Vachon MLS, Lyall WAL, Rogers J *et al.* (1980) A controlled study of self-help intervention for widows. *American Journal of Psychiatry*, 137; 380–384.

Walter C (1980) The mipa: a social belief of peasants. *Revisita Latinoamericana de Psicologia*, 12; 293–312.

White-van Mourik MCA (1989) *The psycho-social sequelae of a termination of pregnancy for fetal abnormality*. MSc thesis, The University of Glasgow, Glasgow.

White-van Mourik MCA, Connor JM, Ferguson-Smith MA (1990) Patient care before and after termination of pregnancy for neural tube defect. *Prenatal Diagnosis*, 10; 497–505.

White-van Mourik MCA, Connor JM, Ferguson-Smith MA (1992) The psychosocial sequelae of a second-trimester termination of pregnancy for fetal abnormality. *Prenatal Diagnosis*, 12; 189–204.

Zinner ES (2000) Men about it: the marginalization of men in grief. *Illness, Crisis and Loss*, 8(2); 181–188.

18 THE HUMAN SIDE OF CARERS

Jennifer Wiggins

INTRODUCTION

> *... it should not be our bodies, families and patients who have to bear the brunt of our undigested emotions.*
>
> (Brien and Fairbairn, 1996)

Clinicians working in prenatal diagnosis inevitably deal with distressing and ethically fraught dilemmas. The multidisciplinary team which consists of doctors, nurses, midwives, ultrasonographers and genetic counsellors has many roles to fulfil: diagnosing abnormality; presenting information about the diagnosis, prognosis, testing options and risks; offering and performing termination and providing support for couples making difficult decisions.

The organization for whom these clinicians work and the clinicians themselves have a responsibility to ensure that pressures of work do not interfere with their professional standards and do not cause them personal, physical or emotional harm.

The responsibility of the employing organization to protect its staff from harm includes having both proactive and reactive strategies in place to minimize harm and to alleviate the effects of harm caused by the work. In addition to any legal requirements, it is in the interest of the employing organization to protect its staff, in order to maintain good quality patient care and to ensure that the organization handles its resources efficiently.

Staff working within prenatal diagnosis/fetal medicine also have to take responsibility for their own wellbeing. Poor mental, emotional and physical health will affect the quality of patient care and will increase the burden for co-workers. Individuals who choose to work as carers, in any field, have a responsibility to ensure their practice is safe for both themselves and their clients. Various governing and voluntary bodies encompassing health care professions have codes of practice and ethical frameworks that clearly place responsibility on the individual practitioner to safeguard their own health.

Ironically, working within the hierarchical structure of the National Health Service (NHS) may make it difficult to ask for or expect this kind of help. There is a tacit assumption that people should be able to manage their work, and it is often perceived as a weakness rather than a sign of maturity if someone requests additional support. 'It is difficult to admit to our willingness to subsume our own needs to those of others/the organization, even if doing so makes us sick' (Wright, 2001).

Once there is recognition and acceptance of the requirement for self-care, there are a variety of resources one can turn to for help: personal therapy, clinical supervision, peer support, mentoring, appropriate training and numerous stress management techniques. By taking responsibility for self-care, health professionals can work towards protecting themselves from the potentially damaging interactions inherent to working in fetal medicine, thereby enhancing the quality of service to clients and gaining a sense of self-worth and pride by realizing their professional potential.

WORKING IN PRENATAL DIAGNOSIS

Working in prenatal diagnosis in any country where termination of pregnancy is legal means one is invariably involved in some way in terminations. Abortion work presents ethical problems for every health care worker, regardless of their personal ethical beliefs. Even for those who strongly believe in a woman's right to choose abortion, there will be some cases that trouble them more than others. Studies of professional attitudes towards abortion indicate that ambivalence and distress are common problems for health care workers (Brien and Fairbairn, 1996). For staff, the work means one is exposed regularly to dilemmas and decisions regarding a baby's life, prognosis and death and to the impact of observing the parents' fears, hopes, disappointment, anger and sadness.

THE PREGNANT COUNSELLOR

Effects on relationship with women

Working in the field of prenatal diagnosis involves special circumstances that can affect the client–counsellor relationship. Pregnancy is not a sickness and is, after a point, a public matter. It is not uncommon for the pregnant patient to have a clinician who is also visibly pregnant. Ironically, the clinician may be regarded as 'healthy' and the patient as 'ill'. It is difficult to think of a parallel situation in other fields of medicine. Whether this creates a negative or positive impact depends on the client's situation and immediate concerns, and on the counsellor's situation, attitude and skills in dealing with the overlap in the personal/professional relationship. A small study (Mueller et al., 1998) into the relationship between pregnant genetic counsellors and prenatal patients found that, for the most part, genetic counsellors felt that their pregnancy enhanced the counsellor/client relationship, in spite of the fact that the boundaries of the relationships were blurred. Counsellors reported they were more likely to be asked personal questions about their pregnancies and their choices for prenatal testing. In general, the counsellors felt their pregnancy gave them more insight and empathy. They were happy to answer personal questions, as they found it helped to build rapport and fostered the relationship. A further study looking at attitudes of genetic counsellors towards their own pregnancies supports these findings (Aronson-Goldberg et al., 1998). Many counsellors reported that having a pregnancy and children had improved their ability to counsel their patients and identify with the difficult decisions they face.

Effects on counsellors' own pregnancy experiences

Interestingly, Aronson-Goldberg *et al.* (1998) also found that while 58% of these pregnancies occurred in genetic counsellors under 35 years of age and only one of those had a high-risk screening test result, 76% of the women opted for prenatal karyotyping. Ninety one per cent of respondents said that their profession had affected their decisions about prenatal testing and their anxiety levels, because they had a more profound understanding of the disabilities that could occur in an unborn baby.

When the counsellor has a problem pregnancy

The issue may be different for the counsellor who has personal experience with tragedy in pregnancy. Consider the counsellor who has a disabled child, suffers from infertility, has had a miscarriage, lost a pregnancy following an invasive prenatal test, had a stillborn baby or a neonatal death or had a termination for medical or social reasons. In what way will these personal experiences affect someone who works in prenatal diagnosis? Will the information they provide be unintentionally biased by their own experience; will they be able to provide appropriate emotional support and assistance as determined by the client's needs? Will the counsellor be able to differentiate between her own pregnancy/baby/decision/loss and the client's experience? Personal therapy, supervision, peer and managerial support are all tools that can help clinicians in these difficult situations to work effectively in spite of their personal experiences.

OCCUPATIONAL STRESS

One does not need to have suffered a relevant personal tragedy to find working in the field of prenatal testing difficult. The sheer volume of work, the time pressures and repetitive nature of the caseload and the daily loss of hope can combine to create a stressful work environment. This stress is inherent to the job and is, to some extent, inevitable. However, if this stress is compounded by an unsupportive or hostile work environment, clinicians may find themselves frustrated in their attempts to care adequately for patients, co-workers and themselves.

THEORETICAL FRAMEWORKS FOR LOOKING AT STRESS

There are many different definitions of stress and theories about how people respond to it. Hans Selye defined stress as a consequence of the interaction between the stimulus and the response to that stimulus. He differentiated between eustress, a positive response, and distress, a negative response (Selye, 1956). This research was the first to demonstrate a link between stress and illness.

The cognitive theory of stress, from which the definition for occupational stress has been developed, emphasizes the way individuals appraise stressful situations. It describes stress in terms of a transaction between an individual and their environment. Research by Lazerus and Folkman (1984) supported the concept that in order to understand the 'stress coping process' the potentially stressful situation needs to be considered together with the individual's coping techniques and emotional reactions, because they are interdependent. According to this perspective, stress is only experienced when situations are appraised as exceeding one's resources (Healy, 2000). Along the same lines, stress has also been described in terms of the effect it has for an individual; if someone perceives a situation to be challenging, threatening or harmful, it can disrupt their ability to function smoothly (Clegg, 2001).

Arnold *et al.* (1995) defined occupational stress as any force that pushes a psychological or physical factor beyond its ranges of ability, producing strain within an individual. The UK Health and Safety Executive defined occupational stress as 'The reaction people have to excessive pressure or other types of demands placed upon them. It arises when they worry they can't cope' (Health and Safety Executive, 1999).

CAUSES OF STRESS FOR HEALTH CARE PROFESSIONALS

Response to pressure varies with the individual, and the pressure depends in large part on the situations in which the individual is involved. It can be useful to assess how distressing a situation is by considering its component parts. Mehrabian and Reed (1969) suggested a formula for determining the severity of any given problem situation:

Severity = Distress x Uncontrollability x Frequency

So, working conditions that are not inherently distressing can still be stressful if there is a recurring problem over which the individual has no control. In general, harmful levels of stress are most likely to occur in situations where pressures accumulate or are prolonged. If employees feel trapped or unable to exert any control over the demands made on them, this can increase their stress levels (Harris, 2001). The Nuffield report on improving the health of the NHS workforce found that certain work factors can protect people in vulnerable situations; for example having more control at work and greater social support enables greater tolerance of high workload (Williams *et al.*, 1998).

There is no shortage of studies assessing the causes and effects of occupational stress amongst health care workers. A common finding in these studies is that occupational stress is not merely due to the stressful nature of healthcare work with its inherent traumas and tragedies. The working environment itself also causes occupational stress. The most frequently reported sources of stress among nurses are high and pressurized workload that affect their personal life, staff shortages and unpredictability and insufficient time to provide emotional support to patients (Williams *et al.*, 1998). Other studies have also identified common themes which health care staff have reported as causing stress, such as: workload, bureaucratic political constraints, lack of professional latitude, role ambiguity and lack of participation in decision-making (Dolan *et al.*, 1992; Sullivan, 1993; Williams *et al.*, 1998; Shaw, 1999).

The Nuffield Trust report found lower levels of occupational stress in small hospitals with good staff cooperation and communication, adequate performance monitoring, a strong emphasis on training and a relatively large degree of self-regulation and flexibility among staff (Williams *et al.*, 1998). This would seem sensible as these characteristics relate directly to some of the causes of stress identified by health care staff.

THE CONSEQUENCES OF STRESS AMONG HEALTH CARE WORKERS

Occupational sickness is now considered to be a major factor in the high sickness and absence rates amongst nurses (Kunkler and Whittick, 1991) with research showing that health professionals have some of the highest occupational stress ratings (Cooper *et al.*, 1988). A large study (Wall *et al.*, 1997) found that 27% of health care staff reported high levels of psychological disturbance, compared with 18% of working people generally. Not only do these figures translate into worrying trends for the employer in terms of staffing problems and high absenteeism rates, but they also mean that the staff are likely to be suffering poor health due this stress. The average life expectancy for a 45-year-old nurse in the UK is 26.1 years, only one year more than miners working underground (Clegg, 2001). Nurses have been shown to have higher than average levels of smoking, alcohol consumption, absence rates and suicide (Hingley and Cooper, 1986).

Interestingly, a study looking at high sick leave rates within the NHS found that the majority of NHS employees surveyed (77%) admitted that they felt guilty about taking time off when they were ill. An even greater majority (85%) said that they would only take time off if they were very ill. Almost 20% of reported sickness or injury absences were attributed to working conditions or work-related stress (Health Education Authority, 1997). The consequences of occupational stress do not just affect the individual health care worker; they also affect the health of other staff who face the strain of manpower shortages and eventually affect the quality of patient care (Clegg, 2001).

Reducing levels of occupational stress and thereby decreasing the level of sick leave would reduce the need for replacement staff, which in turn would save the NHS money. 'In fact, if the NHS could cut down absenteeism by 2.5 sick days per staff member per year, it could save itself £140,000,000 per year' (Williams *et al.*, 1998).

INTERVENTIONS

Most hospitals have occupational health departments to deal with issues around the health and wellbeing of the staff. Some hospitals may also have designated staff counselling services offering personal therapy, supervision, training and group support. The NHS, recognizing it has a duty to deal with the high levels of stress with which its staff are faced, set a target for all NHS staff to have access to counselling services (The NHS Human Resources Framework, 'Working together – Securing a quality workforce for the NHS (2000)) and established guidelines for these services (Department of Health, 2000).

Managing workload through prioritizing and time management, saying 'no' to demands that can't be met, working politically to improve the service and work conditions and taking responsibility for accessing support from peers, through supervision, and through personal therapy may all reduce stress for the individual. Additional training may also help reduce work-related stress by enabling the health professional to deal more effectively with the workload and by increasing their sense of job satisfaction and self-worth (Brien and Fairbairn, 1996).

RESPONSIBILITIES OF THE EMPLOYER

In the UK, levels of staff sickness are higher in the NHS than in the private sector, with occupational stress as a main factor in the levels of absenteeism. (Healy, 2000) This has important implications for the NHS, both in human and financial costs, since evidence indicates that quality patient care is linked to a strong and highly motivated workforce (Royal College of Nursing, 2000). As an employer the NHS has a duty to address this problem and implement plans to reduce levels of work-related stress both to improve working conditions for staff and to improve and safeguard patient care.

The Management of Health and Safety at Work Regulations (Health and Safety Executive, 1999) highlight the need for employers to make suitable and sufficient assessment of health and safety risks to which staff are exposed while at work, including risks arising from stress in the workplace (Clegg, 2001). The recent rise in the number of legal cases against employers also highlights the civil liability they face and requires organizations such as hospitals to monitor the health and wellbeing of employees (Harris, 2001).

REDUCING STRESS IN THE WORKING ENVIRONMENT

Primary prevention of stress has been shown to be more effective than dealing with the symptoms of stress in the individuals. Implementation of organizational changes that serve to increase people's sense of control in their job have been shown to improve workers' mental wellbeing, and self-rated performance while reducing sickness rates (Bond and Bunce, 2001).

In addition to having a sense of control over their own working environment, staff also require good support, open lines of communication and clear guidelines from management regarding their duties and responsibilities. For example, a study of ultrasonographers' experience of giving bad news found that 'staff working in settings where there was a clear protocol specifying how to proceed following disclosure of bad news experience less stress than those working without such a protocol' (Simpson and Bor, 2001).

The Nuffield Trust report on Improving the Health of the NHS workforce (Williams *et al.*, 1998) recommended that staff be given more control over their work and be allowed to participate in decision-making. It also recommended that improvements be made around staff support and communication. In health care there is a correlation between the quality of patient care, staff morale and effective nursing leadership (Manley, 1997).

For an organization to address effectively the issue of stress management, the culture of the organization needs to be examined. Arnold *et al.* (1995) argue that successful action at an organizational level could make staff counselling and stress management unnecessary. There is recognition that, 'where organizations want to benefit from a committed and motivated staff, the impact of management on their health must be considered central to business planning and change management. However, while many organizations reflect this in short term priorities, relatively few take a longer proactive approach' (Health Education Authority, 1998). Unfortunately changes at this level are difficult to implement.

Palliative interventions, such as health promotion schemes, counselling, supervision and training, aim to reduce stress by improving an individual's ability to cope with existing working conditions. These can be effective for those who can access them but are not likely reduce the overall levels of occupational stress within a large organization.

PROFESSIONAL TRAINING

Knowledge

Lifelong learning is essential for safe and effective practice, especially in prenatal diagnosis/fetal medicine where new developments are the only constant in the field. Health professionals who lack knowledge to deal effectively with a situation will find this stressful. Serum screening for Down syndrome is a good example of a common prenatal test, which is inconsistently applied due to a lack of understanding and training. Women's experiences of having serum screening indicate they felt the staff were unclear about the implications of the test and did not explain it properly (Statham and Green, 1993). Studies have shown that health professionals' knowledge of how the test actually works is poor (Sadler, 1997). Midwives are aware of this problem and have asked for more training (Ryder, 1999). This lack of understanding is reflected in midwives' negative view of serum screening (Khalid *et al.*, 1994) and the poor administration of the screening programme (Green, 1994). Access to proper training can improve the service to patients while reducing the stress clinicians feel.

Health professionals involved in fetal medicine also need a good grasp of the abortion laws in their country and to know how their hospital handles the remains of terminations, miscarriages and stillbirths.

Counselling skills

Additional training in counselling skills may be necessary, as basic training in these skills for midwives, nurses, ultrasonographers and other health professionals is often insufficient to meet the demands placed on those working in prenatal diagnosis. Interactions with clients require professionals to provide information in a sensitive way that encourages clients to ask questions and express their emotions. This enables them to make informed choices and gives them a sense of being supported.

Health care professionals are aware of this need, and a perceived lack of communication skills can lead to professional anxiety. The BACP Code of Ethics and Practice (1989) for those who utilize counselling skills in their daily work, states that the practitioner should ensure that s/he has received sufficient training to be able to use them [counselling skills] appropriately and should maintain his/her level of competence. Training in basic counselling skills also provides the health care worker with a frame of reference so they can appreciate their skills, recognize their limitations and feel confident about referring patients elsewhere, thereby ensuring safe practice.

PEER SUPPORT

The value of working within a supportive environment should not be underestimated. Poor social support at work is a key factor affecting levels of staff illness (Williams *et al.*, 1998). In some units there are formal arrangements in place such as a mentoring programme for new members of staff or semi-formal group supervision within a department. However, the degree of informal support usually depends upon the ethos of the specific department and the effectiveness and priorities of the manager for that department. Peer support needs to be non-hierarchical, as senior members of staff also need support and this can be easily overlooked in favour of new staff (Statham, personal communication). Peer support is less constrained by the requirements for patient confidentiality than is support from outside supervisors. Good peer support is an indicator of the quality of communication within the team. Patient care will be enhanced when all clinicians involved in their care are communicating effectively.

SUPERVISION

Clinical or counselling supervision is valuable to the practitioner; its purpose is to 'monitor standards, to develop new insights and skills and to provide personal support' (British Association for Counselling and Psychotherapy [BACP], 1998). Supervision is not to be confused with personal therapy or a management tool. It empowers practitioners through continual professional development and personal support. This in turn is of benefit to the clients, as it is a safeguard against poor practice and compromised professionals. Supervision is widely recognized as an essential part of good practice. This is reflected in the guidelines of many professional bodies in the UK (UKCC, 1995). A Royal College of Nursing report stated that:

> *The use of clinical supervision should be extended. This provides staff with the opportunity to discuss and reflect on their work and allows managers to develop their staff and help them to work effectively within a clinical team. Clinical supervision brings clinicians and supervisors together on a confidential basis to discuss and reflect on practice, with the aim of improving practice, solving problems and increasing understanding of professional issues. It should not be used as a management tool or for performance review.*   (Royal College of Nursing, 2000)

The UK Association for Genetic Nurses and Counsellors (AGNC) Core Competency statement on ethical practice also identifies the need for supervision (www.agnc.co.uk/).

While there is a 'paucity of empirical evidence to support the view that clinical supervision is effective in reducing stress levels' (Clegg, 2001), the ethical principles and humanist theories on which the justification is based are compelling. The BACP's Ethical Framework for good practice in counselling and psychotherapy (2002) highlights the key ethical principles as they apply to competent practice and the importance of supervision. Health care practitioners should be committed to undertaking ongoing professional development so that their practice is up-to-date and relevant (beneficence and self-respect). Services should not be provided when one is unfit, whether through illness or personal circumstances. Professionals need to ensure that their work with patients is not compromised by their own emotional needs (non-maleficence) People should receive the same treatment regardless of their race, gender, religious beliefs, language or ethnic background (justice).

Supervision can address all these issues. It can serve as a tool for monitoring competence by: highlighting training needs, identifying areas of uncovered prejudice, allowing supervisees to assess and acknowledge their own strengths and weakness and empowering supervisees to decline responsibilities which are beyond their scope of knowledge and skills. It can also be useful in helping the counsellor to consider his/her work in the context of the organization and other sources of help for the client. Finally, supervision should help to identify concerns over the standard of a person's work or their physical or emotional wellbeing.

In order for supervision to be effective it needs to be a confidential and professional relationship, separate from the professional's clinical environment. This encourages the frankness that is necessary for successful professional development. The supervisor's role is facilitating the counsellor's skill development, which indirectly benefits the clients, but clinical responsibility remains with the supervisee.

Access to supervision is variable. It may be available through the occupational health department, the clinical psychology department or staff support services or it may not be available at all. It may be offered to all staff, or only a few, depending on their position. It may be free and available during working hours or it may cost money and have to be accessed privately on personal time. Supervision may be arranged on a one-to-one basis or it may be arranged for a group within a department. It may be with someone who is a trained counselling supervisor or it may be with an experienced colleague or co-worker. Although many professional bodies strongly recommend supervision as a concept, very few individuals will be expected to access it as part of their clinical responsibilities. Those who do request it may find it difficult to access and may have to justify why it is necessary.

Some health professionals find the concept of supervision threatening; they may think requiring it is an admission of professional incompetence or personal instability; they may believe insight from others is irrelevant to their practice or may be reluctant to undertake critical analysis of their own competence.

PERSONAL THERAPY

Not everybody would choose to work in prenatal diagnosis/fetal medicine, with all that it entails. A health care professional should have some insight as to how they came to work in this field. 'People are attracted to working in areas that are meaningful to us. Our motives are important and may have significance and influence of which we are unaware' (Brien and Fairbourn, 1996).

Personal therapy gives practitioners the opportunity to explore aspects of their personality and history to give them insight about why they have decided to be a 'carer'. This self-awareness is important as it helps us to protect clients from parts of ourselves that may be harmful if left unexplored. By identifying parts of ourselves with which we are uncomfortable, we are in a better position to be accepting of other people's weak spots.

Therapy may enhance a person's communication and counselling skills, enabling them to work more effectively with clients. It may be useful at various points throughout a clinician's career. Personal circumstances are constantly changing and there are times when one's private life may impact on one's professional duties. Clinicians have a responsibility to monitor how these changes affect their work and take steps to ensure their own safety and that of their clients. The 1998 BACP Code of Practice stated that:

> *Counsellors have a responsibility to themselves and their clients to maintain their own effectiveness, resilience and ability to help clients. They are expected to monitor their own personal functioning and to seek help and or withdraw from counselling, whether temporarily or permanently, when their personal resources are sufficiently depleted to require this.*

CONCLUSION

Clinicians working in prenatal diagnosis face numerous professional challenges that may be stressful. All practitioners have a duty of care to themselves, their co-workers and their patients to ensure that they are emotionally, mentally and physically able to cope with the work and to cope within the system. Job satisfaction and self-esteem are linked with doing a job well. This requires looking after one's self to avoid being damaged by the work. The way one goes about this is dependent on how the work affects them personally. Resources available for self-care may include supervision, peer support and personal counselling. Responsibility rests with the individual clinician to search for the most appropriate assistance, but the onus is on the employer to make provisions for these needs.

Key points

- Both carers and their employers have a responsibility to safeguard the health of the carer in the interests of their clients.
- Whilst carers may feel that being pregnant themselves enhances their relationship with their clients, they may experience anxiety over their own choices because of their understanding of possible outcomes.
- Occupational stress is proportional to how often distress occurs and the control the carer has over their own situation. It is often manifested by high sickness and absence rates.
- Stress in the working environment can be reduced by allowing staff control over their work and participation in decision-making.
- Other interventions that help carers to care for themselves and others include agreed protocols, supervision, lifelong learning to keep knowledge and counselling skills up-to-date, peer support and personal therapy.

REFERENCES

Arnold J, Cooper C, Robinson T (1995) *Work Psychology* (2nd edn). Pitman, London.
Aronson-Goldberg M *et al.* (1998) Attitudes of genetic counsellors towards their own pregnancies. *Journal of Genetic Counselling*, 7(6); 486–487.
BACP (1989) *Code of Ethics and Practice for Counselling Skills*. British Association for Counselling and Psychotherapy, Rugby.
BACP (1998) *Code of Ethics and Practice for Counselling Skills*. British Association for Counselling and Psychotherapy, Rugby.
BACP (2002) *Ethical Framework for Good Practice in Counselling and Psychotherapy*. British Association for Counselling and Psychotherapy, Rugby. *www.bac.co.uk/ members_visitors/public_information/public_code_counsellors.htm*
Bond FW, Bunce D (2001) Job control mediates change in a work reorganization intervention for stress reduction. *Journal of Occupational Health Psychology*, 6(4); 290–302.
Brien J, Fairbairn I (1996) *Pregnancy and Abortion Counselling*. Routledge, London.
Clegg A (2001) Occupational stress in nursing: a review of the literature. *Journal of Nursing Management*, 9(2); 101–106.

Cooper C, Cooper R, Eaker L (1988) *Living with Stress*. Penguin, Harmondsworth, Middlesex. In: (1994) *Prenatal Diagnosis The Human Side* (eds Abramsky L, Chapple J). Chapman & Hall, London, pp. 203.
Department of Health (2000) *The Provision of Counselling Services for Staff in the NHS*. Department of Health, London, catalogue no. 22156. *www.doh.gov.uk/nhscounsel*
Dolan SL, van Ameringen MR, Corbin S *et al.* (1992) Lack of professional latitude and role problems as correlates of propensity to quit among nursing staff. *Journal of Advanced Nursing*, 17; 1455–1459.
Green JM (1994) Serum screening for Down syndrome: experience of obstetricians in England and Wales. *British Medical Journal*, 309; 769–772.
Harris N (2001) Management of work related stress in nursing. *Nursing Standard*, 16(10); 47–55.
Healy CM (2000) Nursing stress: the effects of coping strategies and job satisfaction in a sample of Australian nurses. *Journal of Advanced Nursing*, 31(3); 681–688.
Health and Safety Executive (1999) *Management and Safety at Work Regulations*. Sudbury, Health and Safety Executive, London. *http://www.hse.gov.uk*
Health Education Authority (1997) In sickness and health: health at work in the NHS. Healthlines *www.hawnhs.hda–online.org.uk/*
Health Education Authority (1998) *More Brown Bread and Aerobics: Developing and Sustaining Workplace Health in the NHS*. Health Education Authority, London.
Hingley P, Cooper C (1986) *Stress and the Nurse Manager*. John Wiley, Chichester.
Khalid L *et al.* (1994) The attitudes of midwives to maternal serum screening for Down syndrome. *Public Health*, 108(2); 131–136.
Kunkler J, Whittick J (1991) Stress management groups for nurses. *Journal of Advanced Nursing*, 16(2); 172–176.
Lazerus R, Folkman S (1984) *Stress Appraisal and Coping*. Springer, New York.
Manley K (1997) A Conceptual Framework for advanced practice: an action research project operationalising and advanced practitioner/consultant nurse role. *Journal of Clinical Nursing*, 6; 179–190.
Mehrabian A, Reed H (1969) Factors influencing judgements of psychopathology. *Psychological Reports*, 24; 323–330.
Mueller S *et al.* (1998) The relationship between the pregnant genetic counsellor and the prenatal patient. *Journal of Genetic Counselling*, 7(6); 494.
Royal College of Nursing (RCN) (2000) *Developing a National Plan for the New NHS: Nursing Views on NHS Modernisation in England*. Royal College of Nursing, London. www.rcn.org.uk/professional/ professional_policybriefings_consultation_nhs_plan.html
Ryder H (1999) Prenatal screening for Down syndrome: a dilemma for the unsupported midwife? *Midwifery*, 15(1); 16–23.
Sadler M (1997) Serum screening for Down Syndrome: how much do health professionals know? *British Journal of Obstetrics and Gynaecology*, 104(2); 176–179.
Selye H (1956) *The Stress of Life*. McGraw, New York.
Shaw C (1999) A framework for the study of coping. *Journal of Advanced Nursing*, 29; 1246–55.
Simpson R, Bor R (2001) 'I'm not picking up a heartbeat': experiences of sonographers giving bad news to women during ultrasound scans. *British Journal of Medical Psychology*, 74(2); 255–272.
Statham H, Green J (1993) Serum screening for Down syndrome: some women's experiences. *British Medical Journal*, 307; 174–176.

Sullivan P (1993) Stress and burnout in psychiatric nursing. *Nursing Standard*, 29; 82–88.

United Kingdom Central Council for Nursing, Midwifery and Health Visiting (UKCC) (1995) *Position Statement on Clinical Supervision for Nursing and Health Visiting.* United Kingdom Central Council for Nursing, Midwifery and Health Visiting, London. nmc-uk.org/cms/content/Publications/Position%20statement%20on%20 clinical%20supervision%20for%20nursing,%20etc..asp

Wall TD *et al.* (1997) Minor psychiatric disorder in NHS Trust staff: occupational and gender differences. *British Journal Psychiatry*, 171; 519–523.

Williams S, Michie S, Pattani S (1998) *Improving the Health of The NHS Workforce: Report of the Partnership on the Health of the NHS Workforce.* The Nuffield Trust, London.

Wright S (2001) A Problem shared . . . . *Nursing Standard*, 15(35); 26–27.

Glossary

Allele One of two or more alternative forms of a gene (i.e., there is an allele for type A blood and an allele for type B blood).

Alpha-fetoprotein (AFP) A protein made by the fetus, which is present in the serum of pregnant women and which tends to be found in increased amounts if the fetus has a neural-tube defect and in decreased amounts if the fetus has Down syndrome.

Amniocentesis Withdrawal of a small amount of fluid from the amniotic sac around the developing fetus to enable chromosome, DNA, or biochemical studies to be done.

Anencephaly A specific type of neural tube defect caused by the failure of the upper part of the neural tube to close. This leads to a failure of development of the skull and brain. This malformation is incompatible with extrauterine life of more than a few days.

Anomaly scan A detailed ultrasound scan done for the purpose of looking at the fetal anatomy to enable identification of fetal malformations. Such scans are done routinely at most antenatal clinics in the UK at about 19 weeks of pregnancy.

Ascertainment The identification of individuals or families to be included in a study. The method of ascertainment will affect the results of the study.

Assisted reproduction technology (ART) The name applied to medical techniques used to induce pregnancy. See *in vitro* fertilization (IVF) and intra-cytoplasmic sperm injection (ICSI).

Autosome Any chromosome other than a sex chromosome. Humans have 22 pairs of autosomes.

Base pair A pair of nucleotides (adenine–thymine, cytosine–guanine) in DNA. The order of the base pairs in a gene determines the sequence of the amino acids that are assembled to form the protein coded for by that gene.

Blastocyst An early preimplantation stage of embryonic development in which the cells of the developing fetus and placenta are arranged in the form of a hollow ball.

Carrier An individual who does not manifest a condition but who carries a gene for it and can therefore pass this gene on to offspring who may under certain circumstances exhibit the condition.

Chorionic villus sampling (CVS) The sampling of tissue from the developing placenta (chorionic villi) in order to do chromosome or DNA studies. The sample can be obtained trans-abdominally or trans-vaginally.

Chorionicity The status of twins with regard to the outer membrane surrounding them (the chorion). A shared chorionic membrane (monochorionic) indicates monozygotic (identical) twins, while separate chorions (dichorionic) leave the question open. Chorionicity can often be determined on ultrasound scan early in pregnancy.

Chromosome A rod-shaped body made of DNA found in the nucleus of every cell in the body (with the exception of mature red blood cells). Chromosomes carry the genes that determine the characteristics of an individual. Humans have 23 pairs of chromosomes in each cell – 22 pairs of autosomes and one pair of sex chromosomes.

Combined testing for Down syndrome A combination of maternal serum screening for Down syndrome and a nuchal translucency measurement done on the same day in the first trimester to calculate the risk for Down syndrome.

Concordance This refers to two individuals (often twins) both having or both not having the same trait (often an abnormality).

Cystic fibrosis A disease of the mucus-secreting glands of the lungs, the pancreas, the gastrointestinal tract and the sweat glands. In the Caucasian population, this is the most common serious disease inherited in an autosomal recessive manner. If both parents are unaffected carriers of the disorder, each pregnancy has a one-in-four chance of being affected.

Cytogenetics The science of examining chromosomes.

Delta F508 The name given to the most common mutation causing cystic fibrosis. In the UK it accounts for about 75% of mutations of the cystic fibrosis gene.

Diagnostic test A test that aims to determine with a very high degree of accuracy whether or not an individual has a particular disorder. This is regarded as the 'gold standard' test in a screening programme.

Discordance This refers to the situation in which two individuals (often twins) are different in respect to a particular trait (for example one has the disorder and the other does not).

Dizygous Twins arising from the fertilization of two different eggs. Genetically such twins are no more alike than any other sibling pair.

DNA Deoxyribonucleic acid, the material of which genes are composed.

Dominant inheritance The mode of inheritance characterized by an individual manifesting a trait for which only one of the relevant pair of genes codes. If a condition is inherited dominantly, it can be passed on from an affected parent to an offspring, even though the other parent does not carry the gene for the disease. Each time an affected person has a child, there is a one in two chance that the child will be affected.

Down syndrome (Trisomy 21) Individuals with Down syndrome have an extra copy of chromosome 21 in each cell. They have varying degrees of learning disability, a characteristic appearance, and often have some congenital malformations (especially cardiac). It is the most common single chromosome abnormality in live born children. The incidence increases with maternal age.

Duchenne muscular dystrophy A disease causing severe progressive muscle weakness and eventual death in affected boys. It is an X-linked disease (carried on the X chromosome). Carrier women are unaffected but their sons each have a one-in-two chance of being affected and their daughters each have a one-in-two chance of being unaffected carriers.

Edwards syndrome (Trisomy 18) Individuals with Edwards syndrome have an extra copy of chromosome 18 in each cell. They usually have lethal congenital malformations, so very few of them survive past infancy, but those who do have severe learning disabilities.

Eugenics Attempts to 'improve' a species either through controlling who does and who does not reproduce or through controlling which of their genes are passed on and which are not.

There is considerable debate (with understandable public concern) as to whether prenatal diagnosis with termination of affected fetuses and screening for carrier status is an attempt at eugenic control.

Familial Conditions that 'run in families'.

Fetal blood sampling The withdrawal of a small amount of fetal blood (usually from the point where the umbilical cord inserts into the placenta) in order to do chromosome, DNA, or biochemical tests on it. It is sometimes called cordocentesis.

FISH (fluorescence _in situ_ hybridization) This is a rapid method of chromosome analysis using a fluorescent label on a specific segment of single stranded DNA, so that under ultraviolet light it can be seen in colour under the microscope. For example, if a fluorescent chromosome 21 label were added to cells, one could see whether there were two labelled chromosomes in each cell (normal) or three in each cell (Down syndrome) This can be done much faster than conventional chromosome analysis, since it can be done on interphase cells (i.e. those that are not in the process of dividing).

Gamete A reproductive cell (ovum or sperm).

Gene The biological unit of heredity. Genes are arranged along chromosomes in the centre of each cell. They are made up of DNA. The precise sequence of the DNA determines the precise nature of the protein for which the gene codes.

Genotype The genetic constitution of an organism. The total of all the genes carried by that person, whether expressed or not.

Genetic markers Normal variations that occur between the chromosomes of different individuals, allowing the identification of the source of a specific part of a particular chromosome (for example, which of the mother's two X chromosomes the fetus has inherited).

Haemophilia A clotting disorder that causes sufferers to bleed easily. It is a genetic defect, and the gene causing it is located on the X chromosome. Carrier women are not affected, but each of their sons has a one-in-two chance of being affected, and each of their daughters has a one-in-two chance of being a carrier.

Haemoglobinopathy Any disease of the blood associated with the presence of an abnormal haemoglobin in the red blood cells. The commonest such diseases are sickle cell anaemia (found most commonly in those of Afro-Caribbean origin) and thalassaemia (more prevalent in those of Middle Eastern, Mediterranean, and Far Eastern origin). These diseases are inherited in an autosomal recessive manner, so that if both parents are unaffected carriers of the gene in question, each pregnancy has a one-in-four chance of being affected.

Heterozygous The condition of carrying two different alleles (versions of the gene) for a particular trait. Unaffected carriers of recessively inherited disorders are heterozygous, as they have one faulty and one normal allele of the gene for that disease state. Individuals with dominant disorders are usually heterozygous and carry one normal allele and one faulty allele for the trait.

Homozygous The condition of carrying two identical alleles (versions of the gene) for a particular trait. Genetic traits that are recessive in character, such as blood group type O, are only manifested when an individual is homozygous for that trait.

Human chorionic gonadotrophin (hCG) A hormone produced by the placenta, which is found in the mother's serum. It tends to be present in increased amounts if the fetus has Down syndrome and in decreased amounts if the fetus has Edwards syndrome.

Huntington disease This is a late onset progressive disease characterized by involuntary movements, dementia and eventual death. It is inherited in an autosomal dominant fashion. When an affected person has a child, there is a one-in-two chance that the child will inherit the gene. Because it is a late onset disease, symptoms are unlikely to occur before the affected person has had children.

Hypoplasia Underdevelopment.

Iatrogenic disease Disease caused by medical investigations or treatments.

Integrated test A two-stage screening test for Down syndrome, in which during the first trimester, maternal blood is screened for PAPP-A and a nuchal translucency scan on the fetus is done. These risk results are combined with the risks calculated from maternal serum screening done in the second trimester and the risk due to the mother's age to give one combined result. In theory, this form of screening gives a much lower false positive rate than other screening tests for Down syndrome.

Interphase A phase in the cell cycle when the cell is not actively dividing and the chromosomes cannot be seen under the microscope using conventional techniques.

Intra-cytoplasmic sperm injection (ICSI) This technique, which can be used in in vitro fertilization, is a method of injecting a sperm directly into the egg. This can be done in the treatment of infertility due to the man having an extremely low sperm count. It is also used when it is necessary to have an embryo that has not been in contact with any other sperm such as when preimplantation genetic diagnosis is being done using the PCR technique.

Inversion The turning around of a part of a chromosome. If no genetic material is gained or lost, the individual should not be affected.

In vitro fertilization (IVF) Fertilization of the egg outside the woman's body. This may be done in cases of infertility or to enable preimplantation genetic diagnosis to be done.

Karyotype An individual's full chromosome complement.

Klinefelter syndrome Males who have an extra X chromosome (47, XXY). These males will be infertile and have a 10–20-point reduction in verbal IQ.

Linkage refers to the phenomenon that genes and genetic markers located close to each other on the same chromosome tend to be transmitted together so that an individual who inherits one of them is likely to have inherited the other.

Marker chromosome A small extra chromosome fragment of unknown origin.

Meiosis The cell divisions that result in the daughter cells having only one chromosome from each chromosome pair. This is the mechanism by which egg and sperm cells are made.

Metaphase A stage of cell division during which the chromosomes are visible under a microscope and can be examined.

Mitosis The cell division that results in the daughter cells having the same chromosome complement as the original cell. This is the mechanism by which all cells other than egg and sperm cells are made.

Monozygous This refers to twins resulting from a split early on in embryonic development so that two individuals develop from one fertilized egg. Such twins are genetically identical and will therefore always be the same sex.

Mosaicism The presence in one individual of two cell lines. One line may be normal and the other abnormal. This can be the result of one abnormal cell division early in embryonic development. The effect on the individual will depend on the ratio of abnormal to normal cells and on the distribution of abnormal cells in the body.

Mutation A change in the gene resulting from an error made when the gene is being copied. It may result in altered gene function, which could render the gene less effective, useless or harmful.

Negative result On a diagnostic test, this means that nothing abnormal has been found (a normal result). On a screening test, this means that the individual screened has been found to be in the low-risk category and not to require diagnostic testing.

Neural-tube defect (NTD) A failure of the neural tube to close at the appropriate time in embryonic development. The main types of neural-tube defects are anencephaly, encephalocoele and spina bifida.

Nuchal translucency A fold at the back of the neck of the fetus that tends to be thicker than usual in chromosomally abnormal fetuses and those with cardiac defects. An ultrasound measurement of the nuchal translucency towards the end of the first trimester can be combined with the mother's age-related risk to calculate the risk that the fetus has Down syndrome.

Oestrogen A hormone secreted by the ovaries and the placenta.

Oligohydramnios Too little amniotic fluid around the fetus.

OSCAR This 'one stop clinic for the assessment of risk' uses a combination of maternal serum screening for Down syndrome and a nuchal translucency measurement done on the same day in the first trimester to calculate the risk for Down syndrome.

Patau syndrome (Trisomy 13) Individuals with Patau syndrome have an extra copy of chromosome 13 in each cell. They usually have lethal congenital malformations and so are unlikely to survive past early infancy. If they do survive they have severe learning disabilities.

Perinatal This refers to the time just before, during and after birth.

Phenotype The observable attributes of an individual, produced by the interaction between all their genes and their environment.

Phenylketonuria (PKU) A severe inherited metabolic disorder leading to learning disability. It is due to the inability of the individual to metabolize the amino acid phenylalanine. If it is diagnosed by a simple blood test soon after birth and the infant has a diet low in phenylalanine, learning disability can be avoided to a large extent. It is inherited in an autosomal recessive manner so that if both parents carry the gene, each child they have will have a one in four chance of being affected.

Polyhydramnios An excess of fluid in the amniotic sac.

Polymerase chain reaction (PCR) A technique for causing a segment of DNA to rapidly copy itself millions of times. This enables geneticists to do DNA tests on a sample as small as a single cell. It can be done on interphase cells (those that are not in the process of dividing). While this was developed as a test for single gene disorders, it has now been adapted for the rapid identification of Down syndrome and other selected chromosome anomalies in an amniotic fluid or CVS sample.

Positive predictive value This refers to the chance that a person found to be positive on a particular screening test does actually have the condition being screened for.

Positive result On a diagnostic test this means that an abnormality has been found. On a screening test, this means that the individual has been found to be in the high-risk group and that a diagnostic test will be offered.

Preimplantation genetic diagnosis (PGD) The use of assisted reproductive technology (IVF, ICSI, embryo biopsy) together with genetic techniques (FISH and PCR) to identify unaffected embryos for implantation.

Prenatal exclusion test This is a test that cannot say that a fetus has a condition but can say that it almost certainly does not have the condition. It is used in Huntington disease. The test involves ascertaining whether or not the fetus inherited from the affected grandparent a chromosome from the pair that carries the relevant gene. If the fetus did not, then it almost certainly could not have inherited the disease. If it did, there is a one-in-two chance that it inherited the faulty copy of the gene.

Prevalence The proportion of individuals in a population who have the condition in question at a specified time.

Prior risk This is the risk that an individual is thought to have for developing a particular condition, or having a baby with a particular condition, before further tests are done or before more information becomes available. The prior risk may then be altered in the light of new information.

Progesterone A hormone secreted by the corpus luteum in the ovary that prepares and maintains the uterus for pregnancy.

Recessive inheritance This refers to conditions that are only manifest if both copies of the relevant gene code for that condition. An individual can only be affected with a recessively inherited disorder if both parents carry a gene for the disorder and both of them pass that gene on to the individual. When both partners are unaffected carriers of a recessively inherited disorder, each of their children has a one-in-four chance of being affected with the disorder.

Screening test A test designed to identify those individuals who are at a high enough risk of having a particular disorder to warrant being offered a diagnostic test. A screening test may be an actual test, such as a blood test, or it may be just the asking of a question, such as 'How old are you?'

Sensitivity The proportion of people actually affected with a condition who will be found to be positive on a screening test for that condition. It determines the detection rate.

Serum screening for Down syndrome An antenatal screening test measuring levels of hCG,and alpha-fetoprotein (and sometimes oestriol and inhibin A) in maternal serum (blood without the blood cells or clotting factors). The results of the serum tests are combined with the mother's age-related risk to calculate the risk that the fetus has Down syndrome.

Sex chromosomes The chromosomes that determine the sex of the individual. Females have two X chromosomes and males have one X and one Y chromosome. A girl gets one X from each parent. A boy gets

his Y from his father and his X from his mother.

Sex chromosome anomalies A chromosome pattern with either an extra or missing sex chromosome. See Klinefelter, XYY, Triple X and Turner syndrome.

Sex-linked disorder A disorder that is carried on a sex chromosome. Usually such disorders are carried on the X chromosome, and typically they are manifested only by males since they have only one copy of the X chromosome. They are carried by females who, because of the healthy copy of the gene found on their other X chromosome, are not themselves affected.

Sickle cell disease A recessively inherited severe anaemia found most commonly in people of Afro-Caribbean origin. If both parents are unaffected carriers of the disorder, each of their children has a one-in-four chance of being affected.

Specificity The proportion of people not affected by a disorder who will be found to be negative on a screening test for that disorder. It determines the false positive rate.

Spina bifida A failure of the neural tube to close at the appropriate time during embryonic development, resulting in defective development of the spine and of the spinal cord. This usually means that neural tissue is damaged and the result is at least partial paralysis below the lesion. It sometimes results in hydrocephaly.

Superovulation The maturation of many eggs during one menstrual cycle. This is artificially induced in preparation for in vitro fertilization.

Syndrome A recognized pattern of signs, symptoms or malformations.

Tay–Sachs disease An inborn error of metabolism inherited in an autosomal recessive manner so that if both parents carry the gene, each of their children has a one-in-four chance of being affected. Affected individuals suffer from progressive muscular weakness, paralysis, mental deterioration, blindness and eventual death. Most carriers of the disease are of Ashkenazi Jewish origin.

Teratogen A chemical, drug, virus, toxin or environmental factor (such as radiation or heat) that causes exposed fetuses to have congenital abnormalities.

Thalassaemia A form of severe anaemia that is inherited in an autosomal recessive manner. If both parents are unaffected carriers of the disorder, each of their children has a one-in-four chance of being affected. There are different types of thalassaemia and they vary in severity. It is prevalent in people of Mediterranean, Middle Eastern and Far Eastern origin.

Toxoplasmosis A disease caused by infection with the parasite *Toxoplasma gondii*. A pregnant woman who contracts the illness may not have any symptoms, but it may cause severe neurological damage in an exposed fetus.

Translocation A rearrangement of chromosome material: either parts of two chromosomes have broken off and swapped places (reciprocal translocation), or two whole chromosomes are stuck together (Robertsonian translocation). If no genetic material is gained or lost, the translocation is balanced and should not cause any problems to the individual. However, the carrier of a balanced translocation is at risk of having children with an unbalanced translocation in which there may be some extra or missing genetic material. Such an individual might suffer from severe physical or developmental disability.

Triple X This refers to females with an extra X chromosome, 47, XXX. They have a somewhat reduced IQ (about 10–20 points lower than that of their siblings). They are of normal appearance and are rarely diagnosed postnatally. Fertility is normal.

Trisomy The presence in each cell of three copies of a chromosome instead of a normal pair. In humans, most autosomal trisomies cause spontaneous abortion of the embryo, but trisomies of chromosome 13, 18 and 21 are seen in live births and result in serious disability. Trisomies of the sex chromosomes have less serious consequences.

Trisomy 13 See Patau syndrome.

Trisomy 18 See Edwards syndrome.

Trisomy 21 See Down syndrome.

Turner syndrome This refers to females with only one X chromosome. 98% of Turner syndrome pregnancies miscarry. Some of those who survive have a cardiac anomaly. Without hormone treatment, they do not develop secondary sex characteristics. They are short and infertile. Intelligence is normal, although verbal IQ tends to exceed performance IQ.

Ultrasound scan A visual image produced by bouncing low energy ultrasound waves off an object. It is used for visualizing the fetus *in utero*.

XYY This refers to males who have an extra Y chromosome. They have a somewhat reduced IQ (about 10–15 points lower than that of their siblings). They have an increased chance of behavioural problems. They are of normal appearance and are rarely diagnosed postnatally. Fertility is normal.

APPENDIX 1: USEFUL ADDRESSES

UNITED KINGDOM

(To telephone from abroad, dial 44 and remove first 0 from telephone number.)

Association for Children with life-threatening or Terminal Conditions and Their Families (ACT)

Orchard House, Orchard Lane, Bristol BS1 5DT, UK
Helpline: 0117 922 1556
Admin. and Fax: 0117 930 470
e-mail: info@act.org.uk
Website: http://www.act.org.uk/

Antenatal Results and Choices (ARC) formerly Support Around Termination for Fetal Abnormality (SATFA))

73–75 Charlotte Street, London W1P 1LB, UK
Helpline: 020 7631 0285 (24 hours with out-of-hours emergency number)
Tel: (Office): 020 7631 0280
Fax: 020 7631 0280
e-mail arcsatfa@aol.com
Website http://www.arc-uk.org/

Birth Defects Foundation (BDF)

Martindale, Hawks Green, Cannock, Staffordshire WS11 2XN, UK
Tel: 01543 468888
Fax: 01543 468999
(UK based registered charity, founded by parents, doctors and business people in 1991. BDF's mission is to improve child health, aid families and create awareness of these child health challenges.)

Contact a Family (CAF)

209–211 City Road, London EC1V 1JN, UK
Tel: 020 7608 8700
Fax: 020 7608 8701
Minicom: 020 7608 8702
Helpline: 0808 808 3555 Freephone for parents and families (10am–4pm, Mon–Fri)
e-mail info@cafamily.org.uk
Website http://www.cafamily.org.uk/index.html
(Provides support and advice for families who care for children with special needs, whatever the medical condition of their child.)

Down's Syndrome Association

155 Mitcham Road, London SW17 9PG, UK (For UK mail this is a Freepost address)
Tel: 020 8682 4001

Foundation for the Study of Infant Deaths (FSID)

Artillery House, 11–19 Artillery Row, London SW1P 1RT, UK
General enquiries: 020 7222 8001
Fax: 020 7222 8002
Helpline: 020 7233 2090 (24 hours)
e-mail: info@sids.org.uk
Website: www.sids.org.uk/fsid/

Genetic Interest Group (GIG)

Unit 4d, Leroy House, 436 Essex Road, London N1 3QP, UK
Tel: 0171 704 3141
Fax: 0171 359 1447
e-mail: post@gig.org.uk
Website: http://www.gig.org.uk/
(An umbrella group of voluntary organizations concerned with genetic disorders – can supply addresses of support groups for specific genetic disorders.)

The Miscarriage Association

c/o Clayton Hospital, Northgate, Wakefield, West Yorkshire WF1 3JS, UK
Tel: 01924 200799 (answerphone outside office hours)
Fax: 01924 298834
Website: http://www.the-ma.org.uk

Stillbirth and Neonatal Death Society (SANDS)

28 Portland Place, London W1N 4DE, UK
Helpline: 020 7436 5881 (Answerphone outside office hours)
Office: 020 7436 7940
Fax: 020 7436 3715
e-mail: support@uk-sands.org
Website: http://www.uk-sands.org/

Twins and Multiple Birth Association (TAMBA)
Harnott House, 309 Chester Road, Little Sutton, Ellesmere Port, Cheshire CH66 1QQ, UK
Tel: 0870 121 4000 or 0151 348 0020 (office hours)
Fax: 0870 121 4001 or 0151 348 0765
e-mail: enquiries@tambahq.org.uk
Website: http://www.tamba.org.uk/

USA

(To telephone from the UK, dial 001 before the number.)

National Down Syndrome Society
666 Broadway, New York NY 10012, USA
Tel: (212) 460 9330
Website: http://www.ndss.org/main.html

March of Dimes
1275 Mamaroneck Avenue, White Plains NY 10605, USA
Tel: 888 MODIMES
Fax: 914 997 4763
Website: http://www.modimes.org/

(Aims to improve the health of babies by preventing birth defects and infant mortality through community services, advocacy, research and education.)

Genetic Alliance, Inc.
4301 Connecticut Ave. NW, Suite 404, Washington DC 20008-2304, USA
1-800-336-GENE or info@geneticalliance.org
Hours: 9am–5pm EST
Main office: (202) 966 5557
Fax: (202) 966 8553
e-mail: info@geneticalliance.org
Website: www.geneticalliance.org/
(An international coalition representing more than 300 consumer and health professional organizations with millions of members – all working together to promote healthy lives for everyone impacted by genetics. The Alliance supports individuals with genetic conditions and their families, educates the public and advocates for consumer-informed public policies.)

APPENDIX 2: USEFUL WEBSITES

The following links are from reputable sources, and appeared to give good quality information at the time they were reviewed. However, the editors have not reviewed all the contents of every link, and have no control over content on these links. We would urge you to treat any information obtained from sources on the Internet with caution.

More on the issues of quality control for Internet sites and use of the Internet by patients can be found in the following papers and book:

Gagliardi A, Jada AR (2002) Examination of instruments used to rate quality of health information on the Internet: chronicle of a voyage with an unclear destination. *British Medical Journal*, 324; 569–573.

Eysenbach G, Köhler C (2002) How do consumers search for and appraise health information on the world wide web? Qualitative study using focus groups, usability tests, and in-depth interviews. *British Medical Journal*, 324; 573–577.

Kiley R, Graham E (2002) *The Patient's Internet Handbook*. Royal Society of Medicine Press, London, p. 302.

USEFUL WEBSITES FOR ANTENATAL SCREENING

Amniocentesis and PCR testing
www.amniopcr.com
Antenatal Results & Choices (ARC) www.arc-uk.org
(support group for people making decisions about having antenatal tests and about acting on the results of those tests.)
Antenatal screening information
www.mds.qmw.ac.uk/wolfson
British Society for Human Genetics
www.bshg.org.uk/
Contact-a-Family www.cafamily.org.uk/
(Umbrella group listing many UK patient support groups.)
Down syndrome support groups worldwide
www.nas.com/downsyn/net7.html
Fetal Medicine Foundation
www.fetalmedicine.com
(A charity set up to promote and fund research in fetal medicine.)

General genetics information www.netspace.org/mendelweb
Genetic Interest Group www.gig.org.uk/
(Umbrella group of voluntary organizations concerned with genetic disorders.)
Health Development Agency (formerly Health Education Authority) www.hea.org.uk/
Health Technology Assessment www.ncchta.org
Human Genetics Commission www.hgc.uk.gov/news/
(The UK advisory body on how new developments in human genetics will impact on people and health care. Its remit is to advise on the 'big picture', in particular on social and ethical issues.)
Human Genome Organization www.ornl.gov/hgmis/
Introductory genetics tutorials
www.vector.cshl.org/dnaftb
(Includes videos and animations on DNA)
National Association for Down Syndrome (UK)
www.nads.org
National Down Syndrome Society (USA)
www.ndss.org/main.html
National Electronic Library for Health
www.nelh.nhs.uk/screening
National Institute of Clinical Excellence
www.nice.org.uk
On-line Mendelian inheritance in man
www.ncbi.nlmnih.gov/omim
University of Kansas's Genetics educational resources page www.kumc.edu/gec/geneinfo.html
Unique (formerly the Rare Chromosome Disorder Support Group)
www.rarechromo.org.html/disorders.htm)
(Supports families or individuals affected by rare chromosomal disorders, supplying tailor-made information and links.)

USEFUL WEBSITES FOR PROFESSIONAL STANDARDS

American College of Obstetricians and Gynecologists www.acog.org/
Association of Genetic Nurses and Counsellors (UK) www.agnc.co.uk/
Australian Society of Genetic Counsellors
www.hgsa.com.au/asgc/home.htm/

British Association for Counselling and
Psychotherapy   www.bac.co.uk/
members_visitors/public_information/
public_code_counsellors.htm
Department of Health – The Provision of
Counselling Services for Staff in the NHS
www.doh.gov.uk/nhscounsel/
Health and Safety Executive www.hse.gov.uk/
Human Fertilisation and Embryology Authority
www.hfea.gov.uk/
(A statutory body that regulates, licenses and
collects data on fertility treatments such as IVF
and donor insemination, as well as human
embryo research, in the UK.)
National Screening Committee www.nsc.nhs.uk
(contains useful information on screening)
Royal College of Nursing www.rcn.org.uk/home/
home.html
(Provides policy statements on the working
conditions and conduct of nurses in the UK.)

Royal College of Obstetricians and Gynaecologists.
www.rcog.org.uk
(Contains guidelines and recommendations,
including effective procedures in maternity
care suitable for audit: antenatal screening and
diagnosis.)
Nursing and Midwifery Council (formerly United
Kingdom Central Council for Nursing,
Midwifery and Health Visiting) www.nmc-
uk.org/cms/content/home/
(Guidelines for the practice of these staff in the
UK.)
United States Society of Genetic Counsellors.
www.nsgc.org
(Promotes the genetic counselling profession
as a recognized and integral part of health
care delivery, education, research and public
policy.)

INDEX